D0909373

TECHNIQUES
IN OPHTHALMIC
PLASTIC SURGERY

TECHNIQUES IN OPHTHALMIC PLASTIC SURGERY

Editor

Ralph E. Wesley, M.D.

Director, Ophthalmic Plastic and Reconstructive Surgery
Vanderbilt Medical Center
Nashville, Tennessee

Art Editor

Marcia Egles

Vanderbilt University School of Medicine
Nashville, Tennessee

A WILEY MEDICAL PUBLICATION
JOHN WILEY & SONS
New York • Chichester • Brisbane • Toronto • Singapore

Copyright © 1986 by John Wiley & Sons, Inc.

All rights reserved. Published simultaneously in Canada.

Reproduction or translation of any part of this work
beyond that permitted by Section 107 or 108 of the
1976 United States Copyright Act without the permission
of the copyright owner is unlawful. Requests for
permission or further information should be addressed to
the Permissions Department, John Wiley & Sons, Inc.

Library of Congress Cataloging in Publication Data:

Techniques in opthalmic plastic surgery.

(A Wiley medical publication)
Includes index.
1. Adnexa oculi—Surgery. 2. Surgery, Plastic.
I. Wesley, Ralph E. II. Series. [DNLM: 1. Eye—
surgery. 2. Surgery, Plastic. WW 168 T255]
RE87.T43 1986 617.7'1 85-17813
ISBN 0-471-80439-8

Printed in the United States of America

10 9 8 7 6 5 4 3 2 1

**Dedicated with affection and
appreciation to Rissa Arterberry**

Contributors

Henry I. Baylis, M.D.
Jules Stein Eye Institute
Clinical Professor and Director
Division of Ophthalmic Plastic Surgery
University of California at Los Angeles
Los Angeles, California

Craig E. Berris, M.D.
Clinical Faculty
Department of Ophthalmology
University of California, Davis
Sacramento, California

Charles K. Beyer, M.D.
Clinical Associate Professor
Harvard Medical School
Surgeon, Massachusetts Eye and Ear Infirmary
Boston, Massachusetts

Martin Bodian, M.D.
Ophthalmic Plastic Surgery
State University of New York Medical College
Founding Fellow, American Society of Plastic and Reconstructive
    Surgery
Brooklyn, New York

Stephen L. Bosniak, M.D.
Manhattan Eye, Ear and Throat Hospital
New York Eye and Ear Infirmary
New York, New York

James R. Boynton, M.D.
Clinical Assistant Professor
University of Rochester
Rochester, New York

Glen O. Brindley, M.D.
Assistant Professor
Department of Surgery
Texas A&M University School of Medicine
Scott and White Memorial Hospital
Temple, Texas

Bernice Z. Brown, M.D.
Associate Clinical Professor
University of Southern California Medical School
Doheny Eye Foundation
Children's Hospital of Los Angeles
Los Angeles, California

John A. Burns, M.D.
Department of Ophthalmology
Ohio State University
Columbus, Ohio

Kenneth V. Cahill, M.D.
Department of Ophthalmology
Ohio State University
Columbus, Ohio

Delmar R. Caldwell, M.D.
Professor and Chairman
Department of Ophthalmology
Tulane University
New Orleans, Louisiana

N. Branson Call, M.D.
Director, Oculoplastic Surgery
Veterans Administration Hospital
Salt Lake City, Utah

Charles B. Campbell III, M.D.
Assistant Clinical Professor
Bowman Gray School of Medicine
Surgical Staff
Medical Park Hospital
Forsyth Memorial Hospital
Winston–Salem, North Carolina

Richard P. Carroll, M.D.
Clinical Associate Professor
Department of Ophthalmology
University of Minnesota
Attending Surgeon
St. Paul Ramsey Medical Center
Minneapolis, Minnesota

Richard M. Chavís, M.D.
Clinical Assistant Professor
Department of Ophthalmology
Georgetown University Hospital
Washington, D.C.

William P. Chen, M.D.
Assistant Clinical Professor of Ophthalmology
UCLA School of Medicine
Jules Stein Eye Institute
Harbor–UCLA Medical Center
Torrance, California
Assistant Professor of Ophthalmology
University of California, Irvine
Long Beach, California

John S. Crawford, M.D.C.M., F.R.C.S. (C)
Professor of Ophthalmology
Hospital for Sick Children
University of Toronto
Toronto, Ontario, Canada

Jonathan I. Cutler, M.D.
Assistant Professor of Ophthalmology and Pathology
The Milton S. Hershey Medical Center
Pennsylvania State University
Hershey, Pennsylvania

Richard K. Dortzbach, M.D.
Department of Ophthalmology
University of Wisconsin Medical School
Madison, Wisconsin

Timothy W. Doucet, M.D.
Conroe, Texas

Marcos T. Doxanas, M.D.
Division of Oculoplastic Surgery
Department of Ophthalmology
Greater Baltimore Medical Center
Lecturer in Ophthalmology
Johns Hopkins Hospital
Baltimore, Maryland

Robert M. Dryden, M.D.
Adjunct Associate Professor
Department of Ophthalmology
University of Arizona
Tucson, Arizona

Marcia Egles
Art Editor

Vanderbilt University School of Medicine
Nashville, Tennessee

Frank P. English, M.D., F.R.C.S.
Visiting Ophthalmic Surgeon
Repatriation General Hospital
Brisbane, Australia

Gil A. Epstein, M.D.
Oculoplastic Service Florida Medical Center
Bennett Hospital
Ft. Lauderdale, Florida

William Fein, M.D.
Chairman of Ellis Eye Center
Associate Clinical Professor of Ophthalmology
University of Southern California Medical School
Chairman of Ophthalmology
Cedars–Sinai Medical Center
Los Angeles, California

Joseph C. Flanagan, M.D.
Professor of Ophthalmology
Thomas Jefferson University Medical School
Director of Ophthalmic Plastic Surgery and Orbital Surgery
Wills Eye Hospital
Philadelphia, Pennsylvania

Timothy D.C. Forster, F.R.A.C.S.
Brisbane, Australia

Mark S. Granick, M.D.
Clinical Assistant Professor in Plastic Surgery
University of Pittsburgh
Pittsburgh, Pennsylvania

Arthur S. Grove, Jr., M.D.
Assistant Professor of Ophthalmology
Harvard Medical School
Director of Plastic Surgery
Massachusetts Eye and Ear Infirmary
Boston, Massachusetts

Conrad Hamako, M.D.
Freedom, California

Stanley I. Hand, Jr., M.D.
Assistant Clinical Professor
Department of Ophthalmology
University of South Florida
Tampa, Florida

Weldon E. Havins, M.D.
Las Vegas, Nevada

Michael J. Hawes, M.D.
Assistant Clinical Professor of Ophthalmology
University of Colorado
Denver, Colorado

Sanford D. Hecht, M.D.
Associate Clinical Professor of Ophthalmology
Boston University and Tufts Medical School
Director of Oculoplastic and Lacrimal Services
Boston University Medical School
Boston, Massachusetts
President, Boston Eye Research Institute
Waltham, Massachusetts

Joseph C. Hill, M.D.
Professor Emeritus
Department of Ophthalmology
University of Toronto
Consultant, Toronto General Hospital
Active Staff, South Muskoka Memorial Hospital
Huntsville District Memorial Hospital
Toronto, Ontario, Canada

Albert Hornblass, M.D.
Professor of Clinical Ophthalmology
The State University of New York
Downstate Medical Center
Chief of Ophthalmic Orbital, Plastic and Reconstructive Surgery
Manhattan Eye, Ear and Throat Hospital
Lenox Hill Hospital
New York, New York

Wendell L. Hughes, M.D.
Charter Member, American Society of Ophthalmic Plastic and
    Reconstructive Surgery
Highland Beach, Florida

Jeffrey J. Hurwitz, M.D.
Sunnybrook Medical Center
Toronto, Ontario, Canada

M. Kim Jack, M.D.
Department of Ophthalmology
University of Washington School of Medicine
Seattle, Washington

Arthur J. Jampolsky, M.D.
Director of Smith–Kettlewell Institute of Visual Sciences
San Francisco, California

Calvin M. Johnson, Jr., M.D.
Facial Plastic Surgery

Ear, Eye, Nose and Throat Hospital
New Orleans, Louisiana

Robert E. Kalina, M.D.
Department of Ophthalmology
University of Washington
Seattle, Washington

David F. Kamin, M.D.
Associate Clinical Professor of Ophthalmic Plastic and Reconstructive
  Surgery
Jules Stein Eye Institute and The University of California at Los Angeles
Los Angeles, California

John Kearney, F.R.A.C.S.
Gold Coast Eye Clinic
Queensland, Australia

John S. Kennerdell, M.D.
Professor of Ophthalmology and Neurology
University of Pittsburgh
Chief, Division of Ophthalmology
Montefiore Hospital
Pittsburgh, Pennsylvania

Richard A. Kielar, M.D.
Department of Ophthalmology
Lexington Clinic
Lexington, Kentucky

Roger Kohn, M.D.
Associate Professor
Department of Ophthalmology
UCLA School of Medicine
Los Angeles, California
Chairman Department of Ophthalmology
Kern Medical Center
Bakersfield, California

Joel E. Kopelman, M.D.
Affiliated with The New York Eye and Ear Infirmary
New York, New York

Francis G. LaPiana, M.D., Col. U.S.M.C.
Chief, Division of Ophthalmology USUHS
Director, Ophthalmic Plastic Reconstructive and Orbital Surgery
Walter Reed Army Medical Center
Washington, D.C.

Martin L. Leib, M.D.
Director, Ophthalmic Plastic and Reconstructive Surgery
The Edward S. Harkness Eye Institute

Columbia–Presbyterian Medical Center
Montreal, Quebec, Canada

Bradley N. Lemke, M.D.
Assistant Clinical Professor
Department of Ophthalmology
University of Wisconsin
Madison, Wisconsin

Charles R. Leone, Jr., M.D.
Clinical Professor
University of Texas Health Science Center
San Antonio, Texas

Mark R. Levine, M.D.
Associate Clinical Professor
Case Western Reserve University
Chief, Division of Ophthalmology
Mt. Sinai Medical Center
Director, Oculoplastic Clinics
University Hospitals of Cleveland
Cleveland, Ohio

Robert E. Levine, M.D.
Associate Professor of Clinical Ophthalmology
University of Southern California Medical School
Chief, Eye Section
St. Vincent Medical Center
Los Angeles, California

Richard D. Lisman, M.D.
Assistant Clinical Professor of Ophthalmology
Mt. Sinai Hospital and School of Medicine
Department of Ophthalmic Plastic Surgery
Manhattan Eye, Ear and Throat Hospital
New York Eye and Ear Infirmary
New York, New York

Don Liu, M.D.
Oculoplastic and Orbital Service
Ford Hospital
Detroit, Michigan

Robert H. Magnuson, M.D.
Clinical Professor of Ophthalmology
Ohio State University
Columbus, Ohio

Joseph C. Maroon, M.D.
Clinical Professor of Neurosurgery
University of Pittsburgh

Director, Department of Neurosurgery
Allegheny General Hospital
Pittsburgh, Pennsylvania

Joseph G. McCarthy, M.D.
Lawrence D. Bell Professor of Plastic Surgery
New York University Medical Center
New York, New York

Rodney W. McCarthy, M.D.
Assistant Clinical Professor
Department of Ophthalmology
Medical College of Ohio
Toledo, Ohio

Clinton D. McCord, Jr., M.D.
Clinical Professor of Ophthalmology
Emory University School of Medicine
Atlanta, Georgia

√ **Murray A. Meltzer, M.D.**
Director, Ophthalmic Plastic Surgery
Mt. Sinai Medical Center
Attending Surgeon
Manhattan Eye, Ear and Throat Hospital
Attending Surgeon
Beth Israel Medical Center
Director, Ophthalmic Plastic and Surgery Clinic
Elmhurst General Hospital
New York, New York

James L. Moses, M.D.
Assistant Clinical Professor
The Ohio State University
Mount Carmel Medical Center
Columbus, Ohio

John B. Mulliken, M.D.
Associate Professor of Surgery
Harvard Medical School
Boston, Massachusetts

Thomas C. Naugle, Jr., M.D.
Clinical Associate Professor of Ophthalmology
Tulane Medical School
Director, Ophthalmic Plastic Surgery Service
New Orleans, Louisiana

Russell W. Neuhaus, M.D.
Assistant Clinical Professor
Department of Ophthalmology
University of Texas Health Science Center
San Antonio, Texas

Julius Newman, M.D.
Chairman, Department of Cosmetic Surgery
Graduate Hospital
Philadelphia, Pennsylvania

William R. Nunery, M.D.
Assistant Professor
Director, Oculoplastic Division
Department of Ophthalmology
Indiana University
Indianapolis, Indiana

Jay Justin Older, M.D.
Director, Ophthalmic Plastic Surgery
University of South Florida
Tampa, Florida

Michael Patipa, M.D.
Staff Surgeon
Good Samaritan Hospital
Department of Ophthalmology
West Palm Beach, Florida

Kevin I. Perman, M.D.
Clinical Instructor
Jules Stein Eye Institute
UCLA Medical Center
Los Angeles, California
Consultant, Ophthalmic Plastic and Reconstructive Surgery
Washington Hospital Center
Washington, D.C.

Richard L. Petrelli, M.D.
Assistant Clinical Professor
Department of Ophthalmology
Yale University School of Medicine
Attending Surgeon
Hospital of St. Raphael
New Haven, Connecticut

Jeffrey C. Popp, M.D.
Atlanta, Georgia

Allen M. Putterman, M.D.
Professor of Clinical Ophthalmology
Chief, Oculoplastic Service
Director, Oculoplastic Surgery
Michael Reese Hospital and Medical Center
Chicago, Illinois

Oscar M. Ramirez, M.D.
Instructor in Plastic Surgery

Johns Hopkins University
Baltimore, Maryland

R. Bruce Ramsey, M.D., C.M., F.R.C.S.(C)
Assistant Professor
McGill University
Director, Oculoplastic Service
Senior Ophthalmologist
Montreal General Hospital
Montreal, Quebec, Canada

Peter Randall, M.D.
Chairman, Department of Plastic Surgery
University of Pennsylvania Medical School
Philadelphia, Pennsylvania

J. Earl Rathbun, M.D.
Associate Clinical Professor, Ophthalmology
University of California
San Francisco, California

Peter A. Rogers, M.B., B.S., D.O., F.R.A.C.O., F.R.A.C.S.
Visiting Ophthalmic Plastic Surgeon
Sydney Eye Hospital, Leckriner
Department of Ophthalmology
University of Sydney
Sydney, Australia

Joseph W. Sassani, M.D.
Assistant Professor, Ophthalmology and Pathology
The Milton S. Hershey Medical Center
Hershey, Pennsylvania

David H. Saunders, M.D.
Assistant Clinical Professor of Ophthalmology
Southwestern Medical School
President, Medical City Hospital
Dallas, Texas

Arthur J. Schaefer, M.D.
Clinical Professor of Ophthalmology
Assistant Clinical Professor of Otolaryngology
State University of New York at Buffalo
Director of Ophthalmic Plastic Surgery at Erie County Medical Center
Chief of Ophthalmology
Sisters of Charity Hospital
Director of Ophthalmic Plastic Surgery
Buffalo General Hospital
Buffalo, New York
Chief of Ophthalmology
St. Joseph's Intercommunity Hospital
Cheektowaga, New York

Fred Schwarz, M.D.
Chief of Staff
Providence Hospital
Columbia, South Carolina

David Sevel, M.D., Ph.D.
Division of Ophthalmology
Scripps Clinic Medical Group
LaJolla, California

John W. Shore, M.D.
Chairman, Department of Ophthalmology
Wilford Hall U.S.A.F. Medical Center
San Antonio, Texas

Norman Shorr, M.D.
Associate Clinical Professor
Jules Stein Eye Institute
Beverly Hills, California

Hampson A. Sisler, M.D.
Fellow, American Society of Ophthalmic Plastic and Reconstructive
    Surgery
New York, New York

Robert G. Small, M.D.
Professor of Ophthalmology
The Dean A. McGee Eye Institute
University of Oklahoma
Oklahoma City, Oklahoma

✓ **Byron Smith, M.D.**
Lecturer, Department of Ophthalmology
University of Pennsylvania
Philadelphia, Pennsylvania
Consultant, Ophthalmic Plastic Surgery
Manhattan Eye, Ear and Throat Institute
Consultant, New York Eye and Ear Infirmary
Clinical Professor of Ophthalmology
New York Medical College
New York, New York

David B. Soll, M.D.
Professor and Chairman
Department of Ophthalmology
Hahnemann University
Director, Department of Ophthalmology
Frankford Hospital
Philadelphia, Pennsylvania
Chairman, Department of Ophthalmology
Rolling Hills Hospital
Elkins Park, Pennsylvania

Orkan G. Stasior, M.D.
Clinical Professor of Ophthalmology
Albany Medical Center
Chairman, Department of Ophthalmology
The Child's Hospital
Albany, New York

Charles M. Stephenson, Jr., M.D.
Clinical Professor (Oculoplastics–Orbital)
Loma Linda University School of Medicine
Loma Linda, California
Associate Clinical Professor
University of California at San Diego
School of Medicine
San Diego, California
Senior Consultant
Mericos Eye Institute
Scripps Memorial Hospital
La Jolla, California

Ido Sternberg, M.D.
Head, Division of Oculoplastic Surgery
Shaare Zedek Hospital
Jerusalem, Israel

John V. Van Germet, M.D.
Spokane, Washington

Ralph E. Wesley, M.D.
Director, Ophthalmic Plastic and Reconstructive Surgery
Vanderbilt Medical Center
Nashville, Tennessee

Eugene O. Wiggs, M.D.
Associate Clinical Professor of Ophthalmology
University of Colorado Health Sciences Center
Denver, Colorado

T. David I. Wilkes, M.D.
Director, Ophthalmic Plastic and Reconstructive Surgery Service
Department of Ophthalmology
University of Arkansas for Medical Services
Little Rock, Arkansas

Robert B. Wilkins, M.D.
Clinical Associate Professor
Department of Ophthalmology
University of Texas Medical School
Houston, Texas

Neal P. Wittels, M.D.
Attending Plastic Surgeon

St. Lukes–Roosevelt Hospital
New York, New York

Christine L. Zolli, M.D.
Associate Clinical Professor
University of Medicine and Dentistry of New Jersey
Newark, New Jersey
Assistant Surgeon
Wills Eye Hospital
Philadelphia, Pennsylvania

Preface

Techniques in Ophthalmic Plastic Surgery provides innovations and shortcuts for better results in surgery of the eyelids, orbit, and lacrimal apparatus. Each chapter identifies a specific problem and illustrates a technique with which the surgeon can avoid complications and make the surgery proceed more smoothly.

This book is for ophthalmologists, plastic surgeons, and otolaryngologists who treat ophthalmic plastic and orbital disorders. The procedures vary from the common eyelid procedures, such as chalazion surgery, to orbital explorations, which require the assistance of a neurosurgeon.

Each part generally begins with the less difficult procedures that are most helpful to the less experienced surgeon or to the resident in training. However, less experienced surgeons may find the parts illustrating difficult procedures and specialty techniques of benefit to their problem patients. The procedures described herein should be attempted based on the surgeon's level of experience. Some procedures are best accomplished with the help of a colleague in ophthalmology, plastic surgery, otolaryngology, or neurosurgery.

Most procedures come from members of the American Society of Ophthalmic Plastic and Reconstructive Surgery, although other highly qualified plastic surgeons, otolaryngologists, and ophthalmologists have graciously shared their expertise.

This book supplements other traditional textbooks on ophthalmic plastic surgery. I hope those who read this book will find the same satisfaction that I have found in solving problems in ophthalmic plastic surgery.

Ralph E. Wesley

Acknowledgments

I wish to acknowledge the authors who have allowed us in this book to look over their shoulders and share their surgical techniques.

This book could not have been published without the work of Marcia Egles in preparing and coordinating the artwork. As with so many projects from Vanderbilt and Nashville Veterans Medical Center, Ann Reese and Mary Margaret Alsobrook Peel have illustrated procedures and offered advice and encouragement at all phases of the project. The artwork of George Card, Nancy Snyder, and Lee Brent will always be treasured.

Annette Riddle prepared manuscripts, corresponded with authors, and processed the thoughts and words of this volume. John and Tim Wesley provided assistance with the numerous mailings. Judy Jackson, Gail Oakes, Brenda Ursery, and Annie Hendrix have assisted in countless ways.

Dr. J. Patrick O'Leary provided the idea and motivation for this book. Ray Moloney and Robin Lazrus of John Wiley & Sons have nurtured this project at all phases.

My wife, Julia, has unselfishly helped in so many ways.

Ralph E. Wesley

Contents

TECHNIQUES IN OPHTHALMIC PLASTIC SURGERY

GENERAL TECHNIQUES

PART I

1

Subconjunctival Chalazion Surgery

Christine L. Zolli

INTRODUCTION

Soft chalazions can be removed with incision and curettage. But with larger granulomas, the hard, dense, long-standing mass is best treated with total excision. With the subconjunctival chalazion excision technique, the complete chalazion is excised; the conjunctiva is preserved; the lump is immediately gone, and healing proceeds from a surgical incision rather than with smoldering, inflammation of absorbing residual granulomatous material.

TECHNIQUE

Wide infiltration with 2% lidocaine, with or without epinephrine, prevents pain from the chalazion clamp. The chalazion clamp is tightened to prolapse the chalazion into the ring of the clamp on the conjunctival side. A vertical incision—perpendicular to the lid margin—should be carried through the conjunctiva, overlying the highest bulge of the chalazion with a number 11 Bard–Parker blade (Fig 1.1), stopping at least 4 mm short of the lid margin. Incising the lid margin could cause a lid notch.

The scalpel blade or blunt-tipped Westcott scissors are slipped under the conjunctiva on each side of the incision to undermine and separate the underlying granuloma. Undermined conjunctiva retracts sideways, exposing the bulk of the chalazion (Fig. 1.2).

Resection of the chalazion should start at the posterior end—farthest from the lid margin (Fig. 1.3). The chalazion is grasped with toothed forceps and lifted. To prevent buttonholing of the eyelid skin, blunt Westcott scissors can incise and bluntly undermine a plane between the chalazion and the orbicularis muscle.

The dissection is carried around the chalazion, with the last excision adjacent to the lid margin. With this method, the chalazion can be re-

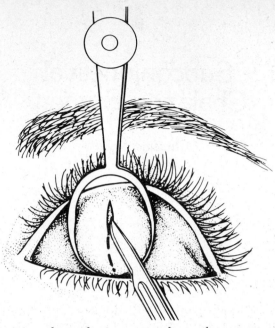

Figure 1.1 Incision through tarsus no closer than 4 mm to lid margin.

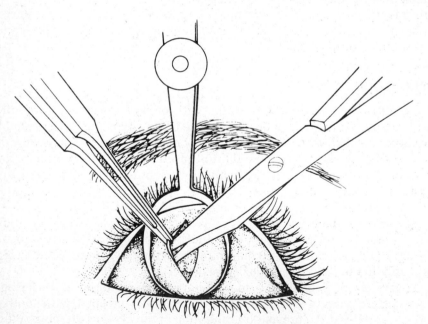

Figure 1.2 Retraction of conjunctiva to expose chalazion.

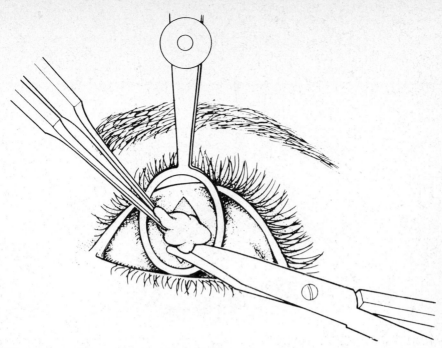

Figure 1.3 *Dissection starting farthest from lid margin.*

moved in one piece, but good results can be obtained in a piecemeal excision as long as removal of the total chalazion is accomplished. Figure 1.4 shows the smooth surface of the orbicularis muscle lining the floor of the wound, and the firm, white tarsus along the lateral edges after chalazion removal.

After excision, the conjunctiva should be brushed back over the wound, the clamp removed, and pressure applied to the lid for hemostasis. Cautery may be used when bleeding does not cease promptly. An antibiotic is instilled in the eye, and a patch is placed and left for several hours after surgery.

Subconjunctival chalazion surgery takes slightly more time than incision and curettage, but the patient has immediate evacuation of the inflammed tissue.

With chalazions that involve the lid margin, the incision should be horizontal rather than vertical and should split the gray line so the soft gelatinous material can be scrapped off with curets. A resection of lid margin tissue might cause a lid deformity.

BIBLIOGRAPHY

Abrahamson IA Jr: Chalazion. *General Practioner* 38:83, 1968.

Bohisian GM: Chalazion: A clinical evaluation. *Ann Ophthalmol* 11:1397, 1979.

Sen DK: Surgical treatment of "collars-stud" chalazion. *Am J Ophthalmol* 70:4356, 1970.

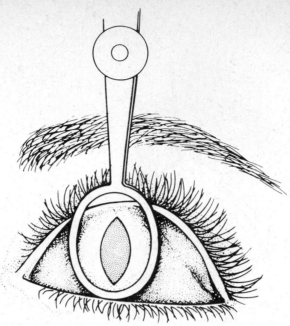

Figure 1.4 Smooth surface of orbicularis muscle after removal of chalazion.

2

Modified Chalazion Surgery Technique

Norman Shorr
Joel E. Kopelman

INTRODUCTION

With standard chalazion surgery, a chalazion ring clamp is placed over
the tarsal plate (Fig. 2.1); a scalpel blade is used to make vertical and
perhaps horizontal incisions (Fig. 2.2) through the tarsal plate; the meibomian glands and their contents are removed, and then the clamp removed.
On removal of the clamp, suffusion of blood into the wound occurs,
which may persist even after a patch is placed on the eyelid.

Our technique helps to alleviate this common, troublesome problem.

TECHNIQUE

Chalazion surgery is carried out as described above. Instead of removing
the chalazion clamp immediately after curettage, the screw is only
loosened on the clamp to allow the blood to effuse slowly into the wound
(Fig. 2.3). Once blood has filled the field, the clamp is retightened in order
to maintain hemostasis (Fig. 2.4).

The clamp is left for approximately 10 minutes while the surgeon perhaps examines another patient. During this period, clot formation occurs.
The clamp is removed. The patient leaves the treatment room with hemostasis and a "bloodless" eye.

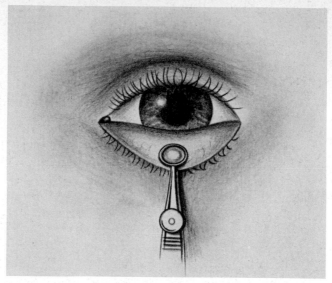

Figure 2.1 Chalazion clamp in place.

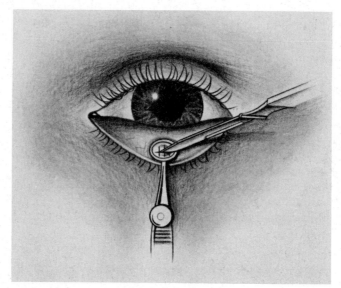

Figure 2.2 Incisions into chalazion.

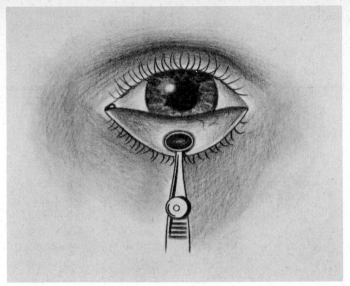

Figure 2.3   Chalazion clamp loosened for blood to fill defect.

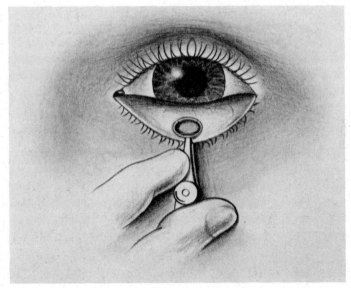

Figure 2.4   Clamp retightened thus allowing blood to clot.

3

Absorbable Suture Technique for Lateral Tarsorrhaphy

Ralph E. Wesley

INTRODUCTION

Patients with exposure keratitis and facial palsy frequently need increased eyelid closure for ocular protection. The absorbable suture technique for lateral tarsorrhaphy allows the surgeon to obtain an estimated 70 to 80% reduction in lagophthalmos without the use of bolsters and complicated dressings.

TECHNIQUE

In a patient with lid retraction, exposure keratitis, or facial palsy, the lid margin for the lateral 4 to 5 mm of each upper and lower lid should be excised (Fig. 3.1A). A double-armed 5-0 Vicryl suture should be placed in a mattress fashion, passing the needles from medial to lateral (Fig. 3.1B) so that the knot (Fig. 3.1C) will be away from the cornea.

The 5-0 Vicryl is tied permanently, and interrupted or running 6-0 plain gut sutures (Fig. 3.1D) are used to close the skin.

No antibiotic ointment or wound care other than normal hygiene needs to be applied as the gut sutures should absorb and slough from the skin surface within a week to 10 days without any cosmetic effect.

The internal 5-0 Vicryl holds the tarsal plates in position to heal forming a stable lateral tarsorrhaphy.

This technique can be performed with lidocaine containing epinephrine at the bedside or as an office procedure. Patients with severe lagophthalmos experience approximately 70 to 80% reduction in the exposure, which frequently tips them back into the comfort zone.

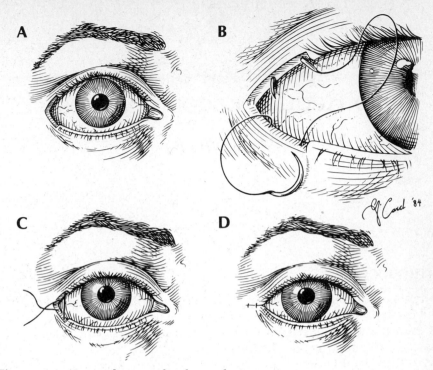

Figure 3.1 Lateral tarsorrhaphy technique.

4

Application of Tape to Reduce Lagophthalmos

Ralph E. Wesley

INTRODUCTION

Patients with facial palsy are particularly vulnerable to exposure keratitis. The eye fails to close due to the orbicularis palsy. The drying is increased by both the widened fissure in normal gaze, as well as by the reduced closure with blinking and during sleep.

A simple application of tape to the eyelid can increase closure enough to provide relief from paralytic exposure keratopathy.

TECHNIQUE

The eye with the facial palsy (Fig. 4.1A) can have the lagophthalmos reduced by pulling the lid downward (Fig. 4.1B) for application of a vertical strip of tape. When the eyelid then opens, the fissure side is reduced (Fig. 4.1C) due to the tape pressing downward.

Benzoin can be applied to the upper lid for the best fixation of the tape. The tape should be applied to override the lid crease, which prevents the paralyzed pretarsal orbicularis muscle from retracting into the orbit by the unopposed levator muscle action.

This technique works best in patients with temporary facial paralysis, such as Bell's palsy. Diligent patients can use this for a prolonged period, especially patients with a prominent orbital rim that tends to hide the appearance of the tape.

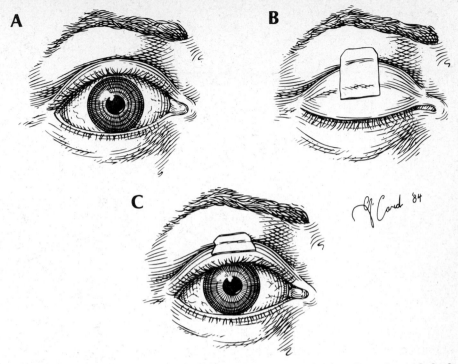

Figure 4.1 Tape applied to force lid downward to reduce lagophthalmos.

5

Steri-Strips
for Suture Tarsorrhaphy

Richard M. Chavis

INTRODUCTION

Closure of the eyelids to prevent corneal and conjunctival exposure may be required with severe proptosis with bleeding into lymphangioma or with conditions such as facial palsy. Conventional methods require the injection of local anesthetics and the placement of sutures through the eyelids.

Steri-strips may be applied to the lids with sutures placed through the tape, eliminating the possibility of inflammation or infection from the sutures and possibly avoiding the use of a general anesthetic with pediatric patients.

TECHNIQUE

Steri-strips are applied horizontally along the upper and lower lids to build up a mound or pyramid of tape with the base at the lid margin. Benzoin can be applied to the eyelid to enhance the adhesion of the base layer to the skin.

Once a bulk of tape has been built up on the upper and lower lids, sutures such as 4-0 silk can be passed through the tape (Fig. 5.1A) and then tied down to bring the lids closed (Fig. 5.1B).

The sutures can be removed at intervals for ocular examination and replaced without the use of anesthesia.

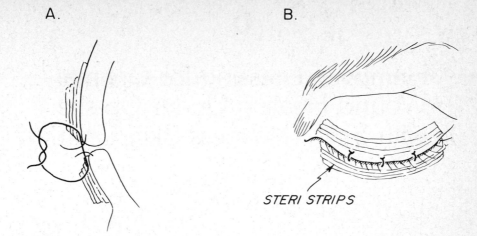

A.

B.

STERI STRIPS

M.M. Alsobrook Peel

Figure 5.1 Eyelid closure with sutures passed through Steri-strips applied to lid margins.

6

Hemovac Dressing for Optimal Wound Healing Under Op-site with Split-Thickness Skin Graft

Oscar M. Ramirez
Mark S. Granick

INTRODUCTION

After harvesting a split-thickness skin graft, a dressing must be applied to prevent hematoma and allow for healing of the donor site. Op-site* is an occlusive, gas-permeable polyurethane film that maintains a moist environment for optimal epidermal regeneration of split-thickness skin graft donor sites.

The technique below provides a continuous suction applied under the dressing to prevent fluid collection, leakage, and soilage of the patient's bedding or clothing and to maintain a closed system.

TECHNIQUE

The vacuum drain is fashioned from a number 21 butterfly needle with the hub of the IV connector removed and a red top vacutainer tube. Holes are placed into the tubing to allow for multiple-draining sites. Ideally the tubing should be at a dependent position for gravity drainage. Op-site is applied, and the tubing is secured with tape. Finally, the needle of the number 21 butterfly needle is inserted into the vacutainer to apply suction (Fig. 6.1)

If large defects are covered with Op-site, the drain can be altered by removing the needle end of the number 21 butterfly needle, using the end of the drain, and securing the IV adapter into the disposable suction bulb.

This system has been used on numerous skin graft donor sites to maintain a clean, secure dressing without hematoma or seroma.

* Registered trademark of Smith and Nephew, Limited, Lochine, Quebec, Canada

16

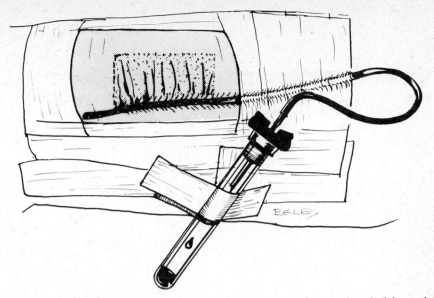

Figure 6.1 *Vacutainer and butterfly maintain clean, dry field under split-skin donor site dressing.*

BIBLIOGRAPHY

Ramarez OM, Granick MS, Futrell JW: Optimal wound healing under Op-site dressing. *Plast Reconstruct Surg* 73:474, 1984.

7

Tarsoconjunctival Biopsy with Disposable Skin Punch

Joseph W. Sassani
Jonathan I. Cutler

INTRODUCTION

Biospy of the upper tarsus can be extremely difficult using conventional blades. A full-thickness biopsy of the tarsus and conjunctiva can be performed easily with a skin biopsy punch to provide tissue for histopathologic sectioning.

TECHNIQUE

With appropriate local anesthesia around the suspected lesion (Fig. 7.1), a skin biopsy punch is applied (Fig. 7.2) and twisted around the lesions that are then elevated with forceps (Fig. 7.3). The base is excised with scissors, and the specimen is submitted for pathologic examination.

To further reduce trauma to the specimen, a suture can be placed a through the specimen after it has been outlined by the biopsy punch. The suture can be used to provide traction as the specimen is amputated at the base. The suture also serves as a means of transporting the specimen to fixative or other container. For safety, the suture needle should be removed. The defect (Fig. 7.4) is allowed to heal by granulation.

The disposable skin biopsy punch comes in various sizes starting at 2 mm in diameter and provides uniform sectioning of the tarsus and conjunctiva in a controlled manner, which can be difficult to accomplish using conventional scalpel blades.

BIBLIOGRAPHY

Sassani JW, Cutler J: A new application for the disposable skin biopsy punch. *Am J Ophthalmol* 92:737, 1981.

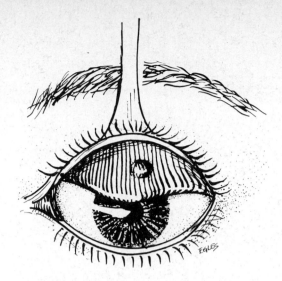

Figure 7.1 Lesion for biopsy on upper tarsus.

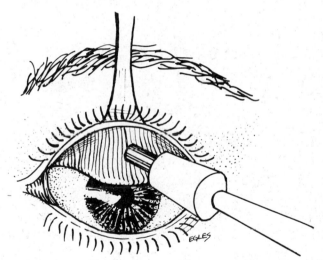

Figure 7.2 Skin punch used to core a biopsy specimen.

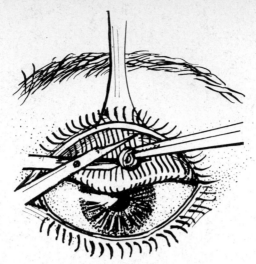

Figure 7.3   Biopsy specimen lifted and snipped free.

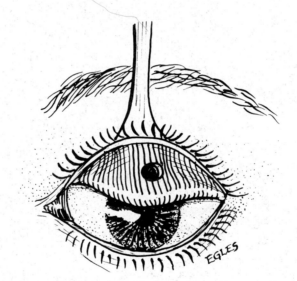

Figure 7.4   Defect allowed to heal spontaneously.

8

Biopsy Techniques
for Eyelid Lesions

Albert Hornblass

INTRODUCTION

Suspicious eyelid lesions should be submitted for histopathologic examination before cryosurgery, electrodesiccation, radiation, or excision. The biopsy specimen should be adequate for a thorough examination; it should contain both normal-appearing skin as well as the suspicious lesion.

TECHNIQUE

When a lesion is large enough to require extensive surgery or is in proximity to a vital area such as the punctum, canaliculus, or globe, an incision biopsy should be performed. A 2.5 to 3.5 mm trephine punch can be used to straddle one side of the tumor (Fig. 8.1A) to include both normal-appearing skin and a portion of the suspicious lesion. The trephine should go deeper than the suspected depth of the lesion to obtain proper tissue for examination.

A horizontal elipse technique can be used with a number 15 Bard–Parker blade to obtain a similar specimen (Fig. 8.1B). With mild cautery or digital compression, bleeding subsides. The biopsy site usually heals well without sutures.

If the biopsy specimen should show malignancy, removal can be accomplished in a facility providing frozen sections to firm histologic margins clear of tumor. With benign lesions, an appropriate excision (Fig. 8.1C) can be performed in the office with a margin of normal tissue.

BIBLIOGRAPHY

Hornblass A: Evaluation and diagnosis of tumors, in Hornblass A (ed): *Tumors of the Ocular Adnexa and Orbit.* St. Louis, CV Mosby, 1979, p 57.

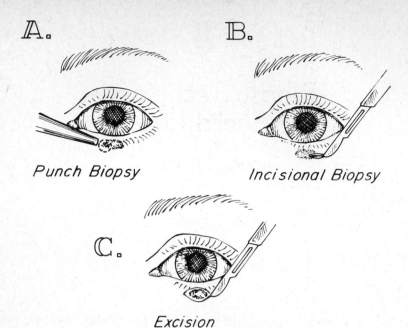

A.

Punch Biopsy

B.

Incisional Biopsy

C.

Excision

Figure 8.1 Suspicious lesions biopsied with skin punch (A) or small elliptical incisions (B) in office. Definitive resection (C) of malignant lesion after biopsy report available. (Hornblass A: Tumors of the Ocular Adnexa and Orbit, ed 1. St. Louis, Mosby, 1979. By permission from C. V. Mosby Company.)

9

Entering the Posterior Orbicularis Space

Allen M. Putterman

INTRODUCTION

The posterior orbicularis space must be entered for eyelid procedures such as levator resection, levator aponeurosis repair, excision of herniated orbital fat with lid crease formation, and biopsy of superior anterior orbital tumors. With the technique below, the surgeon can sever the orbicularis muscle without injuring the levator aponeurosis.

TECHNIQUE

A horizontal incision should be made just through the skin at the level of the desired upper eyelid crease. A 4-0 black silk traction suture is passed centrally through the skin, orbicularis muscle, and superficial tarsus just above the upper eyelid cilia. With gentle traction downward on the suture, a toothed forceps can be used at the superior aspect of the incision to pull outward and upward on the central skin and orbicularis muscle. This traction pulls the orbicularis muscle away from the levator aponeurosis, orbital septum, Müller's muscle, and conjunctiva, which lie deep and surround the globe.

With the central orbicularis muscle properly tented, Westcott scissors are used to incise superiorly and posteriorly to sever the orbicularis muscle and to expose suborbicularis space (Fig. 9.1 top). To expose the potential suborbicularis space further, the orbicularis is severed across the entire eyelid while traction is still applied with the suture below and the forceps above (Fig. 9.1 bottom).

One blade of the Westcott scissors can enter at the central opening of the orbicularis and slide to the extreme of the skin incision. This internal blade can lift the orbicularis muscle outward so that the muscle can be severed from the central opening to the medial and lateral ends, avoiding injury to the levator aponeurosis that lies underneath.

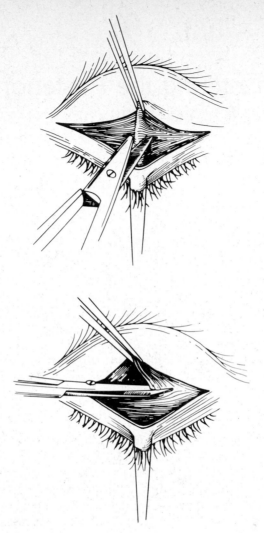

Figure 9.1 Entering the posterior orbicularis space.

With a clean exposure of the suborbicularis space, the levator aponeurosis, orbital septum, preaponeurotic fat, tarsal plate, and Müller's muscle—important anatomic landmarks of the upper eyelid—are more easily identified.

BIBLIOGRAPHY

Putterman AM: Basic oculoplastic surgery, in Payman G, Sanders D, Goldberg M. (eds): *Principles and Practice of Ophthalmology.* Philadelphia, WB Saunders, 1980, p 2266.

10

Scleral Twist Fixation Forceps for Use in Skin Biopsy

Ralph E. Wesley

INTRODUCTION

The goal of cancer surgery is to remove all of the tumor while excising the least amount of normal tissue. Frozen sections should be taken around eyelid tumors, such as basal cell carcinomas, to guarantee that the patient is tumor free before reconstruction.

Most methods involve resection of the tumor followed by excision of thin strips around the tumor for frozen section examination to rule out any unsuspected fingers of tumor extending through the cut surgical margin.

After the tumor is excised, the surgeon may wish to take thin margins around the tumor for the pathologist. The use of toothed forceps for fixation can crush the tissue causing distortion artifact. The technique described below allows the surgeon to excise a thin strip around the wound using firm fixation without damage to excised tissue.

TECHNIQUE

Once a tumor has been excised and peripheral sections are desired, a twist scleral forceps can be inserted into the margin to allow for fixation and manipulation while the surgeon performs his excision. The sharp points penetrate the tissue without crushing or damaging the cells, providing for the best possible pathologic examination while providing the surgeon good control (Fig. 10.1).

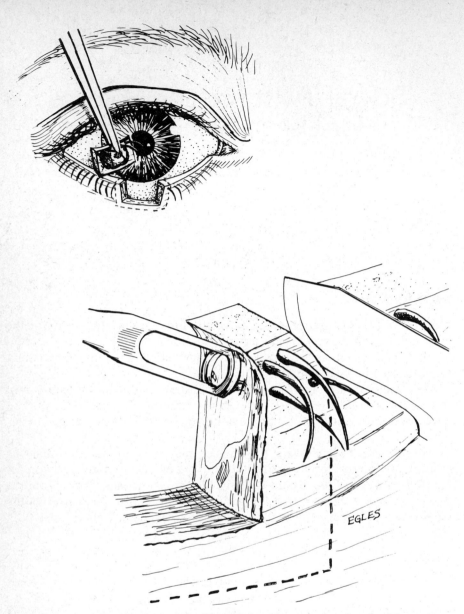

Figure 10.1 (Top) Area marked by dashed lines to be checked for tumor. (Bottom) Twist fixation to obtain margins for frozen sections.

11

Removal of Subcutaneous Tissue from Full-Thickness Skin Grafts

Ralph E. Wesley
Marcia Egles

INTRODUCTION

Full-thickness skin grafts provide better correction of contractures and defects around the eyelids than Z-plasties and flaps. The rich vascularity of the eyelids provides nourishment for full-thickness grafts if subcutaneous tissue has been removed from the graft before placement.

Poor fixation of the graft while trimming subcutaneous tissue from beneath the graft can be frustrating and lead to buttonholes in the graft or leave residual subcutaneous material that can make the final appearance irregular.

With this technique, the graft can be trimmed uniformly in a controlled manner.

TECHNIQUE

Full-thickness skin grafts are most frequently taken from the upper eyelids, the retroauricular area, or preauricular area due to the match and viability of the skin. To remove subcutaneous tissue, the graft should be draped with the skin or epithelial surface against the index finger, fixed with the thumb and third finger, leaving the depths of the graft exposed and on stretch. The surgeon then has good visualization to excise subcutaneous tissue with the other hand while applying a firm pressure against the base of the graft with the scissors during excision (Fig. 11.1).

This technique provides a uniform graft trimmed of all subcutaneous tissue for the maximum viability of the graft.

27

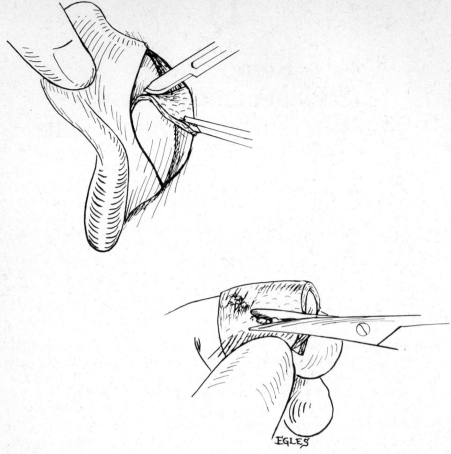

Figure 11.1 Method of fixate skin graft while excising subcutaneous tissue.

12

Maintaining the First Knot in Instrument Tying

Neal P. Wittels

INTRODUCTION

The first knot thrown during instrument tying frequently fails to maintain proper tightness unless the surgeon uses special techniques, such as tying a surgeon's knot or a granny knot, locking the first knot using silk instead of nylon, or having an assistant hold the first knot with a pair of forceps or a clamp. Loosening the first knot can interrupt the surgeon's rhythm, leading to frustration during an eyelid or orbital procedure.

With the technique below the surgeon can maintain tension on the first knot during instrument tying until the second throw is placed to maintain proper suture tension permanently.

TECHNIQUE

The suture is placed in the usual manner, and the first knot tied squarely (Fig. 12.1A). The end should be separated leaving a small end approximately 3 cm in length pointing upward, if possible. The long end of the suture is grasped 10 cm from the knot with a thumb-index pinch. The ring finger then divides the length in two by pushing against the pull of the thumb-index pinch. Tension is thus maintained on the suture with the thumb-index finger pull against the ring finger push.

While maintaining this tension, a loop of suture is produced around the needle holder tip between the ring finger and the thumb-index fixation of the suture (Fig. 12.1B). This should be accomplished by the needle holder sliding additional suture under tension through the thumb-index pinch. Once the loop has been made, the small end of the suture is grasped with the instrument.

Tension is now transferred from the long end to the small end of the suture by pulling on the small end with the needle holder along the skin surface (Fig. 12.1C). With tension on the small end of the suture, the

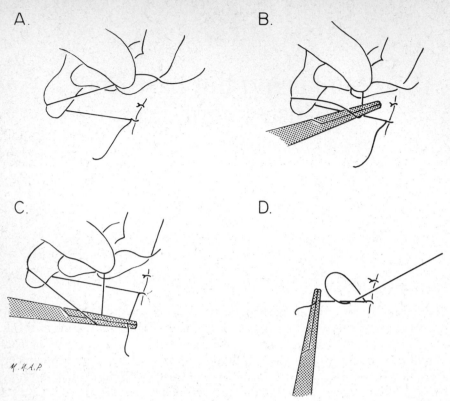

Figure 12.1 (A) Tension maintained on long end of suture. (B) Tension maintained while instrument forms loop. (C) Instrument places short end on stretch. (D) With tension on short end the longer loop is secured for permanent knot tension.

tension can then be released from the long end, and the second square knot can be tied down thus maintaining the original tension on the wound edges (Fig. 12.1D).

BIBLIOGRAPHY

Wittels NP: Maintaining the first knot in instrument tying. Ann Plast Surg 12:483, 1984.

13

Method to Prepare Split-Thickness Ear Cartilage for Use in Ophthalmic Plastic Surgery

Byron Smith
Richard D. Lisman

INTRODUCTION

Ear cartilage has numerous uses in ophthalmic plastic surgery (1–4), such as lowering eyelids in thyroid eyelid retraction, correction of trichiasis, eyelid reconstruction, and with anophthalmic sockets.

Patients implanted with full-thickness cartilage have thickened, roughened, and unsightly lids. The patients have been unhappy with the firmness and appearance of the lid.

Attempts to thin the grafts can result in fragmentation of the halves during preparation, as the full-thickness cartilage is a difficult substance to deal with free hand.

With the technique below, cartilage can be prepared in a precise, meticulous, uniform manner to ensure optimal reconstructive results (5).

TECHNIQUE

To provide ear cartilage for the use in ophthalmic plastic surgery, an outline of the portion of ear cartilage to be harvested is made on the anterior surface of the antihelix of the ear with methylene blue. Towel clips are used to mark the extremities of the outlined cartilage graft with the points placed through and through in order to guide the surgeon in his dissection, which will be performed on the posterior surface of the ear.

The skin on the posterior surface of the ear is hydraulically dissected from the muscle with an injection of lidocaine or saline. The ear is folded forward such that the two towel clips mark the extent of the incisional site. Methylene blue can be used to mark a mildly curvilinear incision between these two towel clips; 2% lidocaine with epinephrine is injected for hemostasis and to separate skin from the donor site.

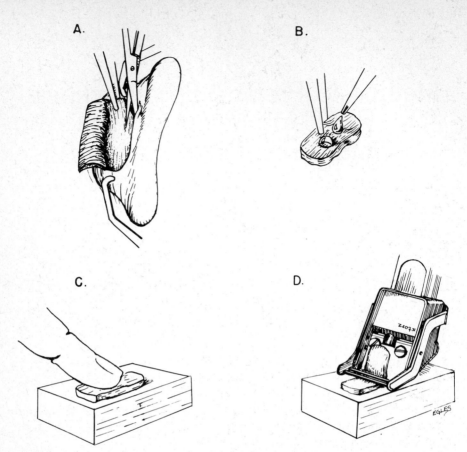

Figure 13.1 *Method to trim ear cartilage with mucotome.*

Skin incision should be made and carried down to the cartilage where a graft is taken in a one-to-one proportion to a desired defect (i.e., if the lid is to be lengthened 4 mm, a 4-mm-wide graft should be taken as opposed to eye bank sclera, which is frequently taken in greater ratios). After incision into the cartilage, the graft should be handled with spring scissors (Fig. 13.1A). Skin should be dissected off the graft with attempts made to leave the skin intact.

The cartilage will curl and retract when dissected from the ear, which makes implantation difficult. Cyanoacrylate glue should be placed on the anterior surface of the graft (Fig. 13.1B) and bonded firmly to a cutting board (Fig. 13.1C). The glue can be obtained from hardware stores and sterilized with gas before surgery.

In 1 or 2 seconds, the cartilage bonds to the cutting board. A uniform, precise graft can be taken using a Castroviejo mucotone set at 4 mm to shave off a thin slice of graft (Fig. 13.1D). A firm hand should be applied to the mucotone with constant pressure while shaving off the graft. A typical graft of 1 to 1.2 mm in thickness can be halved using a 0.5 mm or 0.6 mm setting of mucotone.

The surgeon should normally implant only the piece of cartilage that has not come into contact with cyanoacrylate glue. If the other piece must also be implanted, the cartilage can be separated from the board leaving the layer of glue behind.

The new thin piece of cartilage has the flexibility of eye bank sclera without the increased bulk. When split with this technique, the graft is less friable and is much easier to handle. Though ear cartilage grafts are generally more desirable than composite nasal cartilage grafts, the Castroviejo mucotone set at 0.4 mm can also be used to trim nasal cartilage grafts.

REFERENCES

1. Smith B, Lisman RD: Eyelid tumors: Resection and reconstruction. *Perspect Ophthalmol* 5:183, 1981.
2. Hughes WL: *Reconstructive Surgery of the Eyelids.* St. Louis, Mosby, 1954, p 116.
3. Smith B, Lisman RD: Cosmetic correction of eyelid deformities associated with exophthalmos. *Clin Plast Surg* 8:777, 1981.
4. Baylis, HI: Under-correction, lengthening and use of ear cartilage in eyelid lengthening, in: *Symposium on Surgical Management of Thyroid Ophthalmopathy.* Proceedings of the Annual Meeting of the American Academy of Ophthalmology, 1980.
5. Smith B, Lisman RD: Preparation of split-thickness auricular cartilage for use in ophthalmic plastic surgery. *Ophthalmic Surg* 13:1018, 1982.

14

Safe Eyelid Bandages

Glenn O. Brindley

INTRODUCTION

A pressure bandage has a great effect in reducing eyelid edema and ecchymosis while protecting the wound. However, blindness secondary to orbital bleeding, while rare, can be associated with blepharoplasty. Eye pads prevent the surgeon from checking the patient's pupil and visual acuity postoperatively to rule out severe but unusual complications.

With this technique, the patient can have the benefit of pressure bandages and the safety of adequate eye examination.

TECHNIQUE

After blepharoplasty or other eyelid surgery has been completed (Fig. 14.1), eye pads are cut in half, length wise, placed over the wound (Fig. 14.2), and taped in place (Fig. 14.3). The tape and the eye pads are positioned such that the patient can still see; thus, the eyes can be examined

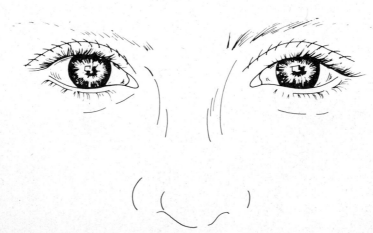

Figure 14.1 Eyelids after surgery

34

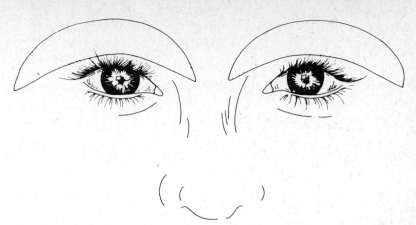

Figure 14.2   Eye pads cut in half placed on wound.

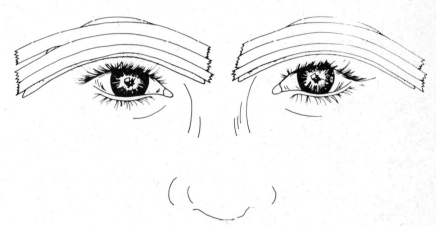

Figure 14.3   Bandage permits eye examination.

and the visual acuity determined. The bandage can be used on the brows, upper eyelids, or lower eyelids. This has been a safe method of using pressure dressings for any eyelid surgery.

15

Multiple Z-plasty for Correction of Scar Contracture at Mucous Membrane Donor Site

Henry I. Baylis
Norman Shorr
Russell W. Neuhaus

INTRODUCTION

A full-thickness mucous membrane graft from the mouth may be required to replace deficient conjunctiva. Complications of the donor site are not common, but can occur with larger grafts. In some instances, severe submucosal scar formation with cicatricial mucous membrane bands and webbs can form such that the patient may be unable to open his mouth fully or to wear his or her dentures (Fig. 15.1).

Multiple Z-plasties and excision of submucosal fibrotic scar tissue provides a method for handling such contracture complications.

TECHNIQUE

A line is drawn with methylene blue along the main force of the scar contracture, and then multiple Zs are drawn along the edges in the usual fashion (Fig. 15.2). The Z's are then incised and mobilized. With appropriate retraction, the submucosal scar tissue (Fig. 15.3) should be excised to release the tension on the oral tissues. Finally, the Zs are transposed to break up and elongate the main line of contracture (Fig. 15.4).

Complications from full-thickness mucous membrane donor sites are not common, but the employment of both steps of this technique, multiple Z-plasty and submucosal scar excision, provides an effective method for correction of the complications.

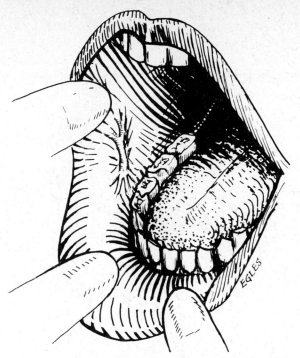

Figure 15.1 Vertical scar contracture at mucous membrane donor site.

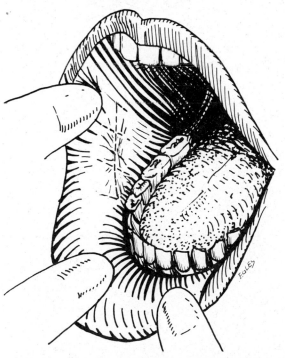

Figure 15.2 Contracture broken up with multiple Z-plasties.

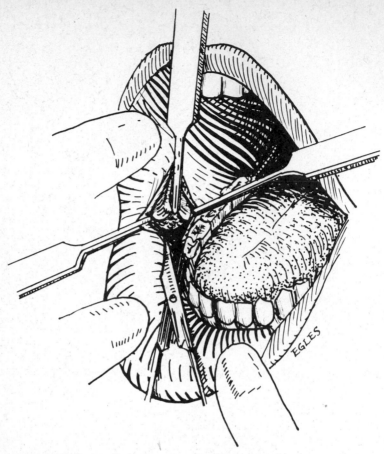

Figure 15.3 Z-plasty flaps retracted, submucosal scar excised.

BIBLIOGRAPHY

Callahan MA, Callahan A: *Ophthalmic Plastic and Orbital Surgery*. Birmingham, Aesculapius Publishing Co., 1979, pp 134–141.

McCord CD Jr: *Oculoplastic Surgery*. New York, Raven Press, 1981, pp 327–347.

Neuhaus RW, Baylis HI, Shorr N: Complication at mucous membrane donor sites. *Am J Ophthalmol* 93:643, 1982.

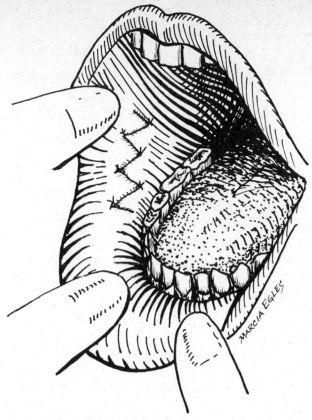

Figure 15.4 Multiple Z-plasty flaps transposed for release of scar contracture.

16

Modification of Lateral Tarsorrhaphy Technique

John S. Crawford

INTRODUCTION

Lateral tarsorrhaphy can be effectively used to protect an exposed cornea with endocrine exophthalmos or exposure keratopathy, to keep lid tissue from contracting following eyelid surgery, to improve the appearance when surgery for lid retraction has been inadequate, to shorten a palpebral fissure that is too wide, or to elevate a drooping lower lid.

Problems in producing a tarsorrhaphy include (1) raw surface may not be held in exact apposition, creating a small lid adhesion that will not hold; (2) inadequate raw surface may not create an adequate adhesion; (3) the use of bolsters or buttons creates an unsightliness during healing for 2 weeks, which requires the patient to wear a patch.

This technique creates a firm lateral tarsorrhaphy, which is cosmetically pleasing.

TECHNIQUE

The size of the tarsorrhaphy depends on the amount of closure required. The lid border is excised for an amount corresponding to the desired size, leaving a 1 mm strip of epithelium near the lashes, and extending to the posterior edge of the lid. A horizontal incision is made in the center of the denoted area so that as the lid borders are pulled together, a larger raw area is created to make a stronger adhesion (Fig. 16.1A).

Two 6-0 plain gut sutures are placed in the posterior edges of the lids to hold the raw areas in exact apposition (Fig. 16.1B). Two 4-0 Vicryl or Dexon sutures are used as matrix sutures with one being tied above and the other below. Small skin incisions are made at the point of exit of these sutures so that the knot is buried, and then 6-0 gut sutures close the wound.

These mattress sutures hold the lids in position for an adequate time for

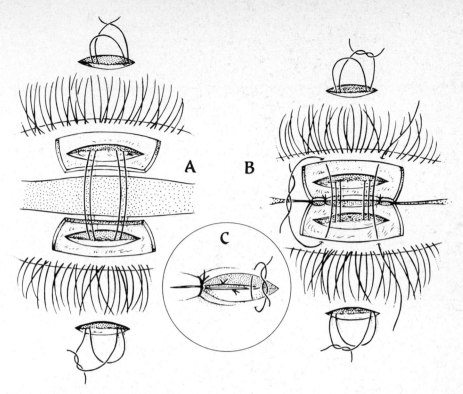

Figure 16.1 Technique for lateral tarshorrhaphy.

the tarsorrhaphy to heal. Two 6-0 plain gut sutures are placed into the anterior edges of lids (Fig. 16.1C) as further assurance that the raw edges will remain aligned, thus the patient does not need to wear a patch over the eye during the healing process.

BLEPHAROPLASTY AND BROW LIFT

PART II

17

Use of Iris Retractor for Removal of Protective Contact Lens After Eyelid Surgery

Ralph E. Wesley
Marcia Egles

INTRODUCTION

The use of an opaque scleral lens during eyelid surgery prevents inadvertant ocular injury and reduces the discomfort from bright operating lights. Difficulty in removing the lenses at the end of the operation can cause pain for the patient during removal, and a scrape of the epithelium can result in a corneal abrasion. Some lenses have been modified with hooks and handles for easy removal, but these lenses are bulky and do not allow for a natural positioning of the lids during surgery.

With the use of a readily available iris retractor, the lenses can be removed without danger or ocular injury.

TECHNQUE

Corneal anesthetic drops are inserted, and a +43.00 diopter opaque scleral lens is used during surgery. At the end of the operation an iris retractor* is inserted into the inferior cul-de-sac until the edge of the iris retractor snaps beneath the contact lens (Fig. 17.1). Now the retractor can be used to pull the inferior edge of the lens upward and outward over the lower lid thus allowing the contact lens to pop outward.

After a long procedure, additional corneal anesthetic drops should be placed before removal to eliminate any discomfort for the patient.

*Storz Instruments No E-0764.

45

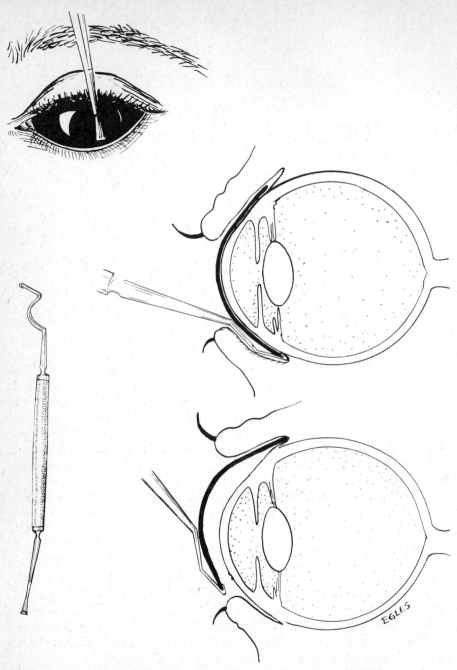

Figure 17.1 Iris retractor used to remove opaque contact lens atraumatically after eyelid surgery.

18

The Surgical Correction
of the Oriental Eyelid

Marcos T. Doxanas

INTRODUCTION

The distinctive clinical appearance of the oriental eyelid comes from a poorly defined eyelid crease, resulting in a full or thickened eyelid. In the oriental eyelid, an inferior extension of the orbital septum fuses with the levator aponeurosis near the eyelid margin (Fig. 18.1). By contrast, in the occidental eyelid, the orbital septum fuses with the levator aponeurosis above the superior tarsal border, creating a lid crease.

The inferior extension of the orbital septum in the oriental eyelid permits the preaponeurotic fat or orbital fat to extend onto the anterior tarsal surface, creating the full appearance. The inferior extension of the orbital septum also blocks the superficial extension of the levator aponeurosis, which creates the occidental eyelid crease. In addition, the brow fat pad may extend inferiorly into the oriental upper eyelid. The technique of oriental eyelid revision described below corrects these distinct anatomic features.

TECHNIQUE

A modification of an upper eyelid blepharoplasty is performed. The eyelid crease is marked approximately 8 to 10 mm above the eyelid margin. Using the "pinch technique," the redundant skin is measured and marked. After installation of the local anesthetic, the skin is then removed. A strip of orbicularis muscle approximately one-half the width of the skin incision is removed along the entire horizontal extent of the upper eyelid (Fig. 18.2A). The excised orbicularis muscle should be at the level of the desired eyelid crease. The orbital septum is then incised, and the preaponeurotic fat is prolapsed (Fig. 18.2B).

Since the orbital septum inserts on the anterior tarsal surface, an abundance of fat is available for careful excision. Debulking the oriental eyelid,

47

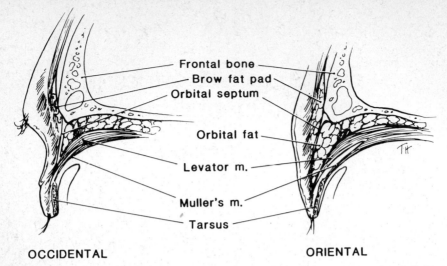

Frontal bone
Brow fat pad
Orbital septum

Orbital fat

Levator m.

Muller's m.

Tarsus

OCCIDENTAL   ORIENTAL

Figure 18.1 *Attachment of septum to levator aponeurosis and differences in fat pads cause different appearance to oriental and occidental eyelids.*

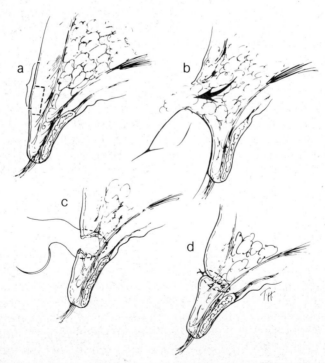

a

b

c

d

Figure 18.2 *Creation of eyelid crease in oriental eyelid. (Reprinted with permission. Ophthalmic Surgery [in press].)*

by removing a strip of orbicularis muscle and preaponeurotic fat, facilitates the formation of an eyelid crease. Following adequate hemostasis, the skin incision is closed with interrupted sutures. Deep epitarsal tissues are incorporated into the skin closure, which enhances the eyelid crease (Fig. 18.2C,D).

This modification of a standard upper eyelid blepharoplasty produces long-term, satisfactory results in converting oriental- to occidental-appearing eyelids.

19

Triangular Skin-Muscle Excision for Safe Lower Lid Blepharoplasty

Ralph E. Wesley

INTRODUCTION

The greater risk of complications and the lesser potential for dramatic cosmetic result makes a safe technique for lower lid blepharoplasty extremely important.

The technique below allows the surgeon to provide a refreshing look to the lower eyelids while minimizing the chance of postoperative ectropion.

The principal of this technique is to provide primarily a lateral stretch of skin and muscle to the lower eyelid to eliminate wrinkles and redundant skin caused by aging and a sagging orbicularis muscle. This avoids the tightening effect from excision of vertical skin that reduces the chances of ectropion or the precipitation of a dry eye in an otherwise asymptomatic patient.

TECHNIQUE

The skin of the lower eyelid should be bunched laterally with a forceps (Fig. 19.1, upper left) to determine the amount of lateral pull needed to reduce wrinkles and refresh the lower eyelids. An equalateral triangle is then drawn, as shown, (Fig. 19.1, upper right) and excised with a number 15 Bard–Parker blade and Westcott scissors.

The subciliary blepharoplasty flap is then developed starting laterally with scissors piercing underneath the orbicularis muscle and carrying the incision from lateral to medial (Fig. 19.1, middle left). The point of the triangle is then closed with a skin suture and excess vertical skin carefully trimmed (Fig. 19.1, middle right). Caution should be used to make sure that the patient has a very minimal amount of vertical skin excised.

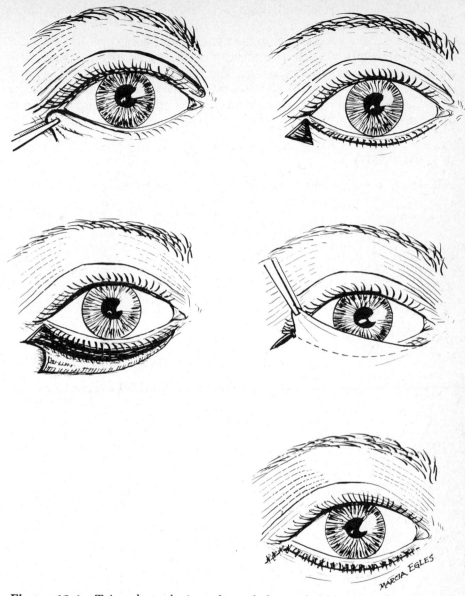

Figure 19.1 Triangle technique for safe lower lid blepharoplasty.

The patient should be directed to look up with mouth agape to put the lower lid on maximum stretch. The surgeon should trim away minimum amounts of lower eyelid skin and orbicularis muscle until adequate vertical skin has been resected. Normally, only 1 to 2 mm of excision laterally are required. Medially, much less is required in the central portion. Even a millimeter of excision may be adequate, as the flaps contract some postoperatively for additional tightening and smoothing of the lower lid.

Finally, the lid is closed (Fig. 19.1, bottom right) with interrupted sutures.

This technique works well in the patients in whom complications can be most disasterous, such as the very demanding younger patients with minimal lower lid dermatochalasis. The less experienced surgeon should start with smaller triangles and less skin excision and should err on the side of safety rather than in an over zealous attempt toward maximum blepharoplasty.

BIBLIOGRAPHY

McCord CD Jr: Techniques in blepharoplasty. *Ophthalmic Surgery* 10:40, 1979.

20

Correction of Ectropion After Lower Blepharoplasty

Ralph E. Wesley

INTRODUCTION

Ectropion can occur after blepharoplasty despite meticulous technique. In patients in whom spontaneous resolution of the ectropion is in doubt or a waiting period unsatisfactory, lateral canthal tendon tightening provides an office method for immediate correction.

TECHNIQUE

The eyelid with ectropion after blepharoplasty (Fig. 20.1A) should be injected with local anesthesia with epinephrine. An incision should split the upper and lower lids down to the periosteum, out 1 cm through the skin (Fig. 20.1B). Westcott scissors disinsert remnants of the lower canthal tendon so that the lid is freed (Fig. 20.1C).

The lid should be pulled up to determine the amount of tightening necessary to return the lid into position against the globe (Fig. 20.1D). After excision of the excess lid, a permanent or absorbable suture can be passed through the cut edge of the tarsus and attached upward and inside the orbital rim to the periosteum (Fig. 20.2A,B), and tied with the knot buried (Fig. 20.2C). For skin closure 7-0 silk can be used (Fig. 20.2D).

With this technique, the surgeon can alleviate the patient's fear that the lid may not return to a normal position, or can hasten that healing process. This procedure corrects the overwhelming majority of ectropion after blepharoplasty, though some severe cases may need skin grafts.

BIBLIOGRAPHY

Anderson RL, Garde DD: The tarsal strip procedure. *Arch Ophthalmol* 97:2192, 1979.

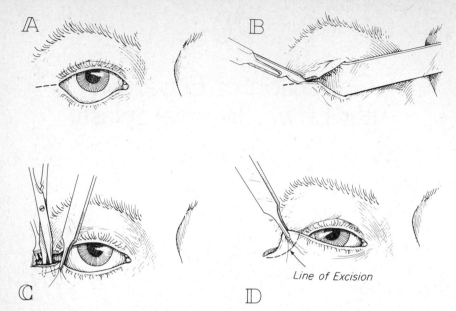

Line of Excision

Figure 20.1 *Correction of ectropion after blepharoplasty.*

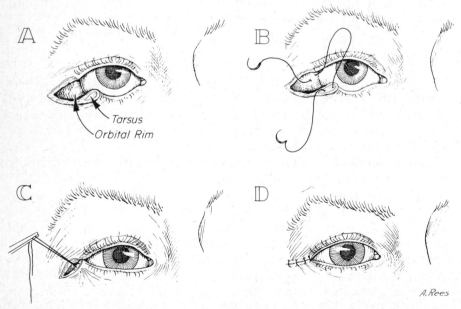

Tarsus
Orbital Rim

A. Rees

Figure 20.2 *Lateral canthal lid tightening.*

Ousterhout DK, Weil RB: The role of the lateral canthal tendon on lower eyelid laxity. *Plast Reconst Surg* 69:620, 1982.

Schaefer AJ: Lateral canthal tendon tuck. *Ophthalmol* 86:1879, 1979.

Wesley RE, Collins JW: McCord procedure for ectropion repair. *Arch Otolaryngol* 109:319, 1983.

21

Conjunctival Incision for Herniated Orbital Fat

Fred Schwarz
Peter Randall

INTRODUCTION

In lower eyelid blepharoplasty, an incision is usually made beneath the cilia for the removal of herniated fat pads and excess skin. In cases of herniated fat pads without excess skin, such as younger patients, a skin incision can be avoided through the use of a conjunctival approach for the removal of herniated orbital fat.

TECHNIQUE

The technique below allows for the graded removal of fat without a skin incision. After lower eyelid infiltration with a small amount of 1% lidocaine with 1:200,000 epinephrine, a conjunctival incision can be made with scalpels or scissors just below the tarsus (Fig. 21.1), where the conjunctiva and orbital septum are closely approximated and can be simultaneously incised. The width of the incision should be approximately three-quarters the distance between the punctum and the lateral canthus.

Retraction sutures or rakes through the free edge of the conjunctiva inferiorly and the tarsus superiorly facilitate exposure. With blunt scissors, a plane of dissection into the orbital septum can be followed to the orbital rim, and then the three orbital fat compartments can be located; the overlying septum can be pierced (Fig. 21.2) with scissors, and the excess fat in each compartment can be removed by separating, clamping, and cauterizing the fat. Care should be used to avoid amputating the conjunctiva cul-de-sac or injuring the inferior oblique muscle.

As with the subciliary approach, the amount of fat to be removed can be judged by external pressure on the globe. Excessive removal of fat can result in a sunken appearance. Inadequate removal may leave an unsightly cosmetic appearance.

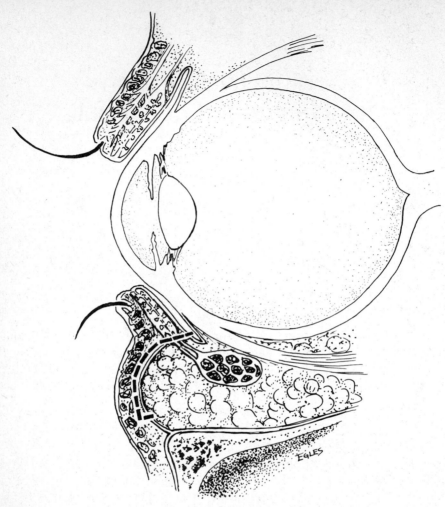

Figure 21.1 *Conjunctival incision carried anterior to septum.*

Once the appropriate amount of orbital fat has been removed, hemostasis is obtained and the conjunctiva is closed with a 6-0 plain gut suture (Fig. 21.3). No sutures are placed through the orbital septum.

This technique avoids any scar on the external skin surface. The procedure can be used for primary fat removal in blepharoplasty or as a refinement for a previously performed blepharoplasty. Traditionally, a second skin incision for touch-up work in lower lid blepharoplasties has been avoided.

BIBLIOGRAPHY

Schwarz F, Randall P: Conjunctival incision for herniated orbital fat. *Ophthal Surg* 11:276, 1980.

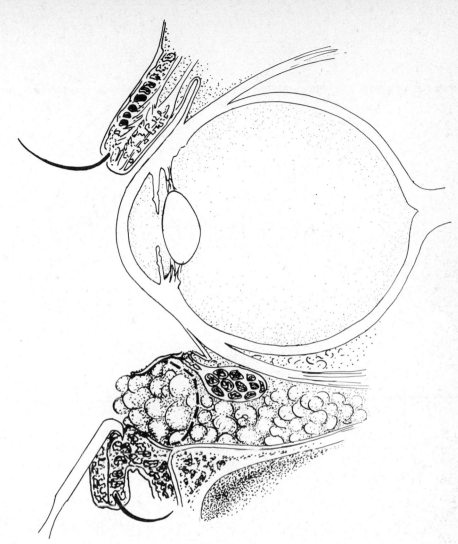

Figure 21.2 Septum opened to remove fat.

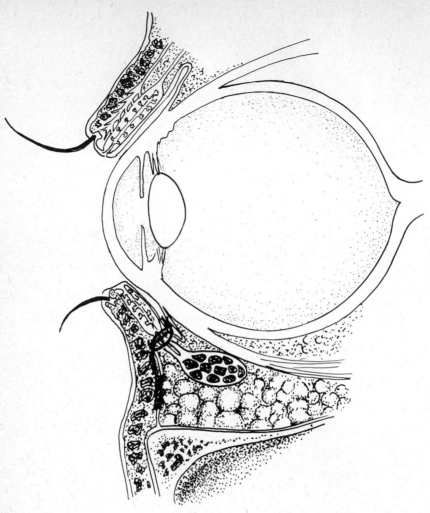

Figure 21.3 Closure of conjunctiva. (Reprinted with permission. Ophthalmic Surgery 11:276–279, 1980.)

22

Nonsurgical Correction of Ectropion After Blepharoplasty

Ralph E. Wesley

Lower eyelid blepharoplasty can cause ectropion resulting in both an irritated eye and an irritated patient. Though ectropion usually resolves, the patient may demand immediate relief.

Frequently, ectropion after blepharoplasty can be corrected immediately by removing the sutures, separating the wound, and allowing the defect to close by secondary intention.

TECHNIQUE

The sutures in the lower eyelid with ectropion after blepharoplasty (Fig. 22.1A) should be removed. The wound should be separated with a cotton-tipped applicator until traction on the lower lid is released and the ectropion corrected (Fig. 22.1B).

The raw area should be covered daily with a steroid-antibiotic ointment. Nearly always, the area heals without noticeable scar (Fig. 22.1C).

This technique works well with mild to moderate ectropion. With severe skin shortage or marked laxity, a lid-tightening procedure must be employed (see Chapter 20).

Ectropion does not always occur from excessive removal of skin. Some patients develop the outward rolling lid margin from eyelid edema. Other patients have prolonged orbicularis muscle weakness from the injection of long-acting anesthetics such as bupivacaine. Both such patients experience spontaneous resolution of ectropion. But an occasional patient develops ectropion despite good lid turgor and proper skin removal.

A generous separation of the wound with this technique is recommended for best results as the free skin-muscle flaps tends to advance spontaneously toward the lid margin.

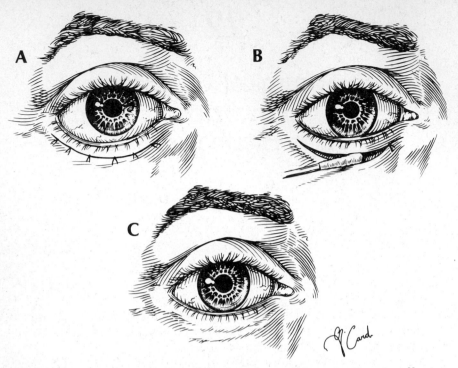

Figure 22.1 Early suture removal and wound separation to alleviate ectropion after blepharoplasty.

23

Simultaneous Treatment of Lower Eyelid Dermatochalasis and Abnormal-Appearing Skin

Allen M. Putterman

INTRODUCTION

Lower eyelid blepharoplasty patients may have not only excess skin and bulging fat but also an abnormal skin quality or pigmentation, usually over the nasal one-half or two-thirds of the lower eyelid (Fig. 23.1A). The conventional lower blepharoplasty removes the more normal skin temporarily and stretches the abnormal nasal skin in that direction, which may worsen the appearance of the lower eyelid.

The technique below allows the surgeon to remove excessive abnormal skin nasally and cover the defect with temporal skin, leaving a more pleasing appearance.

TECHNIQUE

In patients with crinkly nasal eyelid skin, pulling the lower eyelid nasally with the finger provides a simple method to determine suitable candidates for this procedure preoperatively (Fig. 23.1B). The improvement in quality and color of the skin as more normal temporal skin diffuses throughout the eyelid provides a reasonable facsimile of the expected postoperative results. Conversely, if drawing the skin temporally with the finger worsens the appearance of the lower eyelid skin, the standard blepharoplasty approach should be avoided.

An incision is drawn 1.5 to 2 mm below the lashes of the lower eyelid, beginning nasally and extending 2 to 3 mm past the lateral canthus. The line then continues in a horizontal direction in one of the temporal laugh lines for 1 cm. At the nasal aspect of this line, a second line is directed in an inferior, temporal, oblique direction, approximately 1.5 cm (Fig. 23.1C). With local infiltration of 2% lidocaine with epinephrine for anesthesia and hemostasis and with a scleral lens for ocular protection, an

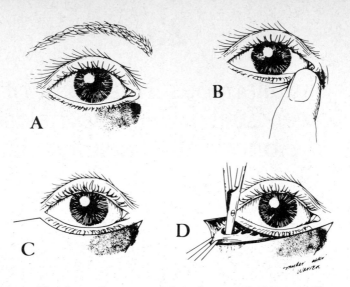

Figure 23.1 *Blepharoplasty to excise abnormal skin nasally.*

incision is made as marked. Then a Westcott scissors is used to dissect the lower eyelid skin from orbicularis muscle (Fig. 23.1D).

The skin flap, normally dissected to the inferior orbital rim (Fig. 23.2A), can be extended inferiorly for more exaggerated cases of dermatochalasis. The orbicularis oculi muscle can be opened across the entire eyelid just above the inferior orbital rim so that orbital fat that prolapses easily, with gentle pressure on the globe, can be clamped with a hemostat, excised, and cauterized.

With the slightest tension nasally and superiorly, the lower eyelid skin flap is pulled to fill the curvature of the nasal lower eyelid convexity (Fig. 23.2B). With the patient's gaze directed upward, the skin that drapes past the incision can be excised (Fig. 23.2C). If the patient is unable to gaze upward because of sedation or general anesthesia, pressure can be applied to the globe through the upper eyelid, which elevates the lower eyelid to a level similar to that achieved by an upward gaze.

A small triangle of skin should be excised vertically above the horizontal infralash incision, and a slightly larger triangle of skin should be excised nasally (Fig. 23.2D). The closure is accomplished with a continuous 6-0 black silk suture from the nasal end of the eyelid down the oblique incision, and then a second suture is run along the eyelid in a nasal to temporal direction (Fig. 23.2E).

Postoperatively, the patient uses an ice compress for 24 hours. With removal of orbital fat, vital eye signs are checked every 15 minutes for 2 hours to avoid possible blindness from retrobulbar hemorrhage. The skin sutures are removed 4 days postoperatively.

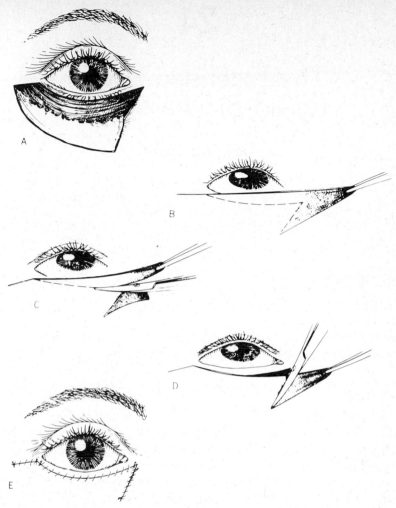

Figure 23.2 Skin excision nasally leaves normal skin.

BIBLIOGRAPHY

Katzen L, Karvelis J: Anesthesia, analgesia, and amnesia, in Putterman AM (ed): *Cosmetic Oculoplastic Surgery*. New York, Grune & Stratton, 1982, pp 89–97.

Putterman AM: Simultaneous treatment of lower eyelid dermatochalasis and abnormal-appearing skin. *Am J Ophthalmol* 96:6, 1983.

Putterman AM: Surgical treatment of lower eyelid dermatochalasis, herniated orbital fat, and hypertrophic orbicularis: A skin flap approach, in Putterman AM (ed): *Cosmetic Oculoplastic Surgery*. New York, Grune & Stratton, 1982, pp 117–133.

Putterman AM: Temporary blindness after cosmetic blepharoplasty. *Am J Ophthalmol* 80:1081, 1975.

24

The Extended Lower Eyelid Blepharoplasty

Robert G. Small

INTRODUCTION

Some patients with blepharochalasis have festoons, or "double bags," with a sagging of the lower eyelid away from the globe. The conventional lower eyelid blepharoplasty is not adequate to correct this deformity. The technique below is designed for these patients.

TECHNIQUE

A lower eyelid subciliary incision extends 1 cm past the lateral canthus. The skin edges are elevated for the incision. The opening of the incision is facilitated by placing the scissors beneath the orbicularis muscle, then the skin incision is completed with sharp scissors.

The skin muscle flaps are dissected to the zygoma. Retraction of the flaps by an assistant with the dissection (Fig. 24.1, upper left). Then, 1 cm of temporal oval of skin muscle flap is excised. Care is taken not to excise excess skin from the lower eyelid. The patient is instructed to open the mouth widely and look up to put the tissues of the midface on a maximum stretch.

The dissected skin is then draped over the lower eyelid, and the excess is marked for excision. Preferably, too little rather than too much skin should be excised from the lower lid. Additional skin can be excised at the lateral extension. Some contraction occurs in the lower eyelid skin during healing (Fig. 24.1, upper right).

To tighten the lower lid, a wedge excision or lateral canthoplasty is performed (Fig. 24.1, middle left). A mattress suture is placed through the skin muscle flap (Fig. 24.1, middle right) into the lateral orbital periosteum (Fig. 24.1, lower left). The skin is closed (Fig. 24.1, lower right).

This operation is used when a standard lower blepharoplasty will not suffice. Dissection of a skin muscle flap down to the zygoma combined

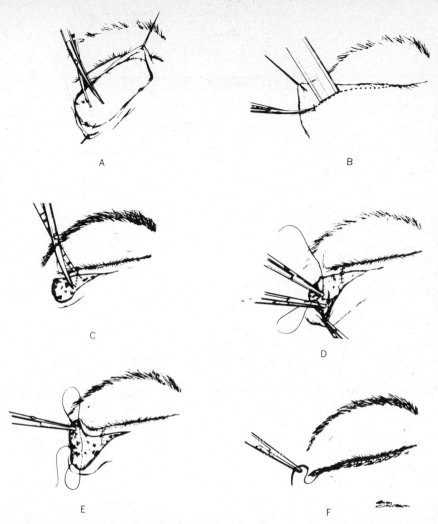

A

B

C

D

E

F

Figure 24.1 Extended lower lid blepharoplasty for festoons. (A) Skin muscle flap dissected to zygoma. Skin edges held up throughout. (B) 1-cm temporal oval of skin-muscle flap excised. (C) Wedge resection of lower eyelid. (D) Deep dermal-orbicularis mattress suture of 3-0 braided nylon. (E) Mattress suture completed in periosteum of lateral orbit. (F) Skin closure.

with a periosteal fixation suture is the basis for the extended lower lid blepharoplasty. This eliminates festoons, or bag-on-bag deformities, not corrected by a conventional blepharoplasty.

BIBLIOGRAPHY

Small RG: Extended lower eyelid blepharoplasty. *Arch Ophthalmol* 99:1402, 1981.

25

Midforehead Lift

Calvin M. Johnson, Jr.

INTRODUCTION

The procerus, frontalis, and corrugator muscles create permanent creases in the glabellar and forehead skin giving the eyes an aged, tired, crowded appearance not corrected by blepharoplasty.

The direct brow lift can effectively elevate and shape brow tissues, but leaves a scar at the brow-forehead juncture and fails to correct the glabellar deformity. The coronal forehead lift can be used satisfactorily except in problem cases, such as patients with male pattern hairline, thinning hair, or patients with a high hairline.

In patients with deep midforehead creases, the midforehead lift can correct brow ptosis and glabellar furrows while hiding the incision in natural skin lines.

TECHNIQUE

The upper incision should precisely follow a forehead crease, though asymmetric and slightly irregular, so the final scar mimicks the crease rather than a surgical incision (Fig. 25.1). The vertical dimension of the incision should reflect the desired amount of elevation of the brow and glabellar tissues.

With an over correction 0.5 to 1 cm desirable to allow for postoperative sagging (the upper blepharoplasty should follow the midforehead lift since less skin excision after the forehead lift will be required). After the incision (Fig. 25.2), skin flaps are elevated inferiorly to the supraorbital rims and superiorly for 0.5 cm, staying just above the tightly adherent underlining musculature.

A transverse incision should be carried through the frontalis muscle and fascia 3 to 4 cm superior to the nasal root, but no more laterally than the supraorbital notches (Fig. 25.3). Through this incision, a flap is dissected inferiorly to the nasal root and medial supraorbital rims in a plane just above the periosteum (Fig. 25.4).

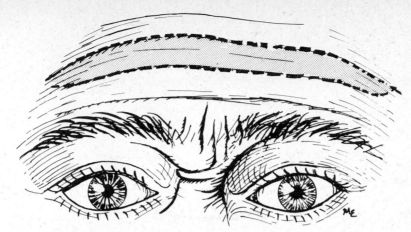

Figure 25.1 *Midforehead lift in natural crease.*

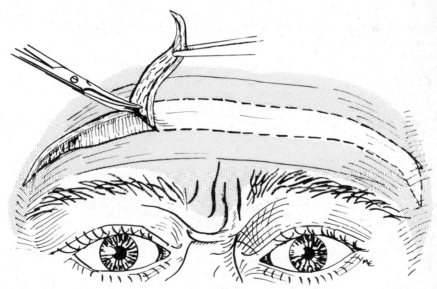

Figure 25.2 *Skin undermined in shaded area above and below incisions.*

The medial ends of the corrugator muscles are identified and isolated to avoid injury to the supraorbital and supratrochlear nerves and vessels. Then, 1 cm of corrugator muscle should be resected bilaterally. The procerus can be divided horizontally with an electrocautery cutting unit.

Superiorly, the dissection is carried in the subgalea plane to the level of the hairline through the horizontal frontalis incision made earlier (Fig. 25.5). As with a coronal forehead lift, the frontalis muscle and fascia are incised horizontally from the undersurface in one or two locations, corresponding to horizontal forehead creases (Fig. 25.5). The incisions should

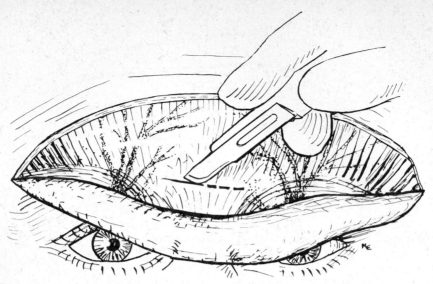

Figure 25.3 Incision through frontalis muscle should avoid supraorbital nerves and vessels.

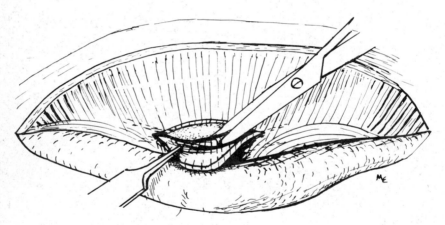

Figure 25.4 Dissection just above periosteum provides access to corrugator and procerus muscles.

not extend laterally beyond the pupils to preserve lateral frontalis function.

A narrow segment of frontalis muscle and fascia may be excised (Fig. 25.6), and the edge is sutured with 4-0 clear nylon sutures to elevate the glabellar and medial brow tissues.

The upper margin of the orbicularis muscle is also tacked superiorly in three or four locations to the underlying, unyielding fascial tissue with 4-0 clear nylon sutures (Fig. 25.7).

The skin can now be closed with 4-0 clear nylon interrupted sutures in

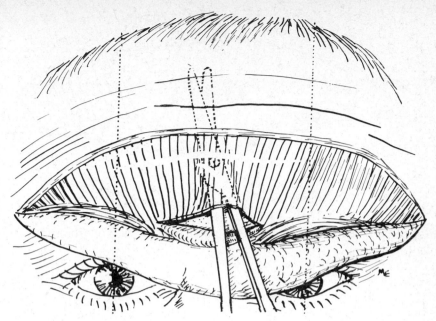

Figure 25.5 *Frontalis muscle incisions shown within pupillary lines.*

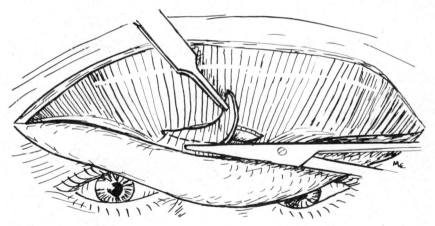

Figure 25.6 *Strip of frontalis excised.*

the dermis, and either running, locking, or simple 5-0 nylon sutures for the skin (Fig. 25.8). A light pressure dressing should be applied, and the sutures should be removed in 3 days; at which point, the wound should be splinted with Steri-strips.

The initial overcorrection should settle in 3 to 4 weeks with complete maturation of the scar in approximately 6 months.

This technique uses deep forehead furrows, primarily in men and older women to provide correct access to correct brow ptosis and glabellar furrowing. Meticulous attention to the technique helps to lessen the chances of damage to supraorbital nerves or vessels.

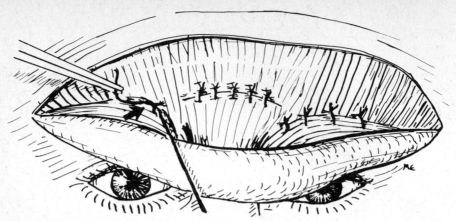

Figure 25.7 *Closure of frontalis incision and fixation of orbicularis muscle.*

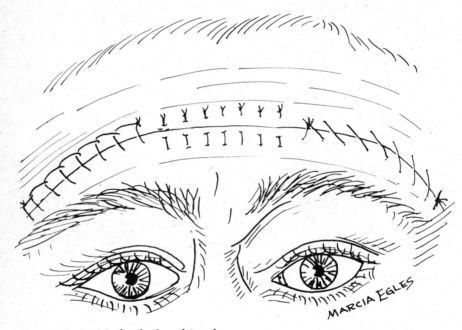

Figure 25.8 *Methods for skin closure.*

BIBLIOGRAPHY

Brennan HG: Management of the ptotic brow. *Otolaryngol Clin Am* 13:272, 1980.
Johnson CM Jr, Waldman SR: Mid-forehead lift. *Arch Otolaryngol* 109:155, 1983.

26

Modifications of Midforehead Lift Incisions

Calvin M. Johnson, Jr.

INTRODUCTION

Variations in the midforehead lift (see Chapter 25) incision can allow the surgeon flexibility in correcting different patterns of brow ptosis when correcting glabellar frown lines.

TECHNIQUE

The upper incision should follow precisely a natural skin line. The lower incisions can be drawn to correct localized brow ptosis. With larger elipses drawn laterally (Fig. 26.1), overcorrection will be obtained in that area. When brow ptosis is primarily centrally (Fig. 26.2), the area of greatest excision should be performed in the midline.

In patients without such deep furrows, a broken incision can be used (Fig. 26.3) to make the healing scar less conspicous since broken patterns are less recognizable as surgical scars.

BIBLIOGRAPHY

Johnson CM Jr, Waldman SR: Mid-forehead lift. *Arch Otolaryngol* 109:155, 1983.

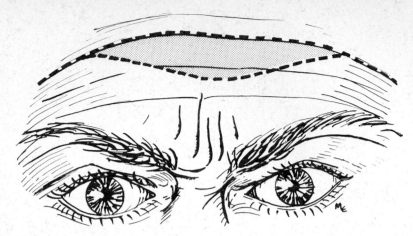

Figure 26.1 Incision for midline brow ptosis.

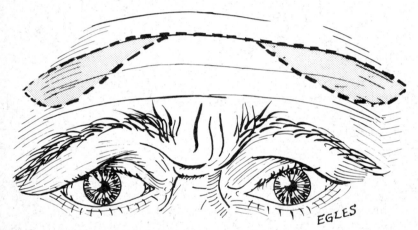

Figure 26.2 Incision for lateral brow ptosis.

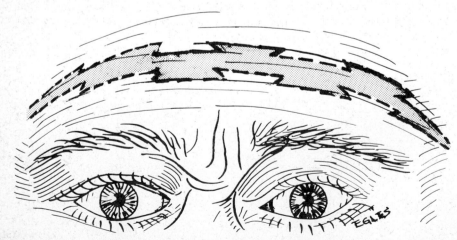

Figure 26.3 Broken geometric incision to hide midforehead incision.

72

27

Coronal Brow Lift for Correction of Brow Ptosis in Forehead Wrinkles

Kevin I. Perman
Henry I. Baylis

INTRODUCTION

Patients frequently come to the surgeon's office requesting upper lid blepharoplasty who actually have a significant degree of forehead and brow ptosis contributing to their problem. Surgically removing all of the apparent excess skin would cause the disasterous complication of attaching the eyelids to the eyebrows.

The direct brow lift, the traditional approach to correction of brow ptosis, can create several problems, including scarring above the brow, failure to eliminate wrinkles in the forehead and glabellar regions, and forehead hypesthesia from frontal nerve injury.

The coronal approach hides the incision behind the hairline and elevates the entire forehead, brows, and glabellar region.

With this technique, the incision behind the hairline allows the forehead to be split into two lamella, with the skin and subcutaneous tissue anteriorly and the frontalis muscle and galea aponeurotica in the posterior portion. The frontalis muscle is interrupted, thus allowing for the passive elevation of the forehead, and the corrugator supraciliary muscles and proceurus muscles are dissected for elimination of vertical forehead wrinkles.

TECHNIQUE

Local infiltration of 0.5% lidocaine with epinephrine (1:200,000) for anesthesia and hemostasis should be used whether the procedure is under local or general anesthesia. The injection should be performed at the level

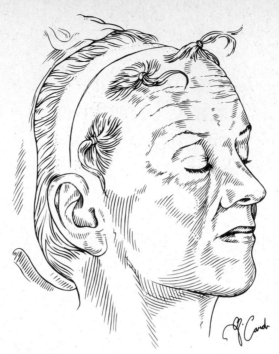

Figure 27.1 *Coronal brow lift incision.*

of the eyebrows to block the supraorbital and supratrochlear nerves. The proposed incision line is infiltrated superficial to the galea.

The incision is carried from the root of the helix of the ear, extending superiorly, and paralleling the frontal hairline to a corresponding point of the opposite ear after the hair in the area has been curled and firmly fixed with rubberbands (Fig. 27.1). The scalp incision should be 5 to 8 cm behind the midfrontal hairline. Hemostatis at the flap margin can be obtained with electrocautery and Rainey clips. The forehead flap is elevated with a combination of scissor and digital dissection to the supraorbital ridges without entering the orbital cavities (Fig. 27.2). A dissection superficial to the periosteum should avoid danger of injury to the temporal branches of the facial nerve.

The corrugator supraciliary muscles are separated from the superior orbital neurovascular bundles, and approximately 0.5 cm is excised from each boney origin. A strip of frontalis muscle of approximately 1 cm in width is excised from beneath the main portion of the flap (Fig. 27.3). Each proceurus muscle is identified and dissected from the nasal bones.

The brow should be detached with blunt dissection from the orbital rims to allow for brow and forehead elevation; then, approximately 2 to 3 cm of flap is resected. The amount to be resected is determined by advancing the flap onto the wound. The forehead flap is trimmed and sutured (Fig. 27.4) with 3–0 Prolene in small segments to reduce bleeding. Staples may be used on the external surface.

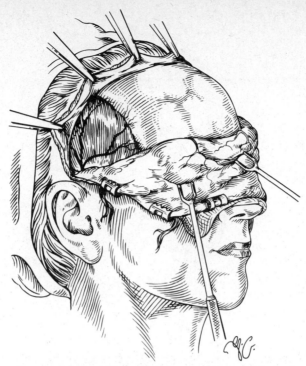

Figure 27.2 Forehead flap dissected to superior orbital rims.

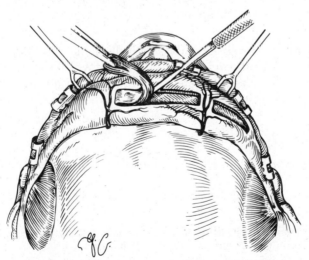

Figure 27.3 Excision of frontalis muscle strips.

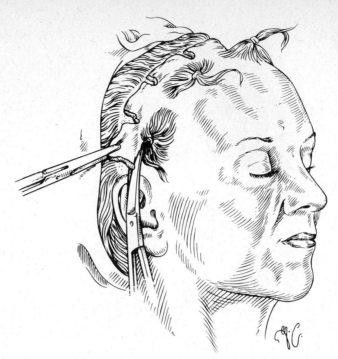

Figure 27.4   *Resection of excess forehead tissue. (Fett DR, Sutcliffe RT, Bayliss HI: The coronal brow lift. Am J Ophthalmol 96:751–754, 1983. Published by The American Journal of Ophthalmology. Copyright by The Ophthalmic Publishing Company.)*

Complications, though unusual, include hematoma, flap necrosis, facial motor nerve injury, and numbness. The brow lift should be performed before the blepharoplasty to determine the appropriate amount of skin for blepharoplasty.

BIBLIOGRAPHY

Fett DR, Sutcliffe RT, Baylis HI: The coronal brow lift. *Am J Ophthalmol* 96:751, 1983.

LeRoux P, Jones SH: Total permanent removal of wrinkles from the forehead. *Br J Plast Surg* 27:356, 1974.

Rees TD: Aesthetic plastic surgery. Philadelphia, Saunders, 1980.

Vinas JC, Caviglia C, Cortinas JL: Forehead rhytidoplasty and brow lifting. *Plast Reconstr Surg* 57:445, 1976.

28

Thin-Haired Coronal W-Plasty Incision

Julius Newman

INTRODUCTION

The coronal forehead lift provides correction of brow ptosis and furrowing of the forehead secondary to prominent frontalis, corrugator, and procerus musculature without the prominent incisions of the direct brow procedures. Camouflaging of the incision is particularly enhanced if the incision is beveled in the direction of the hair follicles with minimal loss of hair along the margins of the scar.

Problems arise in patients with thin hair or in patients in whom the scar widens and becomes noticeable. Further, with enough hair loss, abnormal parting of the hair to non-hair-bearing scar tissue can occur. The coronal brow lift has previously been contraindicated in patients with thin hair.

The coronal W-plasty incision can be used in these problem patients to provide a more pleasing result.

TECHNIQUE

The hair is parted along the planned incision and tied in corn rows; a small area of the scalp is shaved. Using a fine marking pen, the W-plasty incision is mapped with 90-degree angled flaps and 1 cm legs (Fig. 28.1). Local anesthesia (2% lidocaine with 1:100,000 epinephrine along the incision line and 0.5% lidocaine with 1:200,000 epinephrine under the coronal flap) is injected.

The W-plasty incision is carried to the level of the galea with a scalpel. The separate galea incision does not follow the W-plasty pattern. The standard coronal lift procedures are followed including the excision of frontalis muscle, transection of corrugator and procerus muscle bands, and the excision of excess scalp individualized to each patient's needs. Care is taken to avoid neurovascular injury.

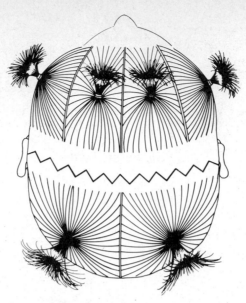

Figure 28.1   W-plasty coronal incision.

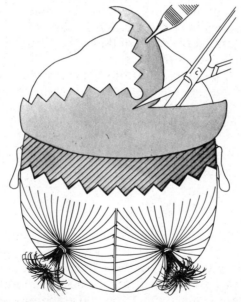

Figure 28.2   Excess scalp removed.

After excess scalp is removed (Fig. 28.2), the anterior border of the incision is serated in a mirror-image W-plasty with 90-degree tips and 1 cm legs to interdigitate with the posterior incision (Fig. 28.3). The edges are then approximated and stapled along each leg using a small staple gun (Figs. 28.4, 28.5). Alternate staples are removed at 1 week, and the remainder are removed on the tenth postoperative day.

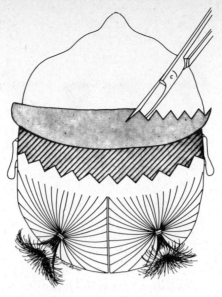

Figure 28.3 *Incision serated to match W-plasty.*

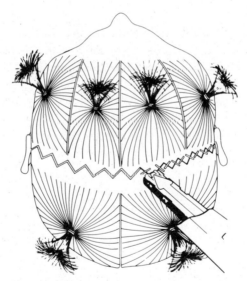

Figure 28.4 *Incision stapled.*

The staples leave no track marks, and loss of hair secondary to tension from retention sutures is avoided. A running W-plasty disguises the continuity of the scar to the eye, and any hair loss is less apparent. The points of the W-plasty are occasionally devoid of hair growth. However, the zigzag appearance of the scar allows the remaining hair easily to hide these small areas of denuded scalp.

79

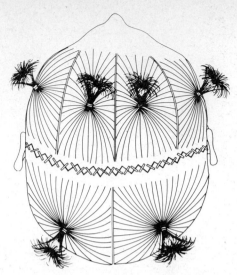

Figure 28.5 *Final W-plasty closure to camouflage incision.*

BIBLIOGRAPHY

Brennan, HG: The frontal lift. *Arch Otolaryngol* 104:26, 1978.

Kaye BL: The forehead lift. *Plast Reconstr Surg* 60:161, 1978.

Liebman EP, Webster RC, Berger AS, et al: The frontal nerve in the temporal brow lift. *Arch Otolaryngol* 108:232, 1982.

Newman J, Dolsky RL, Imber P: Thin haired coronal lift w-plasty incision. *Laryngoscope* 94:407, 1984.

29

Correction of Mild
to Moderate Brow Ptosis
Through Blepharoplasty Incision

Orkan G. Stasior
Bradley N. Lemke

INTRODUCTION

Patients submitting to blepharoplasties frequently need brow elevation. Traditional supraciliary temporal, coronal, or forehead incisions can cause visible scars, paresthesias, and hair loss. Consequently, the blepharoplasty surgeon may avoid elevating the patient's brow and provide a less than optimal postoperative result.

With the technique described below, the surgeon can correct mild to moderate eyebrow ptosis through a blepharoplasty incision.

TECHNIQUE

The amount of eyebrow lift should be determined with the patient in a sitting position and the blepharoplasty incision marked in the upper eyelid crease. With the patient supine, the upper eyelid and brow are infiltrated with 2% lidocaine with 1:100,000 epinephrine. After the incision is performed, sharp dissection should divide the preseptal orbicularis muscle along the entire length of the incision. Dissection should be carried superiorly to separate the orbicularis and frontalis muscle from the underlying tissue (Fig. 29.1).

The underlying tissue initially is the posterior orbicularis fascia, which fades into fatty tissue as the eyebrow and eyebrow fat are approached. The supraorbital nerve branches should be safely avoided if the underside of the frontalis muscle is not dissected more than 2 cm above the eyebrow.

Then, 3-0 nonabsorbable sutures with large needles are used to secure the eyebrow muscle to the frontal bone periosteum (Fig. 29.2). The sutures should be placed approximately 1 cm apart with the middle suture placed at the intended apex of the eyebrow arch.

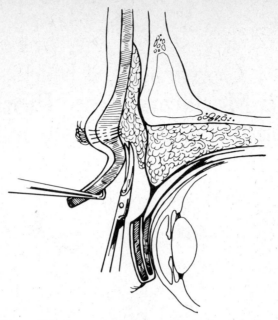

Figure 29.1 Brow lift through blepharoplasty incision.

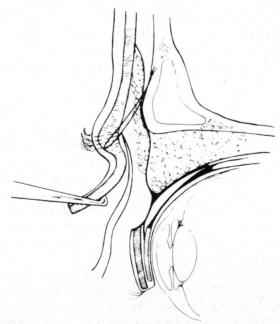

Figure 29.2 Permanent sutures to secure brow muscle to periosteum.

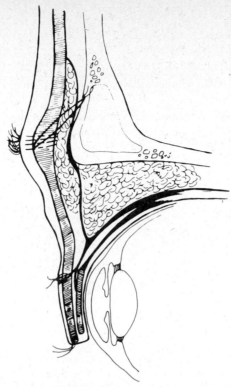

Figure 29.3 *Fixation of brow without loops pulled to tightly. (Reprinted with permission. Stasior OG, Lempke BN: The posterior eyebrow fixation. Adv Ophthalmic Plastic Reconstr Surg 2:193–197, 1983. Copyright by Pergamon Press Ltd.)*

A needle is passed through the eyebrow fat and then securely into the frontal bone periosteum as high as possible. The second pass should be into the thick eyebrow muscle underneath the eyebrow (Fig. 29.3). A single throw should be placed in the central suture, which is then tightened to elevate the brow to the desired level.

The loop does not need to be pulled tight, but the knot should then be locked with 2 or 3 more throws. The remaining medial and lateral sutures are tied in a similar fashion to provide a cosmetically pleasing arch to the eyebrow. Once the eyebrow elevation has been accomplished, the surgeon can then proceed with the blepharoplasty.

This procedure corrects mild to moderate ptosis, leaves no visible scar, and avoids hair loss or parasthesias. An immobile eyebrow does not result after posterior fixation, since the thick eyebrow can pivot over the sutures. The eyebrow height can be adjusted, but the loops should not be tied as tightly as possible.

BIBLIOGRAPHY

Castanares S: Forehead wrinkles, glabellar frown, and ptosis of the eyebrows. *Plast Reconstruct Surg* 31:106, 1964.

Johnson C: The brow lift 1978. *Arch Otolaryngol* 105:124, 1979.

Lemke BN, Stasior OG: The anatomy of eyebrow ptosis. *Arch Ophthalmol* 100:981, 1982.

Stasior OG, Lemke BN: The posterior eyebrow fixation, in SL Bosniak (ed): *Advances in Ophthalmic Plastic and Reconstructive Surgery*. New York, Pergammon, 1983, vol 2, p 193–197.

30

Periosteal Brow Fixation

Robert G. Small

INTRODUCTION

Eyebrow ptosis frequently accompanies blepharochalasis or facial palsy. It also follows facial neurectomy for blepharospasm. A simple skin excision can be used for brow fixation, but the best long-term results are achieved with periosteal fixation. In many patients with eyebrow ptosis, elevation of the lateral half of the brow suffices. The procedure can be performed rapidly with upper and lower blepharoplasty or combined with a facial neurectomy for essential blepharospasm.

TECHNIQUE

A 2.5 cm incision is marked along the lateral one-half to one-third of the eyebrow with the superior curved crescent 1 cm in its greatest vertical height (Fig. 30.1). Full-thickness skin is be excised down to muscle and a crescent of skin is excised. An incision is then carried through all layers to the pericranium. Scissors are used to dissect the skin away from the galea for a short distance (Fig. 30.2).

A 3-0 braided polyester mattress surture is placed through galea/frontalis layer from below upward, as shown in Figure 30.3. The suture is then brought down through the aponeurotic layer (Fig. 30.4). The needle is then passed posteriorly through the pericranium (Fig. 30.5) along the boney skull for about 1 cm and brought out. The needle is passed anteriorly to otain the second bite of periosteum and brought out close to the point where the periosteum was entered (Fig. 30.6). The sutures are drawn up tightly and the brow observed to be at the desired level. The suture is tied securely and the skin closed with running subcuticular 5-0 nylon.

Periosteal fixation of the brow with skin excision reapproximates the eyebrow to its normal position just above the orbital rim. The term "brow

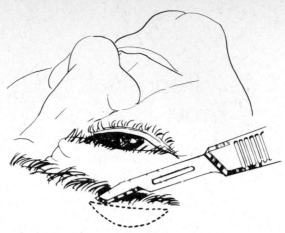

Figure 30.1 Elliptical incision marked in lateral brow.

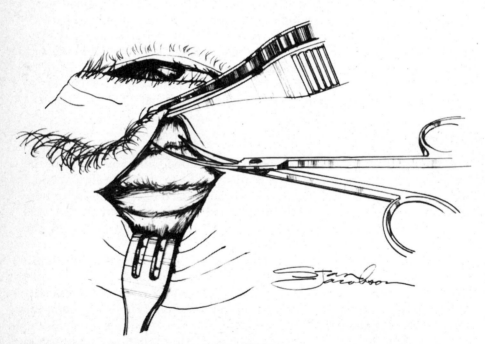

Figure 30.2 Dissection carried to galeal.

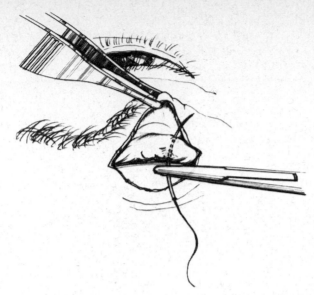

Figure 30.3 Suture from posterior edge of galea-frontalis layer.

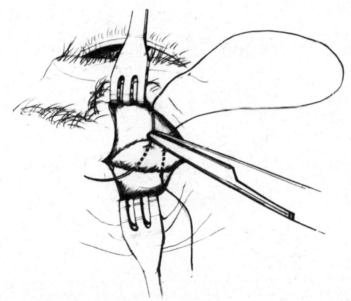

Figure 30.4 Bite through aponeurotic layer.

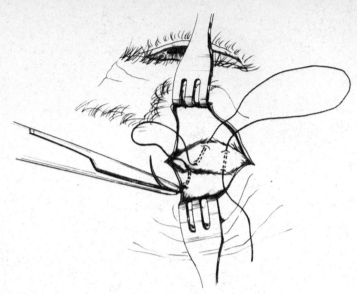

Figure 30.5 Needle posteriorly through pericranium.

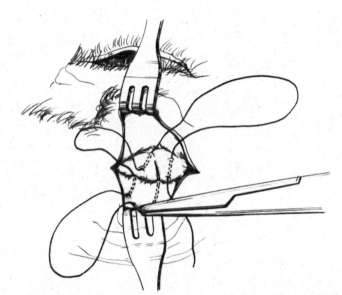

Figure 30.6 Second bite of periosteum for final closure of fixation.

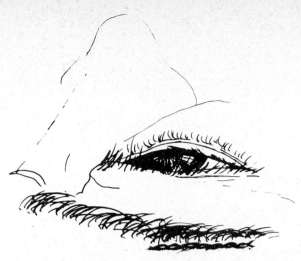

Figure 30.7 *Brow fixation after skin closure. (Reprinted with permission. Small RG: Periosteal fixation in reconstructive blepharoplasty. Adv Ophthalmic Plastic Reconstr Surg 2:89–99, 1983. Copyright by Pergamon Press, Ltd.)*

fixation'' is used, since the brow is not lifted but secured to its normal site (Fig. 30.7). Although the scar from the operation is inconspicuous after a month or two, the procedure is not recommended for young, fair-skinned females.

BIBLIOGRAPHY

Small RG: Periosteal fixation in reconstructive blepharoplasty, in Bosniak SL (ed): *Advances in Ophthalmic Plastic and Reconstructive Surgery.* New York, Pergammon, 1983, vol 2, p 89–99.

ENTROPION AND TRICHIASIS

PART III

31

Suture Repair of Entropion

J. Earl Rathbun

INTRODUCTION

With acute spastic entropion, the lower eyelid turns inward allowing keratinized skin and lashes to rub against the cornea and conjunctiva (Fig. 31.1A). The suture technique for entropion repair can be used to provide immediate relief of the pain and irritation.

TECHNIQUE

One needle of double-armed 5-0 chromic gut suture is passed through the conjunctiva adjacent to the inferior border of the tarsus, then directed inferiorly to engage the disinserted lower eyelid retractors or tuck the dehisced lower eyelid retractors. The needle is passed anteriorly and superiorly to the inferior border of the tarsus. The skin is pulled inferiorly with light traction as the needle penetrates the orbicularis muscle and out the skin just above the inferior tarsal border.

The second needle of the suture is placed in a similar manner 3 mm from the first on the same horizontal plane. The suture is tied as tightly as possible without a bolster. The three sutures are placed in the lateral two-thirds of the eyelid (Fig. 31.1B).

If insufficient correction or overcorrection is obtained, the sutures are replaced varying the technique of passage until the eyelid is in a fully corrected or a slightly overcorrected position. Bringing the sutures out closer to the lid margin gives more correction of entropion, and the lower position gives lesser correction. In congenital epiblepharon, the sutures are placed in the medial one-half or one-third of the eyelid.

The sutures remain in 3 weeks to allow formation of a full-thickness eyelid scar to prevent the anterior lamella (skin and orbicularis muscle) from overriding the posterior lamella (tarsus and conjunctiva). The sutures reattach the disinserted lower lid retractors or tuck any laxity of

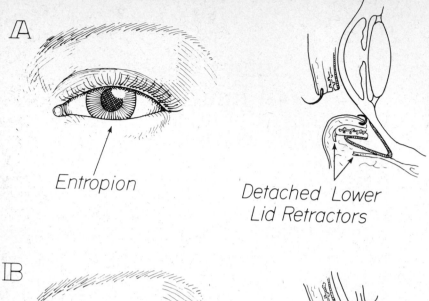

Figure 31.1 Double-armed 5-0 chromic sutures for entropion repair.

lower eyelid retractors. The 5-0 chromic gut creates the necessary inflammatory reaction and fibrosis.

This technique can be applied when entropion complicates eyelid reconstruction, canthoplasties, or entropion repair. The procedure works for acute involutional entropion as well as congenital epiblepharon.

Over correction, resulting in ectropion, can be remedied by the early removal of the sutures and applying massage. If entropion should recur, this technique should not be repeated, but the surgeon should use a procedure that directly corrects eyelid laxity and reattaches disinserted retractors, tucks dehisced retractors, or creates a more definite and wider full-thickness eyelid scar.

BIBLIOGRAPHY

Quickert MH, Rathbun E: Suture repair of entropion. *Arch Ophthalmol* 85:304, 1971.

32

Excision of Skin Elipse
to Correct Entropion
Without Horizontal Laxity

Sanford D. Hecht

INTRODUCTION

The technique below allows the surgeon to correct primary or recurrent entropion that does not involve horizontal laxity by simple skin excision as an office procedure.

TECHNIQUE

An elipse should be drawn with the upper edge 2 to 3 mm from the lid margin with a vertical height between 5 and 11 mm, depending on the degree of skin laxity (Fig. 32.1A). When in doubt, a lesser excision should be performed.

After injecting 2% lidocaine with epinephrine, the incision can be carried out with a 15 Bard–Parker blade. The skin is excised and closed with 6-0 nylon (Fig. 32.1B).

Placing temporary 4-0 black silk sutures in the lower midmargin for upward traction facilitates the marking and excision of skin during the procedure. A corneoscleral lens can be used for ocular protection. Ideally, the elipse should be drawn after the injection of local anesthetic.

When applied to the appropriate cases, this procedure allows for simple, dependable correction of entropion. If applied to a patient with horizontal laxity, this procedure can cause ectropion or retraction of the lower lid, resulting in scleral show.

BIBLIOGRAPHY

Hecht SD: Management of recurrent involution entropion and ectropion surgical failures, in Koch DD, Parke DW, Patten D (eds): *Current Management in Ophthalmology.* New York, Churchhill Livingston, 1983, p 287–288.

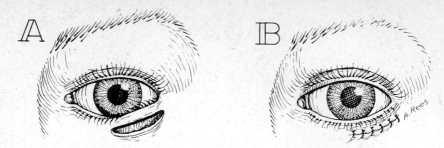

Figure 32.1 Excision of skin (A) to correction entropion (B)

33

Office Repair
of Senile Entropion
with Hyphercation

Robert H. Magnuson

INTRODUCTION

Entropion of the lower eyelid can cause a severe, painful irritation of the eye that needs permanent correction. A hyphercator can be used as a simple method in the office to provide immediate correction of entropion.

TECHNIQUE

The injection of 2% lidocaine into the lower lid with entropion (Fig. 33.1, top) provides anesthesia. A Birtcher hyphercator with a setting of about 75 produces fulguration approximately 1 mm in diameter surrounded by a ring of necrotized epithelium. Approximately 15 punctures can be made just below the lash margin, then an additional 75 to 150 punctures can be made extending down the lower lid (Fig. 33.1, center) until enough epithelial retraction is produced to hold the lashes away from the globe.

If a hyphercator is not available, a high-temperature cautery probe (not the low-temperature model used for cataract surgery) can be used. The procedure takes longer with thermal cautery as the ends of the wire must frequently be cleaned to provide a hot temperature.

This procedure provides immediate relief of entropion (Fig. 33.1, bottom). No patch is required, though the patient should be cautioned that the lid will swell and ooze from the burn for several days. An eschar will form and fall off between the second and third week, but no permanent scar or evidence of the procedure can be found after 4 weeks.

This procedure uses a larger number of less extensive, more superficial punctures than originally described by Ziegler. This procedure is found to be more effective in controlling the senile entropion. The occasional recurrence can be retreated.

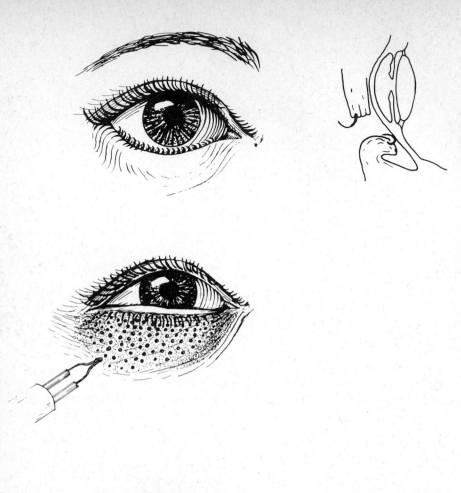

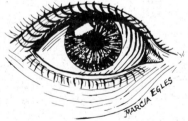

Figure 33.1 *Correction of entropion with cautery.*

BIBLIOGRAPHY

Jones LT, Reeh MJ, Tsujimura JK: Senile entropion. *Am J Ophthalmol* 55:463, 1963.

Magnuson RH: A simple office procedure for the repair of senile entropion. *Ophthalmic Surg* 6:83, 1975.

Schaefer AJ: Senile entropion. *Ophthalmic Surg* 5:11, 1974.

34

Lash Excision
for Lower Eyelid Trichiasis

Richard A. Kielar

INTRODUCTION

Lash excision, described below, is a fast, effective, technically simple procedure that can be performed on an outpatient basis to rid the patient with trichiasis of offending lashes.

TECHNIQUE

In a patient with lower lid trichiasis (Fig. 34.1, top), the lower affected area should be infiltrated with 2% lidocaine with epinephrine for both hemostasis and anesthesia. With a corneal protective lens in place, an incision is made along the gray line using a number 15 Bard–Parker blade. With the Westcott scissors, the skin and orbicularis muscle should be separated from the underlying tarsus for approximately 3 to 4 mm below the lash line. The operating microscope or loops can be helpful in making sure the dissection includes the lash follicles. The section should also be wide enough to include all offending lashes.

Finally, the undermined skin and orbicularis muscle should be excised in a strip approximately 3 mm wide (Fig. 34.1, center). Westcott scissors should be used to undermine the inferior skin edge to release any tension that might pull the lid outward during the postoperative phase.

The bare section should be left to granulate and reepithelialize spontaneously while treated daily with antibiotic ointment.

Hemostasis during the procedure can be facilitated by the use of topical thrombin drops. The use of electrocautery should be avoided as much as possible to avoid producing scar tissue.

Immediately following the procedure, the lid margin appears raw and unsightly. Within a few weeks, the lid will have a normal appearance with correction of the trichiasis.

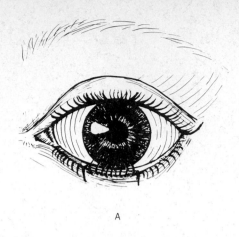

A

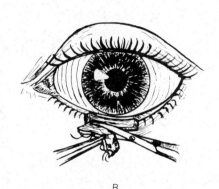

B

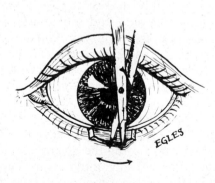

C

Figure 34.1 Abnormal lashes (A) are excised (B). Skin muscle undermined (C) without wound closure.

BIBLIOGRAPHY

Clorfeine GS, Kielar RA: Lash excision in trichiasis. *Ann Ophthalmol* 9:525, 1977.

35

Tarsoconjunctival Trapdoor Flap for Excision of Distichiasis Eyelashes

Richard K. Dortzbach

INTRODUCTION

Distichiasis, a congenital anomaly with an accessory row of eyelashes at the posterior border of the eyelid margin at the location of the meibomian gland openings, requires treatment when the accessory lashes are directed posteriorly, resulting in ocular irritation. Conventional methods of treatment, such as electrolysis or excision by splitting the eyelid margin at the gray line, can lead to complications of trichiasis, entropion, and eyelid margin distortion. The use of buccal mucosa, nasal septal mucosa, and tarsoconjunctival grafts involves complicated surgery.

The tarsoconjunctival trapdoor technique allows for direct microscopic excision of the offending lash follicles without distortion of the eyelid margin.

TECHNIQUE

One or two traction sutures are placed through the upper eyelid margin to help keep the eyelid everted over a Desmarres retractor. Using the operating microscope, the surgeon makes an incision with a scalpel into the tarsoconjunctival surface in a parallel fashion about 2 mm posterior to the eyelid margin in the area of the distichiasis. With the incision carried down to the level of the distichiasis cilia, the scalpel is then directed toward the superior tarsal border in a plane parallel to the abnormal lashes.

The incision is carried far enough to create a tarsoconjunctival trapdoor, which will fully expose the aberrant cilia. Each distichiasis eyelash can be cut near the follicle and then the follicle excised (Fig. 35.1). The remaining shaft of the cilia can be pulled from the eyelid margin. Light

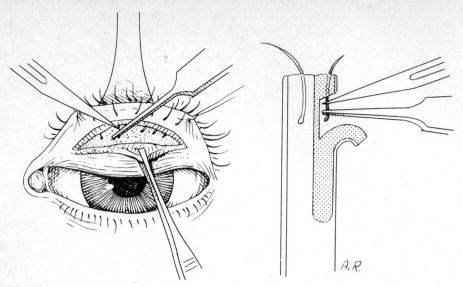

Figure 35.1 *Trapdoor incision to exposure distichiasis follicles.*

cautery can also be helpful in destroying the follicles of the distichiasis eyelashes after the trapdoor is opened.

To close the trapdoor, three double-armed sutures of 4-0 silk are passed through the anterior surface of the tarsoconjunctival trapdoor and then out through the eyelid structures anterior to the trapdoor (Fig. 35.2). Each suture should be tied over a cotton pledget on the skin surface just above the eyelid margin (Fig. 35.3).

The sutures can be removed at 5 days. Nonabsorbable sutures are used to prevent leaving some of the suture in the tarsus, which might cause further inflammatory reaction. The surgeon should be absolutely sure that the sutures do not pass through the posterior tarsoconjunctival surface, which would allow the suture to contact the cornea, resulting in possible corneal abrasion.

I have tried the lid-splitting technique with posterior lamellar cryosurgery: some cases did well, but others developed cicatricial ectropion—all four lids in one patient. While the trapdoor procedure can be rather long and tedious, the main advantage is better preservation of the normal eyelid margin.

BIBLIOGRAPHY

Anderson RL, Harvey JT: Lid splitting and posterior lamellar cryosurgery for congenital and acquired distichiasis. *Arch Ophthalmol* 99:631, 1981.

Dortzbach RK, Butera RT: Excision of distichiasis eyelashes through a tarsoconjunctival trapdoor. *Arch Ophthalmol* 96:111, 1978.

Fein W: Surgical repair for distichiasis, trichiasis and entropion. *Arch Ophthalmol* 94:809, 1976.

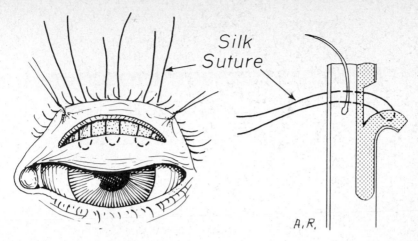

Figure 35.2 *Closure of trapdoor incision.*

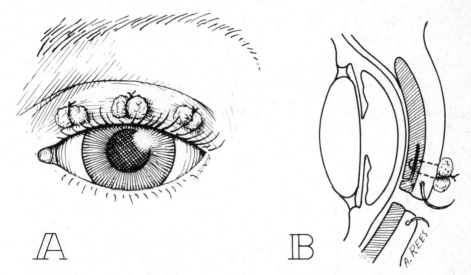

Figure 35.3 *Closure without entropion, trichiasis, or eyelid distortion.*

Scheie HG, Albert DM: Distichiasis and trichiasis: Origin and Management. *Am J Ophthalmol* 61:718, 1966.

White JH: Correction of distichiasis by tarsal resection in mucous membrane grafting. *Am J Ophthalmol* 80:507, 1975.

36

Marginal Rotation Procedure for Correction of Upper-Lid Entropion

Ralph E. Wesley

INTRODUCTION

Rotation of upper eyelid skin and lashes against the cornea with upper eyelid entropion can cause keratitis, pain, irritation, and the threat of corneal ulcer. More severe cases may require grafting of tarsus or cartilage. But the technique below can provide relief of mild upper-lid entropion with a quick, simple, one-stage procedure under local anesthesia.

TECHNIQUE

Under local anesthesia with the protective lens over the eye, the upper eyelid is anesthetized with 2% lidocaine with epinephrine (1:100,000) and hyaluronidase.

An elipse of skin and orbicularis should be excised from the upper lid. The lower incision is carried through the skin and orbicularis muscle down to the tarsal plate approximately 1 to 2 mm from the lashes, and the second incision is made approximately one-third the distance of the tarsal plate.

Once hemostasis has been obtained, the defect should be closed with the technique described below for optimum outward rotation of the lid margin.

Three to four sets of matrix sutures are passed with the initial bite through the skin edge of the lower lid, then carried through with a superficial bite in the tarsus near the superior wound edge, and then out through the skin edge (Fig. 36.1, left).

When the sutures are tied (Fig. 36.1, right) the lashes and lid margin rotate outward away from the cornea (Fig. 36.2). The procedure is effective with milder cases of cicatricial entropion. With progressive disease, the procedure may require reoperation as the lid contracts back onto the

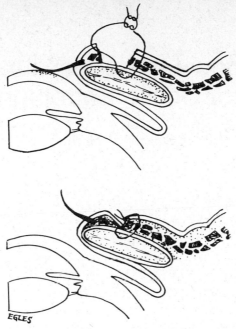

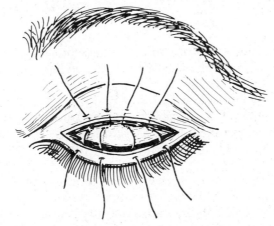

Figure 36.1 Correction of upper entropion. Lower skin edge attached to tarsal plate.

Figure 36.2 Anterior view of suture placement.

cornea at a later date. For more severe cases, tarsotomy and grafting may be required.

37

Bow-Legs Procedure for Senile Entropion

Sanford D. Hecht

INTRODUCTION

Factors associated with senile entropion include insufficiency of the lid retractors, upward movement of the preseptal orbicularis muscle, horizontal lid laxity, and absorption of orbital fat causing enophthalmos. Using the "bow-legs" technique, the surgeon can correct senile entropion with one simple operation.

TECHNIQUE

This technique can be considered a bow-legs procedure, since the incision has the appearance of a person with bowed legs (Fig. 37.1A). To test the maximum horizontal resection, the skin is grasped in the lower tarsal region about 5 to 6 mm below the lid margin with the two toothed forceps separated 7 mm apart. If the forceps cannot be brought together, too large a resection has been planned, and the skin regrasps to 6 mm apart. Conversely, with too much laxity (Fig. 37.1B) the area incised can be increased.

The usual full-thickness resection at the lid margin is approximately 2 to 3 mm, but can vary with the individual. The excision of tissue below the tarsus includes skin, orbicularis, conjunctiva, and retractors to form the lower part of the "V" (Fig. 37.1C).

To facilitate an evenly distributed, tight tarsal closure, the surgeon can place the flat handle of the forceps into the conjunctival cul-de-sac behind the tarsal wound. The needles can penetrate the tarsus and slide along the flat handle and reenter the other tarsal edge of the wound without danger to the globe.

This procedure incorporates nearly all elements believed necessary to correct entropion (Fig. 37.1D): (1) It tenses the lower lid retractor, capsular palpebral fascia, holding the lower tarsus tightly to the globe. (2) It pro-

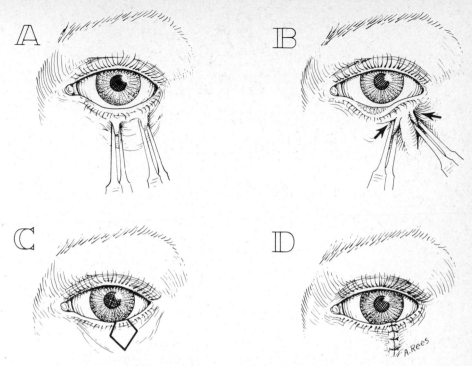

Figure 37.1 Forceps grasp lower lid with laxity entropion (A) to determine size of excision (B) in shape of "bow legs" (C). Final correction (D).

duces a firm skin-orbicularis-tarsal retractor adhesion preventing preseptal orbicularis from overriding the pretarsal orbicularis. (3) It produces a tightening of the orbicularis at the lower tarsus preventing the tarsus from rotating interiorly. (4) It removes an entire section of lid, thus improving the lid globe contact. (5) It uses common eyelid suture technique.

BIBLIOGRAPHY

Hecht SD: Management of recurrent involution entropion and ectropion surgical failures, in Koch DD, Park DW, Patten D (eds): *Current Management in Ophthalmology*. New York, Churchill Livingston, 1983, pp 284–286.

Hecht SD: Bow legs procedure for recurrent and primary entropion. *Ann Ophthalmol* 13:119, 1981.

38

Imbrication of the Lower Lid Retractors for Correction of Senile Entropion

Arthur J. Schaefer

INTRODUCTION

The inferior rectus muscle not only serves as a depressor of the globe, but also retracts the lower lid with force transmitted through the lower lid retractors to the lower tarsus. These retractors consist of an inferior aponeurosis (capsulopalpebral fascia) and the inferior tarsal muscle (Müller's), which are direct palpebral extensions of the capsulopalpebral head of the inferior rectus muscle.

Involutional changes in these lower lid retractors, possibly combined with horizontal tendon laxity, may fail to keep the lower lid in firm contact with the globe, permitting the lid to rotate inwardly as the septal orbicularis muscle contracts and rides up over the tarsal orbicularis—creating a senile entropion.

This technique describes repair of all types of involutional changes in the lower lid retractors to correct senile entropion.

TECHNIQUE

Involutional changes of the lower lid retractors consist of (1) thinning and atony of the retractors, (2) dehiscence of the lower lid retractors, or (3) complete detachment of the lower lid retractors, creating an inward turning of the lid (Fig. 38.1) that can cause severe irritation when the skin or lashes come in contact with the eye. These defects can be corrected by careful dissection and repair of the lower lid retractors.

With local anesthesia, an incision is made horizontally at the base of the tarsus (Fig. 38.2A), and skin dissection is carried through the orbicularis muscle, separating tarsal from septal orbicularis muscle (Fig. 38.2B). A horizontal strip of orbicularis muscle and skin can be excised (Fig. 38.2C). The dissection of the orbital septum from the tarsus is then

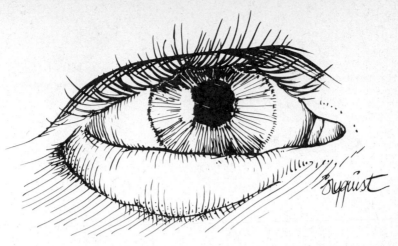

Figure 38.1 Entropion from involutional changes in lower lid retractors.

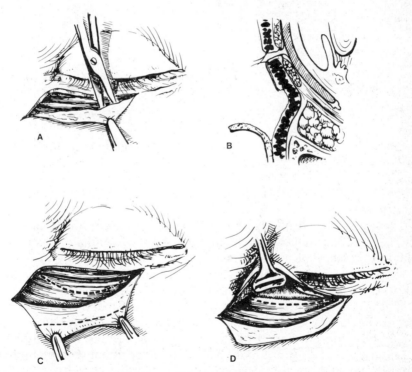

Figure 38.2 Exposure of lower lid retractors and excision of strip of orbicularis muscle.

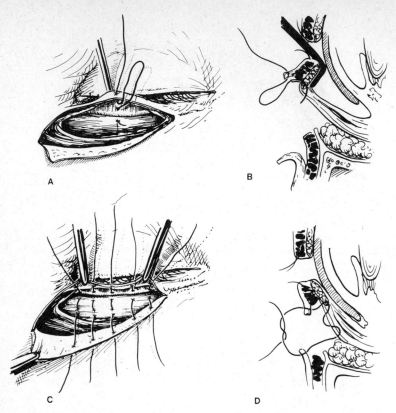

Figure 38.3 *Repair of lower retractors. Muscle hook in cul-de-sac helps rotate base of tarsus outward.*

carried out (Fig. 38.2D) to isolate the lower lid retractors (capsulopalpebral fascia and inferior tarsal muscle).

Repair can be accomplished by passing a needle through the skin (Fig. 38.3A) and through the tarsus facilitated by a tenotomy muscle hook in the cul-de-sac rotating the tarsal base outward (Fig. 38.3B).

Five sets of imbricating sutures are placed (Fig. 38.3C) that include the skin, the base of the tarsus, imbricate the lower lid retractors, and come out through the lower skin incision to be tied externally, as shown in Figure 38.3, in case of thinning of the aponeurosis. Figures 38.4, 38.5, and 38.6 show the placement of the imbricating sutures with a dehiscence (partial disinsertion) in Figure 38.4 with detachment (complete disinsertion in Fig. 38.5) or thinning (attentuation in Fig. 38.6).

With a dehiscence or complete detachment of the aponeurosis from the lower tarsus, the free edge of the retracted aponeurosis should be picked up and the lower imbrication suture passed with a 3 to 4 mm bite below the free edge, which corrects the detachment and shortening of the aponeurosis in one step (Figure 38.7). At the conclusion of the procedure, a base up skin triangle can be excised laterally (Fig. 38.8A) to facilitate horizontal tightening. The sagittal section in Figure 38.8B shows the im-

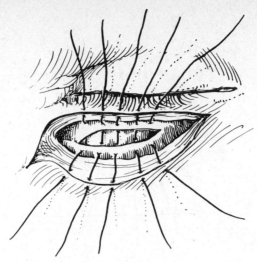

Figure 38.4 Repair of partial disinsertion.

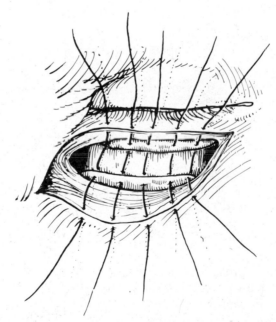

Figure 38.5 Repair of complete disinsertion.

brication of thinned lower lid retractors when a dehiscence or disinsertion does not occur. The final closure is shown in Figure 38.8C.

If the preoperative retraction test (see Chapter 46) indicates horizontal laxity, a lateral canthal tendon tuck should be included with this procedure for effective entropion repair.

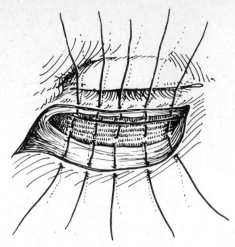

Figure 38.6 Repair with thinning of lower lid retractors.

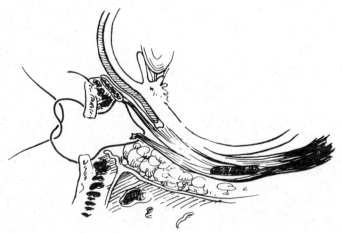

Figure 38.7 Placement of suture to repair lower retractors.

This external approach allows the surgeon to detect the pathophysiology of the lower lid retractors and to correct any of the anatomic variations with one procedure.

BIBLIOGRAPHY

Jones LT, Reeh MJ, Wobig JL: Senile entropion. *Am J Ophthalmol* 74:327, 1972.

Schaefer AJ: Involutional entropion. *Perspect Ophthalmol* 5:137–144, 1981.

Schaefer AJ: Lateral canthal tendon tuck. *Ophthalmol* 86:1878, 1979.

Schaefer AJ: Statistical summary senile entropion surgery. *Ophthalmic Surg* 8:125, 1977.

Schaefer AJ: Variation in the patho-physiology of involutional entropion and its treatment. *Ophthalmic Surg* 14:653–655, 1983.

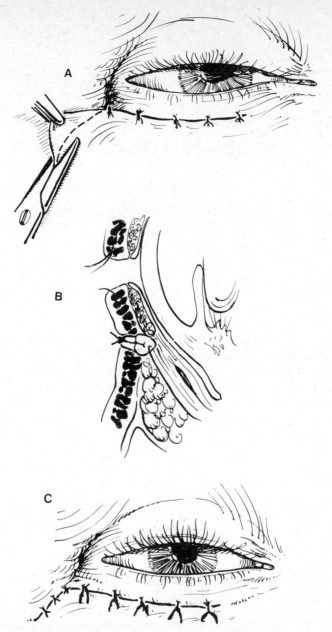

Figure 38.8 Base-up skin triangle excised laterally. Final closure. (Reprinted with permission Ophthalmic Surgery 14:653–655, 1983.)

39

Correction of Cicatricial Upper Eyelid Entropion with Ipsilateral Tarsal Graft

Henry I. Baylis
Conrad Hamako

INTRODUCTION

Numerous procedures have been described for correction of upper eyelid entropion, but long-lasting success generally requires some type of mucous membrane graft to correct severe entropion.

The technique below can correct unilateral or bilateral upper eyelid entropion by using full-thickness tarsus from the ipsilateral eyelid to lengthen the posterior lamellar and rotate the lid margin outward for relief of the constant irritation.

TECHNIQUE

The affected upper eyelid (Fig. 39.1A) should be everted over a bone plate to facilitate an incision 1.5 to 2.0 mm above the mucocutaneous junction for the full length of the tarsus. Only the conjunctiva and tarsus should be incised to avoid the fibers of the levator aponeurosis that attach to the anterior surface of the tarsus.

To harvest the graft, a horizontal scratch line is made on the tarsus outlining an elliptical strip superiorly approximately 3.0 to 4.0 mm in height. A full-thickness tarsal incision along the scratch line is carried out (Fig. 39.1B, middle arrow). With the graft still attached superiorly to the conjunctiva and Müller's muscle, fibers of the levator aponeurosis are bluntly separated from the anterior surface of the tarsal graft. The graft is removed by separating Müller's muscle and conjunctiva from the superior margin (Fig. 39.1B, top arrow).

The graft can be placed in the marginal tarsotomy bed (Fig. 39.1C).

To facilitate suturing, the graft is placed on the lower lid with the conjunctival surface down. The fractured margin of the upper lid is everted to direct the cut edge of the superior tarsus toward the graft. A

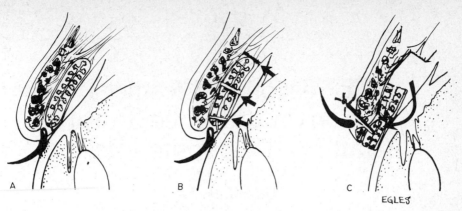

EGLES

Figure 39.1 *Upper entropion corrected with ipsilateral tarsal graft.*

single-armed 6-0 Prolene suture can be passed from skin surface just above the nasal lid margin through the tarsotomy incision and carried in a running fashion with lamellar bites of tarsal tissue and graft tissue. The suture is externalized at the opposite temporally and tied to its nasal end.

Next, a double-armed 6-0 Dexon suture with a small half-curve needle is placed horizontally in a lamellar fashion through the anterior surface of the tarsal graft at its midpoint (Fig. 39.1C). The suture should be placed 1.5 to 2.0 mm from the free margin of the graft with each arm of the suture passed superiorly under the lid margin and then directed downward and passed out through the lash line. An additional set of mattress sutures is placed in a similar manner on either side of this central everting suture. Apparent overcorrection should be noted following surgery.

The donor site need not be sutured. Antibiotic and steroid ointment can be applied, and a firm pressure dressing can be placed over the eye for 6 to 12 hours. The Prolene suture should be removed 6 to 10 days later by cutting one end of the suture at the skin surface and applying firm, steady traction at the opposite end.

The tarsal graft expands the posterior lamellar of the eyelid and prevents inward rotation of the lid margin and lash line. The donor site at the superior tarsus epithelializes without apparent contraction.

This technique avoids suturing the eyelids closed, and all surgery can be performed on a single eyelid.

BIBLIOGRAPHY

Bayliss HI, Hamako C: Tarsal grafting for correction of cicatricial entropion. *Ophthalmic Surg* 10:42, 1979.

Dortzbach RK, Callahan A: Repair of cicatricial entropion of upper eyelids. *Arch Ophthalmol* 85:82, 1971.

Soll DB: *Management of Complications in Ophthalmic Plastic Surgery.* Birmingham, Aesculapius, 1976, p 159.

Tenzel RR: Repair of entropion of upper lid. *Arch Ophthalmol* 77:675, 1967.

40

Correction of Cicatricial Entropion with Free Tarsal Graft from Opposite Eyelid

Henry I. Baylis
Conrad Hamako

INTRODUCTION

Chapter 39 describes a technique whereby a tarsal graft may be taken from an upper eyelid with cicatricial entropion and rotated into a tarsotomy site on the involved eyelid in unilateral or bilateral cases of cicatricial entropion from shortening and scarring of the posterior tarsal conjunctiva lamellar.

In unilateral cases, or with patients in whom adequate mucous membrane on the ipsilateral eyelid may not be present, the technique below can be used for tarsal grafting from the opposite eyelid for correction of cicatricial entropion.

TECHNIQUE

The technique uses the principles described in Chapter 39 to correct entropion of the eyelid in which the posterior portion of the lid is shortened, rotating skin and lashes against the globe (Fig. 40.1A). An incision should be made 1.5 to 2 mm inside the tarsal conjunctival mucous membrane junction of the involved eyelid for the full horizontal length of the tarsus (Fig. 40.1B, arrow).

A graft is then taken from the opposite tarsal plate using the method described in Chapter 39. This graft is then brought over, and the tarsotomy site is opened appropriately. This contralateral tarsal graft can be placed into the defect and sutured with running 6-0 Prolene and mattress sutures described previously to correct the entropion (Fig. 40.1C).

116

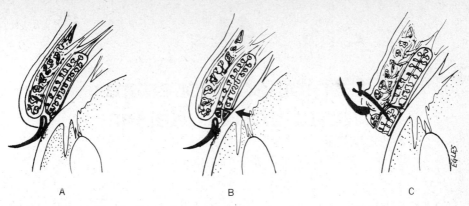

A   B   C

Figure 40.1   Contralateral tarsal graft to correct upper lid entropion.

BIBLIOGRAPHY

Bayliss HI, Hamako C: Tarsal grafting for correction of cicatricial entropion. *Ophthalmic Surg* 10:42, 1979.

Dortzbach RK, Callahan A: Repair of cicatricial entropion of upper eyelids. *Arch Ophthalmol* 85:82, 1971.

Soll DB: *Management of Complications in Ophthalmic Plastic Surgery.* Birmingham, Aesculapius, 1976, p 159.

Tenzel RR: Repair of entropion of upper lid. *Arch Ophthalmol* 77:675, 1967.

41

Combined Procedure
for Entropion Repair

Ralph E. Wesley

INTRODUCTION

The numerous procedures for entropion repair emphasize the need for dependable, effective methods to prevent inward rotation of the lower eyelid. The combined method of lateral canthoplasty and refixation of the lower eyelid retractors, while requiring a thorough knowledge of eyelid anatomy, allows the surgeon to correct entropion permanently.

TECHNIQUE

Using local infiltration anesthesia and a protective lens, a subciliary blepharoplasty-type incision is made beneath the lid and extended 1 cm laterally from the outer canthus (Fig. 41.1A). The skin muscle flap should be carried inferiorly exposing the tarsus, Müller's muscle, and, finally, the capsulopalpebral fascia (Fig. 41.1B).

Interrupted sutures of 6-0 Vicryl reattach the edge of the capsulopalpebral fascia to the inferior border of the tarsal plate (Fig. 41.1C and D). Attaching the fascia superiorly on the tarsal plate will cause an unwanted ectropion.

To eliminate horizontal laxity, the 15 Bard–Parker blade should split the upper and lower lids at the lateral canthus, sweeping down to the periosteum and connecting with the previous skin incision (Fig. 41.2A) while some of protection is provided for the globe. Then, 3 to 4 mm of lateral canthal tendon can be excised with Westcott scissors (Fig. 41.2B). A 4-0 Vicryl mattress suture on a P-2 needle can be used to reattach the cut edge of the lower lateral tarsus to the orbital rim periosteum providing an upward and inward sweep to the lower lid (Fig. 41.2C). Skin closure is accomplished with interrupted 7-0 silk sutures (Fig. 41.2D).

The correction of entropion uses a skin muscle flap to isolate the detached lower lid retractors (Fig. 41.3). The 6-0 vicryl sutures correct the defect of the lower lid retractors, which should transmit force from the

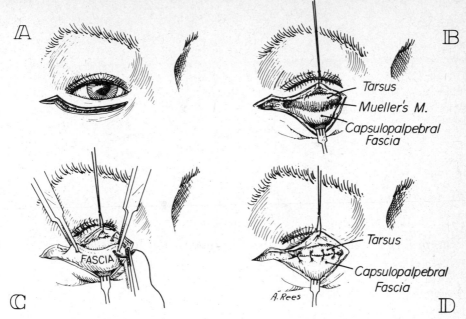

Figure 41.1 Subciliary approach to repair lower lid retractors.

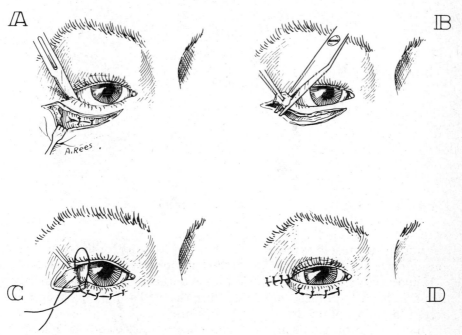

Figure 41.2 Correction of lower lid laxity.

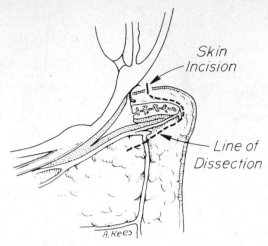

Figure 41.3 Sagittal view: disinsertion of lower lid retractors.

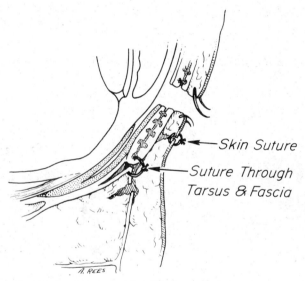

Figure 41.4 Sagittal view: repair of lid retractors.

inferior rectus muscle to the base of the tarsus in order for the lower lid to retract downward when the eye rotates inferiorly (Fig. 41.4).

Hemostasis with this procedure is enchanced by injecting local anesthesia with hyaluronidase and epinephrine as well as the topical application of thrombin drops during the procedure.

This procedure has been uniformly effective in correcting entropion without the problem of recurrences. The method is indicated in cases where recurrent entropion must be avoided, such as before cataract surgery or reoperations and on patients who live a considerable distance from eye care.

BIBLIOGRAPHY

Dryden RM, Leibsohn J, Wobig J: Senile entropion: Pathogenesis and treatment. *Arch Ophthalmol* 96:1833, 1978.

Wesley RE, Collins JW: Combined procedure for senile entropion. *Ophthalmic Surg* 14:401, 1983.

42

Correction of Entropion Following the Cutler–Beard Procedure

Richard P. Carroll

INTRODUCTION

The Cutler–Beard procedure can be used to reconstruct complete upper eyelid defects with a full-thickness flap from the opposing lower lid while preserving the lid margin of the donor lower eyelid. After 6 to 8 weeks, the flap is separated at the level of the intended upper eyelid margin, and the pedicle flap is repositioned down into the donor lower eyelid (Fig. 42.1A).

Because the full-thickness flap advanced into the upper eyelid defect contains little or no tarsus, shrinkage of the posterior lamellar of the reconstructed eyelid sometimes occurs after division of the flap. The resulting cicatricial entropion (Figure 42.1B) can cause severe ocular irritation secondary to fine cilia or keratinized tissue on the margin of the reconstructed eyelid. Adjunct such as lubricants, contact lenses, and cryotherapy may be palliative, but frequently these modalities do not alleviate the patient's symptoms caused by the postoperative cicatricial entropion.

With the technique illustrated below, the entropion may be corrected to provide relief to these patients.

TECHNIQUE

An incision is made with a razor blade knife at the mucocutaneous junction of the involved upper eyelid. The cutaneous edge is then picked up with a fine-tooth forceps, and the skin is dissected off the remaining structures of the reconstructed margin using a razor blade knife. The dissection is continued superiorly approximately 7 mm and then carried across the entire horizontal plane of the eyelid (Fig. 42.2A).

122

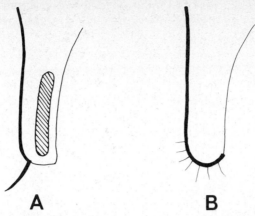

Figure 42.1 (A) Normal lid. (B) Entropion after upper lid reconstruction.

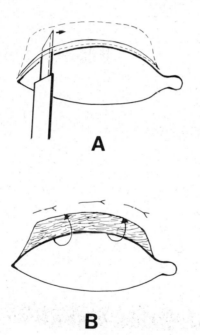

Figure 42.2 (A) Incision at mucocutaneous junction. (B) Sutures placed to correct entropion.

This block of skin and muscle is resected, and 2 mm above the leading anterior lamellar edge three 6-0 silk horizontal mattress sutures are placed through all layers of the eyelid, except the conjunctiva. The remaining eyelid margin tissues are then rotated anteriorly and sutured with a running 6-0 silk suture to the leading edge of the anterior lamellar (Fig. 42.2B). The running suture is removed at 5 days, and the mattress sutures are removed at 10 days.

123

This procedure has resulted in a satisfactory correction of mild cicatricial entropion following upper eyelid reconstruction with the Cutler–Beard procedure.

BIBLIOGRAPHY

Carroll RP: Entropion following the Cutler–Beard procedure. *Ophthalmology* 90:1052, 1983.

Cutler NL, Beard C: A method for partial and total upper eyelid reconstruction. *Am J Ophthalmol* 39:1, 1955.

43

Repair of Cicatricial Entropion with Autogenous Ear Cartilage Grafts

David F. Kamin

INTRODUCTION

Cicatricial entropion of the upper eyelid causes pain, irritation, and blepharospasm resulting in keratitis with the threat of corneal ulceration. With milder cases, rotational techniques can provide relief, but in severe cases, or patients with progressive disease such as ocular pemphigoid, additional tissue must be added to provide for a long-lasting solution.

The technique below uses the easily obtained ear cartilage to reform the posterior lamellar and to correct the cicatricial entropion.

TECHNIQUE

The upper lid should be everted over a Desmarre retractor and the cicatricial tissue dissected (Fig. 43.1) from the upper lid. By dissecting the cicatrix, a bed for the graft is prepared (Fig. 43.2). Towel clips are used to retract the anesthetized ear (Fig. 43.3), so a vertical incision can be made through the posterior ear skin down to the cartilage with a number 15 Bard–Parker blade. The ear cartilage is exposed, and then the appropriate size graft is incised and dissected free from the ear (Fig. 43.4). The donor site from the ear is closed, and the graft is fashioned to fit the defect.

For the proximal edge of the graft (near the lid margin), a running pull-out 6-0 Prolene suture secures the graft into the defect, coming out above the level of the tarsus between Müller's muscle superiorly and the proximal border inferiorly (Fig. 43.5). The distal aspect of the tarsus is then excised and everted with Weiss stitches of 6-0 Dexon (Fig. 43.6).

The addition of the autogenous ear cartilage advances the tarsal plate and enables the distal aspect of the eyelid to be everted when the graft is

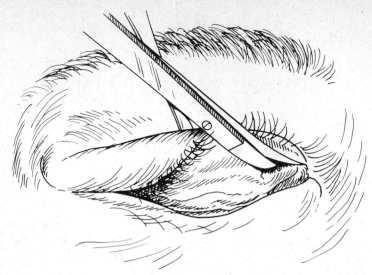

Figure 43.1 Upper lid everted to expose scar tissues.

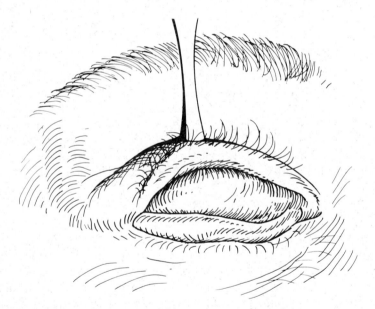

Figure 43.2 Graft bed created by removing cicatrix.

sutured. The Prolene suture (Fig. 43.7) is removed in 2 weeks; Dexon is allowed to absorb.

The grafts provide a firm but malleable backbone to the upper lid. In 6 to 8 weeks the graft will epithelialize. Autogenous ear cartilage, which does not shrink as occurs with eyebank sclera, provides long-lasting correction of entropion.

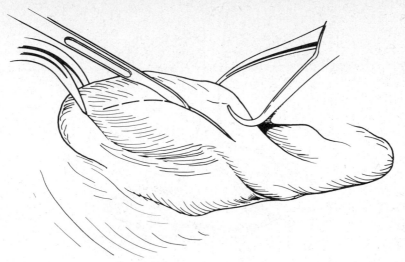

Figure 43.3 Ear retracted to obtain ear cartilage graft.

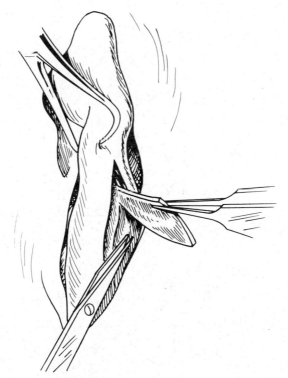

Figure 43.4 Ear cartilage graft excised.

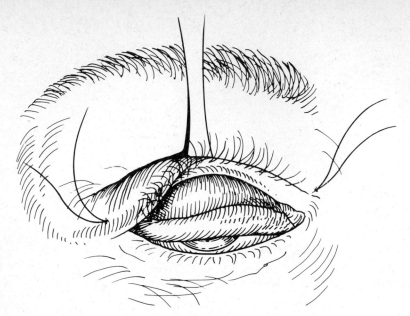

Figure 43.5 Ear cartilage graft sewed with pull-out 6-0 prolene.

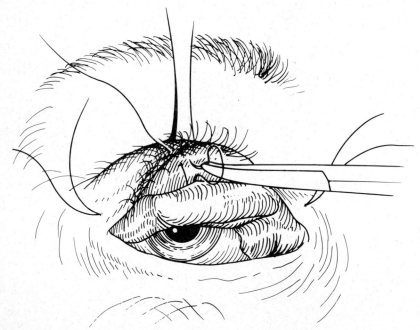

Figure 43.6 Posterior fixed with weiss sutures.

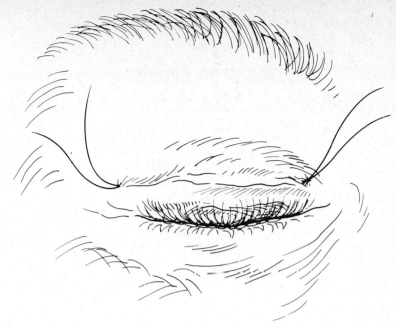

Figure 43.7 Appearance of pullout suture.

44

Tarsal Polishing
and Mucous Membrane Grafting
for Cicatrizing Diseases
of the Eyelids

William P. Chen

INTRODUCTION

Cicatricial diseases of the eyelids such as with Stevens–Johnson syndrome, ocular pemphigoid, and chemical burns can cause pain, photophobia, corneal irritation, and corneal vascularization, decrease in goblet cell densities, metaplasia of the meibomian glands, and keratinization of the conjunctiva, leading to epidermalization, cicatricial entropion, and trichiasis.

Many treatments have been advocated for this distressing disease, including rotational sutures, tarsal rotation, mucous membrane grafting with excision of diseased tarsus, and nasochondral mucosal graft. Tarsal polishing with mucous membrane grafting offers a method to correct the entropion as well as to provide increased goblet cells and perhaps a higher ambient oxygen tension to the precorneal tear film.

TECHNIQUE

The eyelid is infiltrated with 1% lidocaine with 1:100,000 epinephrine. A strip of full-thickness buccal mucous membrane 20 × 40 mm is harvested using a blade and scissors. The graft is cleared of any submucosal fat and is soaked in dilute gentamicin solution.

Two 4-0 silk sutures are placed epitarsally on the skin side, and the lower lid is everted with a cotton-tipped applicator (Fig. 44.1). A 3-mm smooth dermabrading tip on a rotary handle is used to polish the scarred and epidermalized tarsal conjunctiva (Fig. 44.2).

When trichiasis is present, it is necessary to perform a skin muscle recession in the following manner: The lid is split posterior to the gray

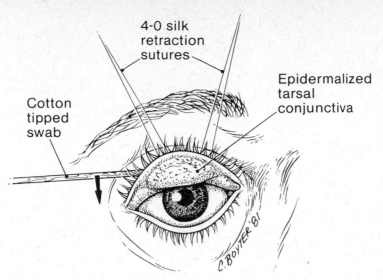

Figure 44.1 Upper or lower lid is everted with 4-0 silk suture.

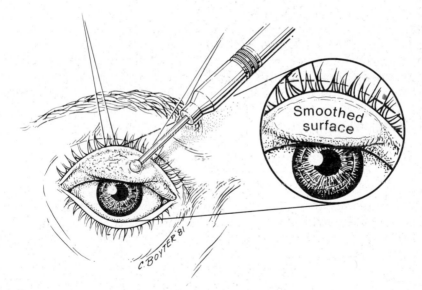

Figure 44.2 Rotary polishing of tarsal conjunctiva.

line using a razor blade and dissected into an anterior skin/muscle layer and a posterior tarsal conjunctival layer. A 1-mm vertical relaxing incision is then made at each end of the tarsus to be advanced, and the skin muscle layer is recessed 2-mm backward from the tarsal margin with further dissection. Lashes turned inward are removed from the posterior lamella.

The two layers are anchored in this position using three 4-0 silk sutures, passing full thickness through the eyelid above the superior edge of

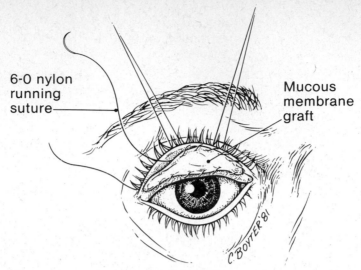

6-0 nylon running suture

Mucous membrane graft

C·BOYTER·81

Figure 44.3   *Graft sutured with 6-0 nylon, knot exteriorized.*

the upper tarsus or inferior edge of the lower tarsus. With the lid marginal abnormality and tarsal surface well polished, the buccal mucous membrane is then trimmed to its proper size and layed along the lid margin and recipient tarsal bed to be anchored with running 6-0 nylon with the suture knot exteriorized (Fig. 44.3).

The graft is allowed to roll over the anterior tarsal surface in cases where skin muscle recession for trichiasis was performed. In most cases, the opposing eyelid requires similar treatment. Intermarginal sutures, using 4-0 silk, are used to spling the grafts along the lid margins with the knots tied on the skin side (Figs. 44.4 and 44.5). Oral antibiotics are given in most cases. The sutures can be removed after 7 days.

Most patients report symptomatic relief of eye pain and irritation and decreased redness and tearing. In certain patients, a decrease in reflex tear secretion with resultant improvement in vision has been noted.

The clinical improvement appears to result from three factors: First, a smooth epithelial lining is interposed between the lid tissue and the cornea, preventing further injury to the cornea. Two, the buccal mucous membrane provides goblet cells and mucin secretion to the precorneal tear film. Three, a healthy mucosal graft possibly provides a higher ambient oxygen tension to the precorneal tear film. The structural, integrity, and support of the eyelid is maintained as the tarsal plate is not excised.

BIBLIOGRAPHY

Arstikaitis MJ: Ocular aftermath of Stevens–Johnson Syndrome. *Arch Ophthalmol* 90:376, 1973.

Beyer CK, Carroll JM: Moderately severe cicatricial entropion. *Arch Ophthalmol* 89:33, 1973.

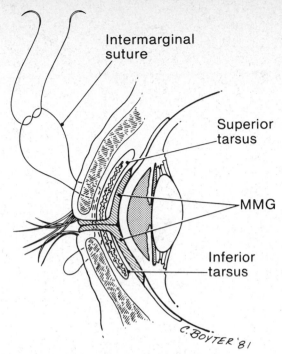

Figure 44.4 *Intermarginal sutures stent graft.*

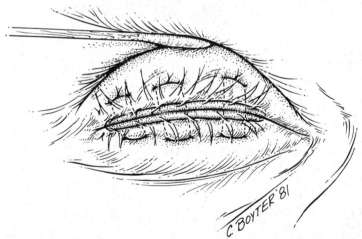

Figure 44.5 *Appearance of eyelids at end of procedure. (Reprinted with permission Ophthalmic Surgery 14:1021–1025, 1983.)*

Hosni FA: Repair of trachomatous cicatricial entropion using mucous membrane graft. *Arch Ophthalmol* 91:49, 1974.

McCord CD Jr, Chen WP: Tarsal polishing in mucous membrane grafting for cicatricial entropion, trichiasis and epidermalization. *Ophthalmic Surg* 14:1021, 1983.

Ralph RA: Conjunctival goblet cell density in normal subjects and in dry eye syndromes. *Invest Ophthalmol* 14:299, 1975.

ECTROPION

PART IV

45

Taping Technique to Correct Ectropion

Ralph E. Wesley

INTRODUCTION

Though permanent surgical correction is the preferred treatment for ectropion, some patients refuse surgery. Others may have a temporary ectropion from Bell's idiopathic facial palsy. Surgery may not be possible in those allergic to local anesthetics, patients with severe bleeding disorders, or patients from mental institutions who will not cooperate.

The tape technique provides a temporary method to correct ectropion without surgery, though some patients have used tape indefinitely.

TECHNIQUE

The ectropion in the involved lid (Fig. 45.1A) can be corrected by placing a strip of tape firmly onto the lower lid (Fig. 45.1B) and then pulling the lid upward and outward with a sweeping motion to be fixated against the globe, as shown in Figure 45.1C. Application of benzoin to the skin before placement of the tape allows for a more prolonged effect.

Ideally, this should be used as a temporary procedure, but some conscientious patients use this technique for years.

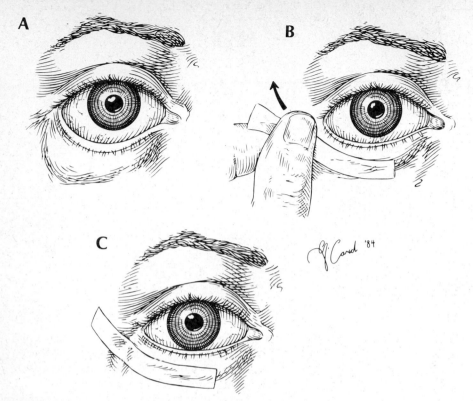

Figure 45.1 Tape method for ectropion.

46

Lateral Canthal Tendon Tuck with Entropion Repair

Arthur J. Schaefer

INTRODUCTION

Senile entropion can be repaired in the overwhelming majority of cases with imbrication of the lower lid retractors. Problem cases can arise with a coexisting relaxation of the lateral canthal tendons. The technique listed below (1) illustrates the retraction test to identify those patients with relaxed canthal tendons and a simple technique to provide for horizontal lid tightening through the lateral canthal tendon tuck.

Entropion failures (2) are associated with lateral and medial canthal tendon laxity. Preoperatively, this can be identified by the retraction test to indicate patients who need not only imbrication of the lower lid retractors (2–3) but also lateral canthal tendon tightening.

TECHNIQUE

The skin of the patient's lower lid should be grasped gently with the index finger and thumb just below the lash border centrally to withdraw the lid from the globe. With good resiliency of elastic tissue in normal patients, the lid should withdraw only 2 to 3 mm from the globe (Fig. 46.1A). With a typical senile entropion, the lid withdraws approximately 10 to 12 mm with gentle traction (Fig. 46.1B). In cases with marked relaxation of the retractors and the lateral and medial canthal tendons, retraction of about 20 to 25 mm occurs (Fig. 46.1C). These patients need correction of the marked horizontal relaxation as an adjunct to imbrications of the lower lid retractors.

To tuck the lateral canthal tendon, the incision along the lower border of the tarsus to imbricate the lower lid retractors can be extended following (see procedure in Chapter 38) the upward curve of the lower lid in the lateral direction to just beyond the lateral orbital rim. The skin and orbicularis muscle must be freed over the lateral canthal tendon and orbital rim to expose the lateral canthal tendon and periosteum beyond the rim.

139

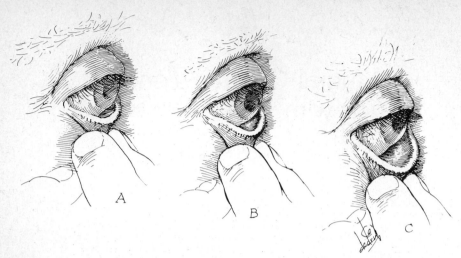

Figure 46.1 Testing eyelid turgor indicates patients that require lateral canthal tendon tuck as well as repair of retractors.

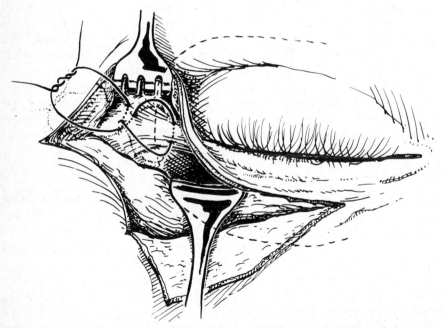

Figure 46.2 Tightening the lower eyelid with lateral canthal tendon tuck suture. (Reprinted with permission. Ophthalmology 87:1013–1018, 1980.)

With the tendon well freed up and exposed, a double-armed 4-0 Supramid suture can be placed in vertical direction through the medial extremity of the lateral canthal tendon. The upper end of the double-armed suture is then passed in a superior-to-inferior direction through the tendon and periosteum at the orbital rim or just beyond, depending on the amount of tightening (shortening) necessary. The other arm is now passed through the tendon and periosteum in an inferior-to-superior direction just lateral to the first arm of the 4-0 Supramid suture (Fig. 46.2).

As these sutures are drawn up, the tendon can be tucked or tightened 10 mm or more. An assistant can aid in drawing the suture up by placing a superior oblique muscle hook in the lateral commissure at the junction of the upper and lower lids to retract the wound laterally, enabling the surgeon to tuck the tendon with ease.

After the tendon is tucked, the surgeon proceeds with the imbrication of the lower lid retractors, as previously described in Chapter 38. The retraction test and the lateral canthal tendon tuck allow the surgeon to identify problem cases of senile entropion that may require more than simple imbrication of the lower lid retractors for successful entropion repair.

The lateral canthal tendon tuck would be contraindicated in marked medial canthal tendon laxity or dehiscence to avoid temporal displacement of the punctum and elongation or tearing of the canaliculus. As the lateral canthal tendon is tucked, the surgeon should simultaneously check the punctum for lateral displacement to indicate medial canthal tendon laxity or dehiscence. In such an instance, the medial canthal tendon should also be repaired.

REFERENCES

1. Schaefer AJ: Lateral canthal tendon tuck. *Ophthalmology* 86:1879, 1979.
2. Schaefer AJ: Senile entropion. *Ophthalmic Surg* 5:33, 1974.
3. Jones LS, Reeh MJ, Wobig JL: Senile entropion. *Am J Ophthalmol* 74:327, 1972.

47

Correction of Medial Ectropion with Medial Canthal Plication

Ralph E. Wesley

INTRODUCTION

Medial ectropion from laxity of the medial canthal tendon can cause tearing and irritation to the eye. The usual methods of horizontal lid tightening may simply pull the punctum to the midportion of the lid when these procedures are applied to medial ectropion.

Direct plication of the medial canthal tendon corrects the pathologic defect and eliminates medial ectropion.

TECHNIQUE

With a razor knife, an incision should be made at the mucocutaneous junction connecting the medial canthal angle a 0.4 mm temporal to the inferior punctum (Fig. 47.1). A thin skin flap should be carefully undermined, and the medial canthal tendon should be identified. The first arm of a double-armed 7-0 suture should be passed vertically through the orbicularis muscle, and with partial thickness, it should be passed through the tarsus. The same arm is then passed in the opposite direction vertically just under the orbicularis muscle, and a second bite should be taken in the reverse direction with that same suture creating a whip stitch.

Both sutures are now passed toward the medial canthus underneath the orbicularis muscle, where each arm passes through the medial canthal tendon anterior to posterior (Fig. 47.2) and tied firmly so the knot and suture is buried. The incision can be closed with 7-0 silk sutures to complete the correction of the ectropion (Fig. 47.3).

The suture connecting the medial end of the tarsus to the medial canthal tendon in effect plicates the stretched tendon restoring the lower lid to a normal physiologic condition. This operation does not involve the removal of normal tissue, but rather involves the repair of the physiologic

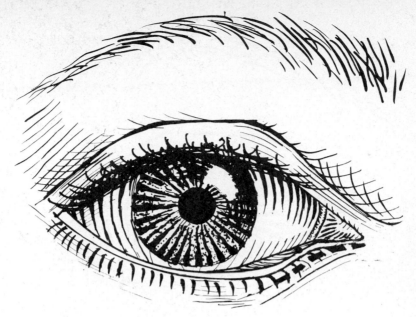

Figure 47.1 Medial ectropion incision.

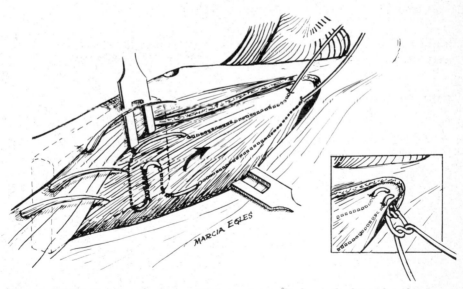

MARCIA EGLES

Figure 47.2 Suture placement to repair medial canthal tendon laxity.

defect. The initial stitch must be placed lateral to the punctum to include a firm bite of tarsus. Passing the sutures under the orbicularis and burying the knot at the medial canthal tendon prevent any irritation or inflammation of the skin.

Preoperative injection of 2% lidocaine with epinephrine (1:100,000)

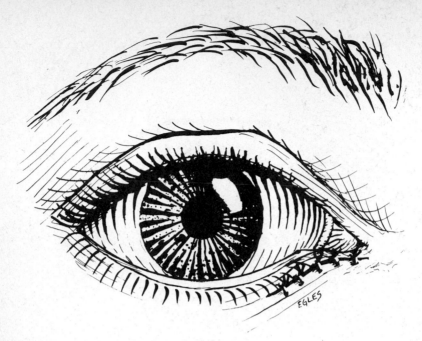

Figure 47.3 *Correction of medial ectropion.*

and the topical application of thrombin drops helps to provide hemostasis and allow the surgeon to avoid electrocautery in this area.

BIBLIOGRAPHY

Katzan LB, Tenzel RR: Canthal laxity in eyelid malpositions, in Bosniak S (ed): *Advances in Ophthalmic Plastic and Reconstructive Surgery.* New York, Pergammon, 1983, vol 2, pp 232, 233.

48

Z-T-Plasty
for Medial Ectropion

Ralph E. Wesley

INTRODUCTION

The lazy-T operation (1) corrects milder cases of medial ectropion using a full-thickness eyelid resection lateral to the punctum to avoid the lacrimal system and a horizontal excision of a spindle of conjunctiva to rotate the medial lid inward. The conjunctival and lid incisions intersect to form a "T" rotated 90 degrees, giving the name *lazy T-operation*.

Many patients with medial ectropion have a shortage of skin. The lazy-T operation excises skin. With the Z-T-plasty, the inward rotation effects of the lazy-T are combined with the Z-plasty on the skin for added correction of the medial ectropion.

TECHNIQUE

A Z-plasty is marked on the lower lid on the affected side that has medial ectropion (Fig. 48.1A). The flaps of the Z-plasty are incised with a 15 Bard–Parker blade and Westcott scissors to expose the inner lamellar of the lid. At this point, a full lid excision is marked as well as a spindle of conjunctiva (Fig. 48.1B). After this has been excised and reapproximated with interrupted 6-0 Vicryl stitches, a "T" rotated on its side can be seen (Fig. 48.1C). This tightens the lid with the full tarsal excision, and the conjunctival spindle helps to rotate the lid inward.

To lengthen the skin, the flaps of the "Z" are then transposed and sutured with 7-0 silk for the final correction of the medial ectropion (Fig. 48.1D).

The Z-T-plasty combines the lid tightening and inward rotating forces of the lazy-T operation with a moderate amount of skin lengthening with the surface Z-plasty.

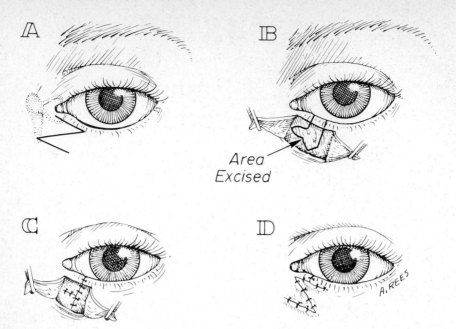

Figure 48.1 Z-plasty (A) relaxes medial ectropion and saves skin excised with usual "Lazy-T" procedures. Flaps retracted (B) for lid tightening and conjunctival shortening (B). After closure internally (C), flaps transposed (D) for better correction of medial ectropion.

REFERENCES

1. Smith B: The "Lazy-T" correction of ectropion of the lower punctum. Arch Ophthalmol 94:1149, 1976.

49

Tarsal (Marginal) Ectropion

Ralph E. Wesley

INTRODUCTION

In tarsal ectropion, the lid has an outward torque, which will not be corrected by traditional lid-tightening procedures. The frustration of recurrect ectropion can be avoided with tarsal ectropion by repairing the lower lid retractors in combination with a lid-tightening procedure.

TECHNIQUE

Lower lid retractors (capsulopalpebral fascia and Müller's muscle) normally transmit force from the inferior rectus to the inferior tarsus on a downward gaze (Fig. 49.1A). With disinsertion of the lower lid retractors (Fig. 49.1B), orbicularis muscle rides under the tarsal plate with a severe outward torquing force causing ectropion. The disinserted lower lid retractors may be identified in the inferior fornix. A small amount of conjunctiva should be excised to allow access to the disinsertion of the lower lid retractors (Fig. 49.1C), and three interrupted 6-0 Vicryl sutures used to reattach the fascia to the base of the tarsus (Fig. 49.1D).

Additional stabilization of the lid can be accomplished by lateral canthal tendon tightening by splitting the upper and lower lids at the lateral canthus (Fig. 49.2A), excising 2 to 3 mm of full-thickness eyelid (Fig. 49.2B), and reattaching the lower lid with a mattress suture, grasping the periosteum inside the orbital rim (Fig. 49.2C). Closure can be accomplished with interrupted skin stitches (Fig. 49.2D).

BIBLIOGRAPHY

Wesley RE: Tarsal ectropion from detachment of the lower eyelid retractors. *Am J Ophthalmol* 93:491, 1982.

Putterman AM, Urist MJ: Surgical anatomy of the orbital septum. *Ann Ophthalmol* 6:290, 1974.

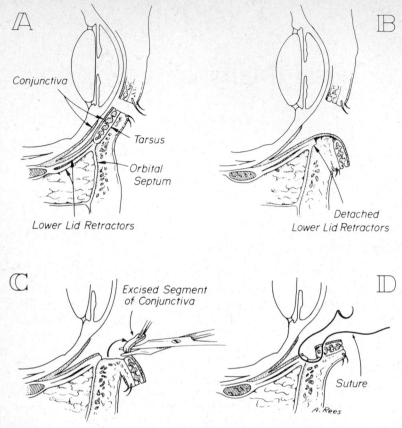

Figure 49.1 (A) Normal eyelid anatomy. (B) Detachment of lower eyelid retractors. (C) Exposure of retractors. (D) Repair of disinsertion of capsulopalpebral fascia and Müller's muscle.

Putterman AM: Ectropion of the lower eyelid secondary to Müller's muscle. Capsulo-palpebral fascia detachment. *Am J Ophthalmol* 85:814, 1978.

Wesley RE, McCord CD Jr, Jones NA: Height of the tarsus in the lower eyelid. *Am J Ophthalmol* 90:102, 1980.

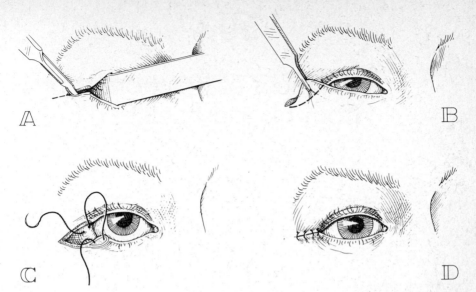

Figure 49.2 (A) Lateral canthototomy. (B) Excision of lateral lid tissue. (C) Attachment of lower eyelid inside orbital rim. (D) After correction of ectropion.

50

Treatment of Epiphora
from Flaccid Eyelids

Joseph C. Hill

INTRODUCTION

When eyelids do not press firmly against the globe the patient may experience gradually increasing epiphora, aggravated by wind or cold weather. The lower eyelid is easily pulled 6 mm away from the eyeball by the examiner. The sag of the lower lid may be noted by comparison to the intercanthal line or by comparison to the medial canthus.

Left unattended, this problem becomes accompanied by a stagnant tear sac, providing a good culture medium for infection to develop. Later, the complication of stenosis and complete occlusion of the lacrimal drainage system can occur.

Most often, the lateral canthal tendon weakness creates the problem. The technique of lateral canthal tendonesis can correct the eyelid abnormality.

TECHNIQUE

To differentiate whether the medial or lower canthal tendon is at fault, the surgeon should observe the amount to which the lateral canthus moves medially when the lower eyelid is pushed toward the nose. This measurement is compared to the movement of the medial canthus when the lower eyelid is pushed away from the nose. The greater movement indicates the tendon with the most laxity.

To correct this deformity with lateral canthal tendonesis, a linear incision (Fig. 50.1A) is made beginning 2 mm from the lateral canthus extending laterally for 2 cm. The skin is undermined, and the orbicularis muscle is split (Fig. 50.1B) to the orbital rim. The periosteum is separated for approximately 1 cm from the orbital rim, and a diamond drill is passed through the bone 7 mm posterior to the orbital rim (Fig. 50.1C), while a periosteal elevator protects the eye from the drill.

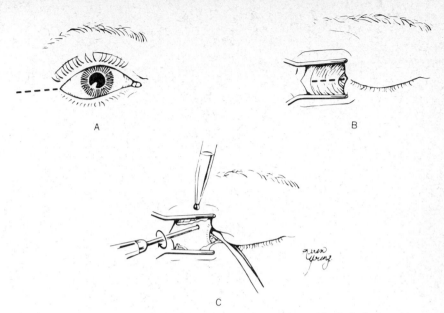

A

B

C

Figure 50.1 *Exposure for correction of lateral canthal defect.*

A 2-0 silk suture is passed through the drilled bone (Fig. 50.2A) after being placed through the tendon in a cross-stitch orthopedic manner (Fig. 50.2B) so the tendon can be pulled into the drilled hole, which should be at least 5 mm to allow for ease of entry of the tendon.

Cautery is applied to the upper and lower mobilized flaps (Fig. 50.2C). Then 5 mm of the separated upper and lower orbicularis muscle is resected, and the 2-0 silks are passed through the orbicularis muscle (Fig. 50.3A). The orbicularis muscle is then closed (Fig. 50.3B), after the silk from the tendon has been passed through the resected muscle.

The tendon is pulled through the bone (Fig. 50.3C), and the silks are then passed through the upper and lower edges of the skin to be secured in place by tying over a 2-0 hole button on the skin surface. The skin can be reapproximated with interrupted sutures, and the tendon suture can be tied over the button to be left in place for 6 weeks (Fig. 50.3D).

This procedure corrects epiphora due to flaccid eyelids.

BIBLIOGRAPHY

Dick MW: Surgical management of orbital tarsal disparity. *Arch Ophthalmol* 75:386, 1966.

Hill JC: Analysis of senile changes in the palpebral fissure. *Trans Ophthalmol Soc UK* 95:49, 1975.

Hill JC: Treatment of epiphora owing to flaccid eyelids. *Arch Ophthalmol* 97:323, 1979.

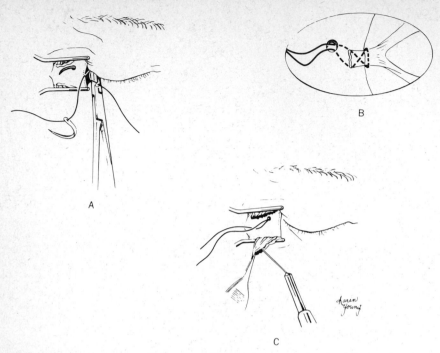

Figure 50.2 *Repair of lateral canthal tendon.*

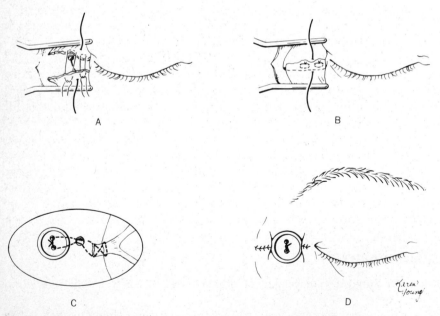

Figure 50.3 *Fixation and closure for repair of lateral canthal tendon.*

51

Ectropion Repair
with Tarsal Rotation Sutures

Roger Kohn

INTRODUCTION

Ectropion from skin shortage or horizontal laxity can be corrected with skin grafts and lid-shortening procedures. In patients with neither horizontal orbital/tarsal disparity nor vertical skin contracture, tarsal rotation sutures provide a simple, effective outpatient method to correct tarsal (mechanical) ectropion.

TECHNIQUE

Local anesthesia is obtained to block the infraorbital nerve on the affected lid (Fig. 51.1). Three sets of 4-0 silk sutures are placed at the medial, central, and lateral quadrants of the lower lid, with the conjunctival entrance and exit sites approximately 4 mm apart.

The needles on the silk are removed and replaced by Trochar 5 surgical needles or the equivalent, to permit deeper penetration. With a plastic surgery needle holder and the concave side of the needle facing away from the globe, the needles are passed vertically with the tip, pointing toward the infraorbital rim in a downward course so the needle enters the tarsus, passes through the inferior aponeurosis and septum to engage the periosteum of the infraorbital rim. The needle tip is allowed to curve outward, emerging through the skin anteriorly or slightly below the level of the infraorbital rim (Fig. 51.2). Sutures are placed approximately 4 mm apart and passed through rubber bolsters (Fig. 51.3).

The three sets of silk sutures should be tied over the rubber bolsters with the tension adjusted according to the desired degree of lid rotation. The placement of temporary knots facilitates the fine tuning of this adjustment. The sutures should remain in place for 6 to 8 weeks, which should give a permanent correction of the ectropion (Fig. 51.4).

The principle behind the tarsal rotation suture is that it employs the

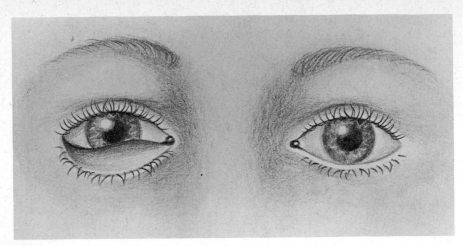

Figure 51.1 Mechanical ectropion.

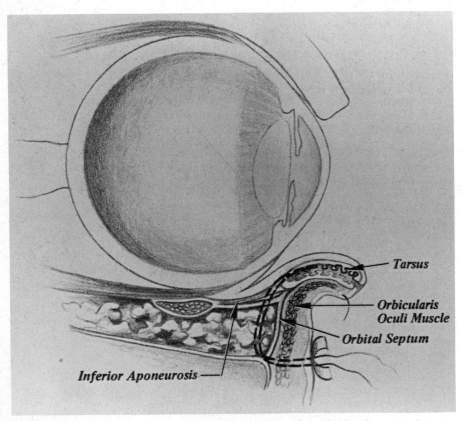

Tarsus

Orbicularis Oculi Muscle

Orbital Septum

Inferior Aponeurosis

Figure 51.2 Suture placement slightly below level of infraorbital rim.

154

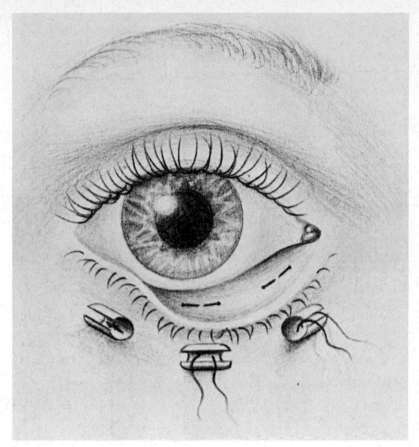

Figure 51.3   Sutures 4 mm apart, passed through rubber bolsters.

firm periosteum of the infraorbital rim as the center of rotation of the pulley system. The resulting torque causes the tarsal plate to intort as the internal eyelid structures are pulled inferiorly to deepen the cul-de-sac.

BIBLIOGRAPHY

Kohn R: Mechanical ectropion repair using tarsal rotation sutures. *Ophthalmic Surg* 10:48, 1979.

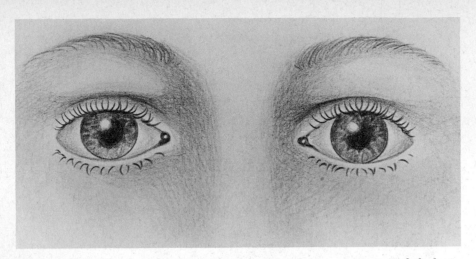

Figure 51.4 Final correction. (Reprinted with permission. Ophthalmic Surgery 10:48–52, 1979.)

52

Combined Z-Plasty and Horizontal Shortening for Ectropion

Allen M. Putterman

INTRODUCTION

A horizontal shortening procedure usually corrects acquired, senile ectropion resulting from horizontal laxity. Cicatricial ectropion from vertical skin loss can be treated with a Z-plasty of the eyelid skin when the vertical shortage is in one eyelid segment, or it can be treated with a skin graft when the shortage is diffuse.

When ectropion occurs from both vertical loss of skin and horizontal eyelid laxity, a horizontal lid shortening procedure or Z-plasty alone frequently leaves some residual ectropion. Correction of this type of ectropion has generally required a pentagonal resection of eyelid tissue combined with a skin graft.

When the skin cicatrix is localized to one-third of the eyelid, the surgeon can use the technique of combined Z-plasty and horizontal shortening to avoid skin grafts. This technique not only treats the horizontal laxity and cicatricial components, but also eliminates the scarred lid segment and any lid margin abnormalities.

TECHNIQUE

An incision should be drawn at the lid margin approximately 6 mm temporal to the eyelid scar contracture, extending 10 mm vertically from the margin where a connecting nasal oblique line is drawn toward the inferior apex of the scar (Fig. 52.1A). The scar can be delineated by palpation and resistance to elevation of the lower eyelid or depression of the upper eyelid.

After local infiltration of lidocaine with epinephrine for anesthesia and placement of a scleral lens for ocular protection, a number 11 Bard—

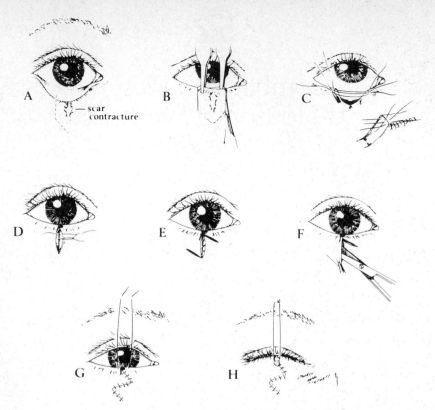

Figure 52.1 *Combined Z-plasty and lid shortening for ectropion. (Putterman A: Combined Z-plasty and horizontal shortening procedure for ectropion. Am J Ophthalmol 89:525–530, 1980. Published by the American Journal of Ophthalmology. Copyright by The Ophthalmic Publishing Company.)*

Parker blade is used to incise full-thickness eyelid over the vertical incision. The blade is passed through the eyelid approximately 4 mm from the lid margin, and then a clean, sharp vertical cut upward is sliced through the eyelid margin. The knife blade is reversed for the full-thickness incision to the end of the vertical line. Westcott scissors is used to excise along the oblique line, terminating beneath the inferior scar apex.

With the contact lens removed, the eyelid is grasped with two forceps several millimeters below the eyelid margin and several millimeters on either side of the incision, to prevent of the incision from being crushed, which might interfere with suturing and healing. The forceps are pulled in opposite directions to overlap lid remnants on each side of the incision (Fig. 52.1B) to produce slight tension. A scratch incision is used to mark the eyelid margin.

With the protective lens replaced, the pentagonal resection is completed similar to the temporal incision. The full-thickness pentagon includes the scarred segment of eyelid.

The lid margin can be closed with three 6-0 black silk double-armed sutures (Fig. 52.1C). Four to six 6-0 Vicryl sutures are passed through the superficial tarsus, pretarsal fascia, and orbicularis muscle to close the vertical incision (Fig. 52.1D).

A Z-plasty is now drawn 60 degrees from the vertical incision for a distance equal to the length of the slightly stretched vertical incision (Fig. 52.1E). Whether the superior or inferior incision is nasal or temporal depends on the skin available for flaps in those directions.

The Z-lines are incised, and the temporal and nasal skin flaps are undermined from underlying orbicularis muscle with sharp pointed scissors (Fig. 52.1F). (Observing the points of the scissors through the translucent skin during dissection prevents buttonholing of the skin and avoids trapping subcutaneous tissue within the flaps.)

The flaps should be transposed, and the skin adjacent to the flaps should be undermined until the flaps can be overlapped with minimal tension. The flaps are then sutured to surrounding skin with interrupted 6-0 black silk sutures (Fig. 52.1G).

A double-armed 4-0 black silk suture is passed on each side of the sutured eyelid margin, entering approximately 4 mm from the eyelid margin through orbicularis muscle and superficial tarsus and exiting at the gray line (Fig. 52.1G). The ends of the suture are passed through the forehead above the central eyebrow in cases involving the lower eyelid and through the central cheek when the upper eyelid requires correction. With the contact lens removed, the suture is tied over small cotten pledgets so the eyelid is stretched with slight tension (Fig. 52.1H).

In 6 or 7 days, the skin sutures are removed. At 12 to 14 days, the eyelid margin and tarsorrhaphy sutures are removed. Then, 2.5 to 3 weeks postoperatively, the patient should begin massaging the lower lid upward, or the upper lid downward, over the incision. The massage is continued for 1 month.

BIBLIOGRAPHY

Putterman AM: Combined Z-plasty and horizontal shortening procedure for ectropion. *Am J Ophthalmol* 89:525, 1980.

53

Temporalis Muscle Transfer for Correction of Recurrent Involutional Ectropion

Stephen L. Bosniak

INTRODUCTION

Inadequate canthal tendon tightening or horizontal lid shortening can cause recurrent ectropion. Overzealous lid shortening without prior tendon plication will cause a noticably smaller horizontal palpebral fissure, the punctum will be displaced temporally, and the ectropion may persist.

A temporalis muscle transposition can be used to support the lower eyelid in cases in which inadequate or misdirected surgery has occurred.

TECHNIQUE

A 4 cm preauricular incision is carried into the scalp behind the hair line overlying the anterior aspect of the temporalis muscle (Fig. 53.1). With the anterior surface of the temporalis muscle exposed, a disposable nerve stimulator is used to identify the terminal branches of the facial nerve, which are superficial and prominent over the malar eminence so that care may be exercised in avoiding these facial nerve branches.

A 1.5 cm wide strip of temporalis muscle with as much fascia and insertional epicranium as possible is developed (Fig. 53.2).

Next, at the medial canthus, a vertical incision 1.0 cm in height straddling the insertion of the medial canthal tendon is made, and the superficial head of the tendon is carefully isolated with blunt dissection. A tunnel beneath the orbicularis muscle and in front of the lower tarsal plate is made from the perauricular incision to the medial canthal incision by undermining with face-lift scissors.

The temporalis muscle-fascia strip is transposed (Fig. 53.3). If the transposed muscle-fascial strip is not long enough to reach the medial canthal tendon, the strip can be lengthened by transposing a lamellar flap of the

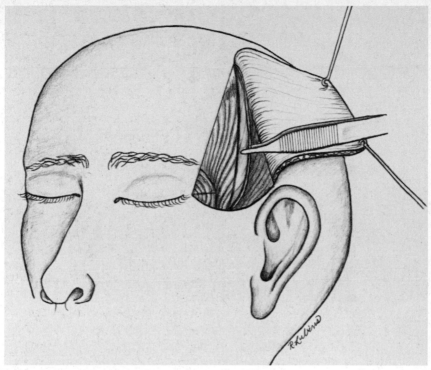

Figure 53.1 *Incision to expose temporalis muscle.*

anterior fascia (Fig. 53.3, upper right insert). The muscle is passed through the suborbicularis tunnel and anchored to the periosteal insertion of the medial canthal tendon with a double-armed Mersilene suture (Fig. 53.3, upper left insert).

Polyethylene tubing from a number 23 butterfly scalp vein set can be placed in the temporalis muscle defect to serve as a drain.

Then, 4-0 chromic sutures can be used to close the temporalis fascia, and 5-0 nylon sutures can be used for the skin. The number 23 butterfly needle is inserted into a vacutainer tube; a pressure dressing with head-roll is applied, and the vacutainer tube is changed daily until no further drainage occurs, and then it is removed. The medial canthal wound is closed with 6-0 nylon. Sutures are removed at 7 days.

This procedure can be used to correct recurrent ectropion as described above. A horizontal lid shortening procedure may be used in conjunction with this method if rotation of the punctum is necessary.

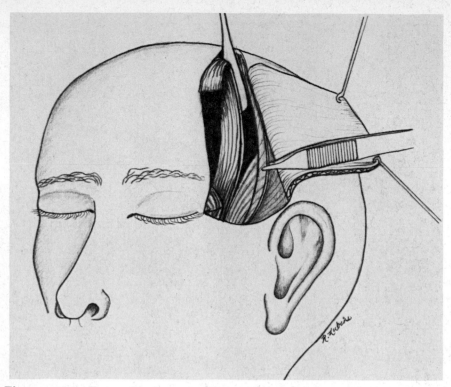

Figure 53.2 Preparing temporalis muscle and epicranium.

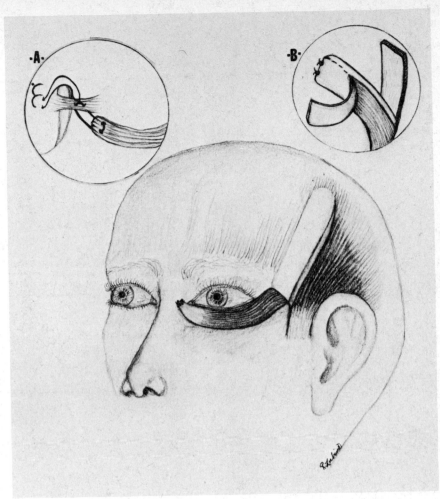

Figure 53.3   Temporalis fascia transposed to correct ectropion.

LACRIMAL

PART V

54

Occlusion of the Punctum with Cyanoacrylate

Albert Hornblass

INTRODUCTION

Occlusion of the punctum can sometimes provide relief from keratitis sicca. The technique described below uses cyanoacrylate (Crazy Glue) for a simple, inexpensive, reversible method of punctal occulusion.

TECHNIQUE

The lower lid should be retracted and the punctum dilated with a punctum dilator (Fig. 54.1A). Cyanoacrylate is placed on a sharp pointed instrument, such as a punctum dilator (Fig. 54.1B), and dropped on the inferior punctum and allowed to settle (Fig. 54.1C).

As soon as the material hardens, a razor blade should be used to shave along the lid margin. The punctum is occluded by the glue remaining in the lacrimal system (Fig. 54.1D).

Care should be taken to avoid glue falling into the conjunctival cul-de-sac. The punctum plug of cyanoacrylate glue can be removed, if needed.

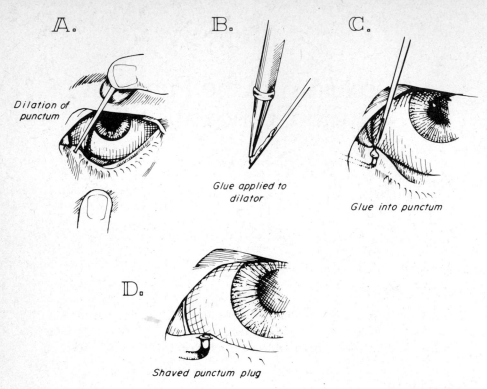

A.

Dilation of punctum

B.

Glue applied to dilator

C.

Glue into punctum

D.

Shaved punctum plug

Figure 54.1 After dilating the punctum (A), cyanoacrylate glue applied to punctum dilator (B). Glue allowed to flow into punctum (C). Excess glue shaved with scalpel leaving punctum plug (D).

55

Application of Thermal Cautery to Relieve Punctal Stenosis

William Fein

INTRODUCTION

Most procedures relieve punctal stenosis and reestablish patency of the lacrimal system with dilation or snipping of the punctum. This technique uses traction produced by cautery to the mucosa and muscle at the base of the lacrimal papilla to pull open the walls of the punctum.

TECHNIQUE

This procedure has been used on the lower puncta in cases in which both the upper and lower puncta are occluded. A minute amount of 1% lidocaine is injected into the area of the punctum, and surgery is performed with a slit lamp or operating microscope.

With the patient's eye directed upward, the lower lid is everted slightly until the punctum is directed toward the operator (Fig. 55.1). A punctum dilator should be used to dilate the punctum and the vertical canaliculus.

Cautery is then applied around the base of the lacrimal papilla (Fig. 55.2) carefully, so the cautery penetrates only through the surface epithelium and just into the muscle layer. Deeper penetration can cause scarring of the connective tissue ring around the punctum or the mucosa lumen, which could cause constriction of the lumen and failure. The thermal cauthery should be the low-temperature type used in cataract surgery as opposed to the high-temperature hand-held cauteries, which would burn the tissue excessively.

The cautery causes retraction of the tissues away from the punctum (Fig. 55.3) to pull the system open. Postoperatively, topical gentamicin can be used, and the patient is treated daily with dilation and irrigation for 1 week and then once weekly for 3 additional weeks.

This procedure has been a simple, highly effective treatment of punctual stenosis, though failures can arise from continuation of the original

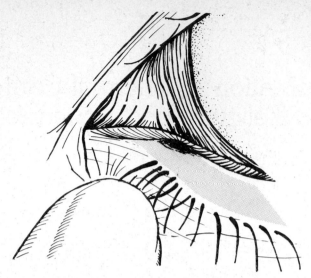

Figure 55.1 Stenotic inferior punctum rotated outward.

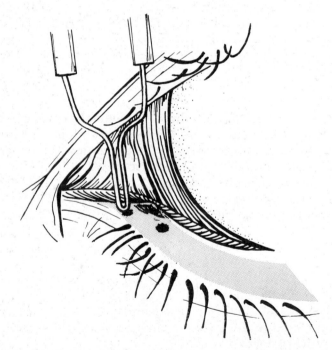

Figure 55.2 Cautery around puncta.

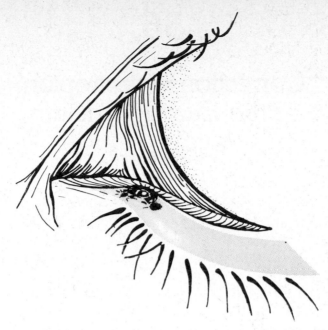

Figure 55.3 *Punctum pulled open by cautery contractures.*

disease process, overtreatment with scar contracture of the punctum, and the existence of obstructions in the lacrimal excretory system at locations other than the external punctum.

BIBLIOGRAPHY

Jones LT: New lacrimal developments, in Mustarde JC, Jones LT, Callahan A (eds): *Ophthalmic Plastic Surgery Up-to-date.* Birmingham, Aesculapius, 1970, p 96.

Veirs ER: Congenital obstruction of the nasolacrimal draining system, in Bevoe AG (ed): *Symposium on Surgery of the Ocular Adnexa.* St. Louis, Mosby, 1966, p 104.

Ziegler SL: Galvano cautery puncture: Ectropion and entropion. *JAMA* 53:183, 1907.

56

Correction of Ectropion of the Eyelid Punctum

Frank P. English
John Kearney

INTRODUCTION

Outward rotation, or ectropion, of the lower punctum can cause persistent tearing. A popular procedure for the correction of punctal ectropion has been the lazy-T technique, which allows the surgeon to correct the deformity with both horizontal tightening and inward rotation adjustments. The lazy-T procedure can be technically difficult and can possibly damage inferior canaliculus. The conjunctival sutures can cause discomfort to the patient, even when tied on the skin surface.

This technique provides a simple, one-stage technique that avoids conjunctival sutures but accomplishes both horizontal tightening and inward rotation.

TECHNIQUE

With infiltration local anesthesia for the middle half of the lower lid and topical anesthesia for the eye, a full-thickness incision should be made lateral to the punctum, extending beyond the lower limit of the tarsal plate. The lateral portion of the eyelid is grasped with forceps to apply tension nasally so the surgeon may estimate the amount of resection required. A full-thickness wedge is then carried out with straight scissors (Fig. 56.1, top). With a carefully planned marginal suture, the surgeon can rotate the nasal flap, eliminating the need for a horizontal resection of tarsus as with the lazy-T procedure.

A bite is taken with a 6-0 silk suture with the point of entry 2 mm from the wound edge. The suture exits in a similar position from the other side with the placement of the suture such that the lateral flap is in a plane posterior to the exit of the medial bite (Fig. 56.1, middle). When the first throw is tied, the medial section rotates posteriorly placing the punctum

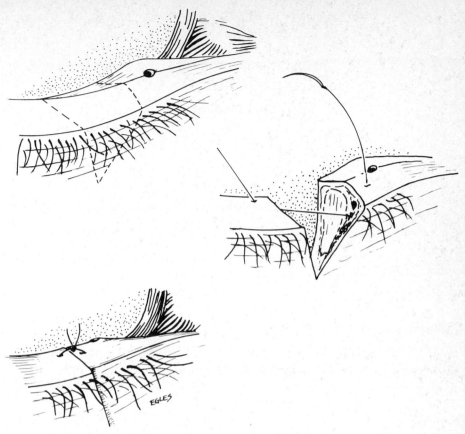

Figure 56.1 *Correction of punctum malposition.*

into the proper position (Fig. 56.1, bottom). A single throw should be placed, as this suture may need to be replaced for the proper adjustment.

Once the proper positioning of the punctum has been achieved, the suture may be tied down permanently. Additional 6-0 sutures are used to close the vertical defect.

Normally, the surgeon uses the gray line for eyelid alignment. The gray line is generally nonexistent in the immediate vicinity of the punctum.

This procedure corrects mild to moderate stages of punctal ectropion. In more severe cases, a horizontal excision of tarsus or conjunctiva can be performed similar to the lazy-T procedure if indicated after placement of the first tie described above.

BIBLIOGRAPHY

English FP, Kearney RJ: Ectropion of the eyelid punctum. *Am J Ophthalmol* 96:805, 1983.

Smith B: "Lazy T" correction of ectropion of the lower punctum. *Arch Ophthalmol* 94:1149, 1976.

57

Management of
Ostium Stenosis
after Dacryocystorhinostomy

John A. Burns
Kenneth V. Cahill

INTRODUCTION

Even after DCR (dacryocystorhinostomy) with silicone intubation, 5 to 6% of patients may develop closure of the ostium. Following a postsurgical asymptomatic period, the patient develops epiphora followed by complete blockage within the first 3 months after surgery.

With the technique below, a functioning lacrimal system can nearly always be created without necessity of DCR revision.

TECHNIQUE

In the supine position in the office treatment room, the site of the ostium can be identified by intranasal examination, noting the silicone tubing along the lateral wall of the nose just anterior to the middle turbinate (Fig. 57.1). With topical anesthesia of 4% cocaine, a von Graefe muscle hook can be inserted into the dimple that was previously the DCR ostium under direct visualization (Fig. 57.2). The hook can be passed to the interior of the lacrimal sac behind the anterior lacrimal crest.

Aggressively, the hook is used to stretch the ostium in all directions. A significant opening will be obvious, and the patient can be irrigated freely. The patient should be reevaluated in 1 week.

If muscle hook dilation is unsuccessful, the ostium can be enlarged to a diameter of at least 5 mm with end-biting rongeurs. Generally, this is performed in the operating room with better equipment and suction and possibly with general or anesthesia standby. The ostium should be enlarged until fluid can be irrigated easily into the nose. New silicone tubing should be inserted and the patient's nose packed with antibiotic ointment impregnated in one-half inch wide cotton tape for the next 5 days.

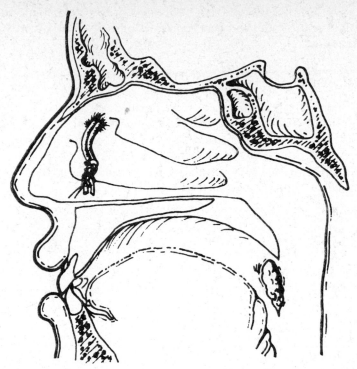

Figure 57.1 Silicone tubing from stenosed DCR ostium anterior to middle turbinate.

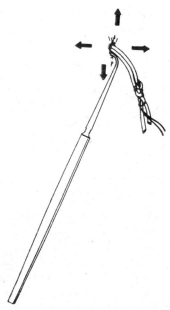

Figure 57.2 Ostium aggressively stretched open with von Graeffe muscle hook.

Nearly 50% of the patients can be treated in the office. These maneuvers virtually eliminate the need for repeating a more involved standard DCR procedure.

BIBLIOGRAPHY

Burns JA: Lacrimal apparatus surgery, in David Dorff, FH (ed): *Atlas of Eye Surgery.* Columbus, Ophthalmology Illustrated, 1978, p 233.

Lindberg JV, Anderson RL, Bumstead RM, et al: Study of intranasal ostium external to dacryocystorhinostomy. *Arch Ophthalmol* 100:1758, 1982.

Welham RA, Henderson PH: Results of dacryocystorhinostomy: Analysis of causes for failure. *Trans Ophthalmol UK* 93:601,1977.

58

Suture Tagging of an Anterior Nasal Mucosal Flap in Dacryocystorhinostomy

Eugene O. Wiggs

INTRODUCTION

During DCR (dacryocystorhinostomy) (Fig. 58.1A), the mucosal flaps out of the rhinostomy can be difficult. The flaps can be easily retrieved from down in the rhinostomy with a small skin hook.

TECHNIQUE

The anterior flap of nasal mucosa used in DCR is mobilized with a knife incision into the nasal mucosa at the posterior aspect of the rhinostomy. Curved pointed scissors complete this portion of the mobilization of the nasal mucosa.

The flaps are difficult to grasp with a forceps, but a small skin hook can be placed into the rhinostomy to retrieve the anterior nasal mucosa flap (Fig. 58.1B). A knife is then used to make vertical cuts in the mucosa at the upper and lower aspects of the rhinostomy while at the same time pulling the flap slightly toward the skin wound with the small double hook.

The hook then engages the anteriorly based flap of the nasal mucosa, allowing easy placement of sutures into the flap (Figs. 58.1B and C).

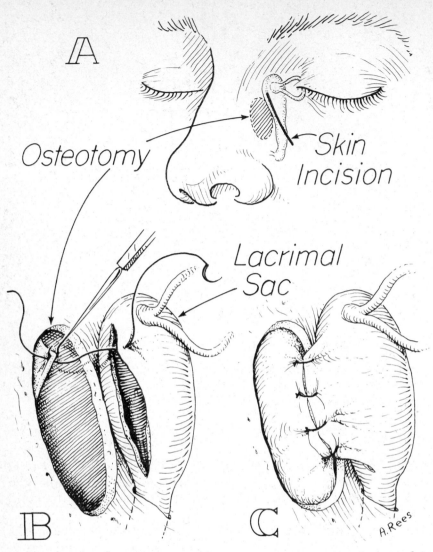

A

Osteotomy

Skin Incision

Lacrimal Sac

B

C

A.Rees

Figure 58.1 During dacryocystorhinostomy (A) skin hook passed into rhinostomy (B) to retrieve anterior nasal mucosal flap (C).

59

Treatment of Obstruction
of the Lacrimal System

John S. Crawford

INTRODUCTION

Most congenital nasolacrimal duct obstructions clear spontaneously within 4 to 6 weeks, or even up to a year, but some never clear. Treatment with topical antibiotic drops may keep the eye free of infection, but obstruction in the lower end of the nasolacrimal duct can result in bacteria entering the lacrimal sac, causing dacryocystitis and subsequent discharge. With continued tearing, a simple probing is carried out. On rare occasions, with more persistent problems, a fracture of the turbinate may be required. If tearing and obstruction cannot be cured by a simple probing, intubation of the lacrimal system may be necessary

When tearing persists after probing was performed without much difficulty, the mucosa may be acting as a valve closing over a portion of the lacrimal draining systems. When two or three probings do not cure the tearing, silicone tubes can be used to stent the entire lacrimal system. The conventional method of inserting silicone tubes (1) can be extremely difficult. The method described below is a simple, effective way to place silicone intubation into the lacrimal system (2–3).

TECHNIQUE

Silicone tubes are passed into each puncta, through the canaliculus, and down the nasolacrimal duct and the ends secured under the inferior turbinate (Fig. 59.1). This is carried out much easier by gluing the ends of the silicone rod onto two wires with knobs on the end. At the lower end of the nasolacrimal duct, the wires are removed from the nose with a special hook, which easily locates the wire under the inferior turbinate (1). The knob on the end of the wire keeps the hook from slipping off as the maleable wire is brought out the nose.

In special cases, the lower end of the nasolacrimal duct is quite small

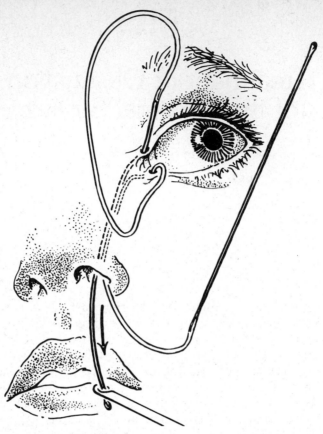

Figure 59.1 Treatment of lacrimal obstructions with silicone tube placement. Special knob on the end of lacrimal wires allows hook to easily locate wire under inferior turbinate and pull out the nose.

and may have a more posterior downward direction such that the wire has to be pulled forward around an acute angle (Fig. 59.2A). The sharp bend may cause the tubing to be pushed off the wire (Fig. 59.2B). To solve this problem, an ear curret is passed over the wire and pushed back into the nose to direct the tubing backward and downward until the silicone tubing is out of the nose (Fig. 59.2C).

Traditionally, the ends of the silicone tubing have been tied together to form a knot. Regardless of the number of throws cast, a child would occasionally pull the loop of silicone tubing at the medial canthus with the knot traveling up the nasolacrimal duct into the lacrimal sac. These multiple throws at the knots would be too large to be worked out the canaliculus for removal.

An improved method of securing the ends of the silicone tubing involves gluing them together with Histoacryl glue while stenting them with a 4-0 prolene suture inserted into the ends of each silicone tube.

The tubes are placed on stretch so that the loop of tubing does not

180

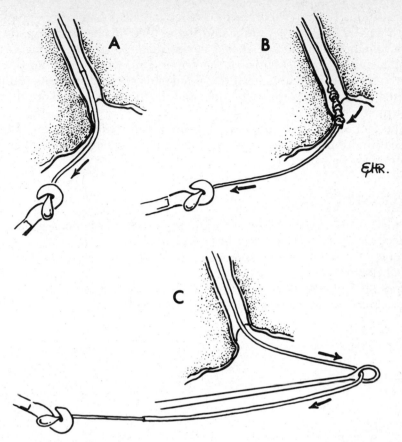

Figure 59.2 A nasolacrimal duct with unusual posterior direction puts stress on tubing during removal (A) such that the silicone may bunch and come off the wire (B). Placing an ear curette over the wire and pushing it posteriorly allows the tubing to be brought down into the nose, it then can be brought forward out of the nostril (C). (Crawford JS: Diseases and plastic surgery of the lids and lacrimal apparatus. The Eye in Childhood Disease. Grune & Stratton, Inc., 1983.)

migrate upward. A pair of mosquito forceps with rubber or silicone tubing over each tip holds the silicone tubing while securing the ends. The gluing is accomplished using approximately a 10 mm length of 4-0 prolene. First, the suture is inserted into the end of one of the tubes, and then a drop of Histoacryl glue is touched to the end of the tubing. Then the remaining end of the prolene is inserted into the other tube and glued similarly in place with Histoacryl glue.

Drawing several drops of Histoacryl into a small plastic syringe and injecting some glue through a 30-gauge needle into the tubing around the prolene facilitates the procedure. Tubes are left in place for approximately 3 to 6 months.

Traditionally, removal of the tubes that have been tied together requires that the child be given a general anesthetic. With this method of gluing the ends together, general anesthesia is not required as the tubing can be grasped with a forceps between the upper and lower puncta and pulled out the upper canaliculus until the glued ends appear. Then the tubing is cut just above the lower canaliculus, and the tubing is pulled out through the upper canaliculus.

The technique above provides a simple method for inserting silicone intubation for treatment of nasolacrimal duct obstruction as well as ease of removal.

REFERENCES

1. Quickert MH, Dryden R: Probes for intubation in lacrimal drainage. *Trans Am Acad Ophthalmol Otolaryngol* 74:431, 1970.
2. Crawford JS: Intubation of obstructions in the lacrimal system. *Can J Ophthalmol* 12:289, 1977.
3. Craft SP, Crawford JS: Silicone tube intubation and disorders of the lacrimal system in children. *Am J Ophthalmol* 94:290, 1982.

60

Infracture of
the Inferior Turbinate
with Periosteal Elevator
in Congenital Nasolacrimal
Duct Obstructions

Michael Patipa
Robert B. Wilkins
Weldon E. Havins

INTRODUCTION

When probing fails to relieve nasolacrimal duct obstruction, silicone intubation has been a popular treatment.

We have found infracturing the inferior turbinate to be a simple, successful, safe, and easy procedure to perform in the small percentage of obstructions that fail to resolve spontaneously or, that have recurred after probing.

TECHNIQUE

Probings with inferior turbinate infracture are performed under general anesthesia with endotracheal intubation. Gauze moistened with a few drops of 4% cocaine should be gently placed beside the inferior turbinate along the floor of the nose using the headlight, nasal speculum, and dressing forceps.

After 3 minutes, the packing can be removed and the dull end of the Freer elevator placed on the lateral surface of the anterior third of the inferior turbinate. With the Freer elevator, pressure should be applied medially so the inferior turbinate is fractured with a gentle rotating motion (Fig. 60.1).

The Freer elevator is then moved posteriorly along the lateral wall of the turbinate, and the posterior two-thirds of the inferior turbinate is

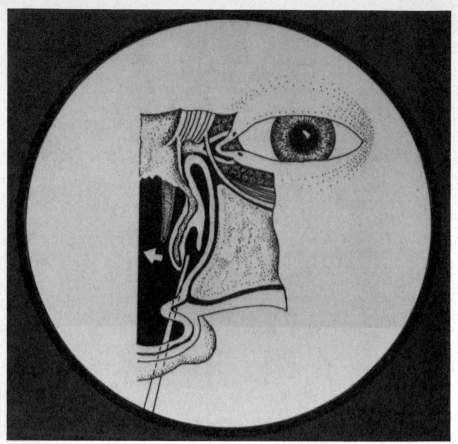

Figure 60.1 *Fracture of inferior turbinate with periosteal elevator. (Reprinted with permission.* Ophthalmic Surgery *14:666–670, 1983.)*

fractured medially. A moderate amount of pressure may be required to infracture the inferior turbinate. A definite "give" can be felt at the moment of infracture. The small amount of bleeding that may occur from the nose usually stops within 2 minutes.

Probing is then performed through the upper canaliculus to the floor of the nose in the routine manner. The probe from the upper canaliculus travels a distance of about 20 to 25 mm. The tip of the probe in the nose should be identified by passing a second probe into the nose and feeling "metal on metal."

If contact of the two probes cannot be verified, the probe down the NLD may be located submucosally along the floor of the nose. The sharp end of the Freer elevator should be scraped against the probe until a metal-to-metal contact occurs and opens the NLD into the nose. Patency should be confirmed with fluorescein-tinged saline irrigated through the upper canaliculus into the nose.

As an alternative method, a Weil lacrimal cannula on a 3 cc syringe with fluorescein-tinged saline can be passed via the upper canaliculus into the lacrimal sac and then down the NLD. A fine-suction catheter passed along the floor of the nose will suction any fluorescein solution. The appearance of fluorescein in the suction catheter confirms patency of the lacrimal system.

Silicone intubation has been traditionally used after probing failures. In addition to the difficulty in passing silicone tubes, complications occur such as persistent tearing, mucoid discharge, partial expulsion of the tube superiorly, and failure. Removal of silicone tubes from beneath the inferior turbinate can be difficult and require general anesthesia.

In patients allergic to cocaine, we recommend 2.5% phenylephrine drops for vasoconstriction. The turbinate fracture should be avoided in children with serious bleeding disorders. We recommend probing in the office for children under 8 months of age. With older children or those who are probing failures, we have found fracture of the turbinate offers a simple, effective method to treat pediatric nasolacrimal duct obstruction.

BIBLIOGRAPHY

Durso F, Hand SL, Ellis FD, et al: Silicone intubation in children with nasolacrimal duct obstruction. *J Pediatr Ophthalmol Strabismus* 17:389, 1980.

Havins WE, Wilkins RB: A useful alternative to silicone intubation in congenital nasolacrimal duct obstructions. *Ophthalmic Surg* 14:666, 1983.

Jones LT, Wobig J: *Surgery of the Eyelid and Lacrimal System.* Birmingham, Aesculapius, 1976, pp 163–167.

Lauring L: Silicone intubation of the lacrimal system: Pitfalls, problems and complications. *Ann Ophthalmol* 24:489, 1976.

Peterson RA, Robb RM: The natural course of congenital obstruction of the nasolacrimal duct. *J Pediatr Ophthalmol Stabismus* 15:246, 1978.

61

Outfracture of the Inferior Turbinate in Persistent Congenital NLD Obstruction

Ralph E. Wesley

INTRODUCTION

In children who have failed to respond to routine lacrimal probing, outfracture of the turbinate nearly always clears them if they have nasolacrimal duct. A simple twist of the inferior turbinate with a hemostat alleviates the obstruction.

TECHNIQUE

One-eighth percent neosynephrine on cotton is packed into the nose of the child with the unsuccessful lacrimal irrigation. A few minutes later the packing is removed. Using a pediatric nasal speculum, a straight hemostat should be advanced into the nose (Fig. 61.1) to grasp the inferior turbinate. The inferior turbinate should be rotated a full 90 degrees by twisting the hemostat (Fig. 61.2).

This turning action should open up the nasolacrimal duct at the inferior portion and allow for adequate drainage. To make sure the child does, in fact, have a nasolacrimal duct, a small tenotomy muscle hook can be placed under the inferior turbinate to isolate the inferior end of the NLD (Fig. 61.3). To prevent a nose bleed, thrombin drops and Gelfoam are packed under the inferior turbinate at the conclusion of the procedure.

If the patient does not have a nasolacrimal duct a DCR can be performed at that time. If an NLD exists, the surgeon should wait a month to see the result of the outfracture, which is almost uniformly successful even in older children and those who have had probings numerous times previously.

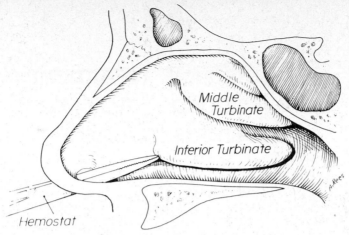

Figure 61.1 Hemostat inserted to grasp inferior turbinate.

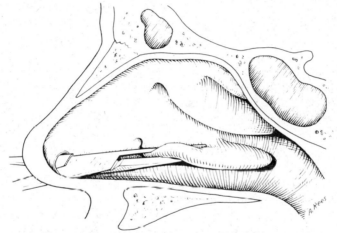

Figure 61.2 Full 90-degree rotation performed.

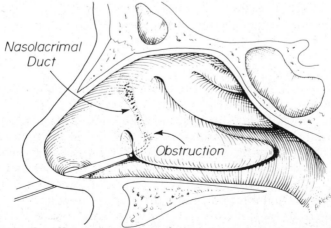

Figure 61.3 Small tenotomy muscle hook used to verify existence of NLD.

187

62

Insufflation Treatment of Occluded Nasolacrimal Apparatus in Children

David Sevel

INTRODUCTION

Traditional probing techniques for treatment of congenital occlusion of the nasolacrimal duct can damage the lining of the nasolacrimal duct (Fig. 62.1) causing permanent scarring. The insufflation technique avoids this complication.

TECHNIQUE

With the child under mask rather than endotracheal general anesthesia, the upper and lower puncta are gently dilated with the puncta dilator. A 27-gauge lacrimal cannula previously sanded to remove and barbs or rough edges is attached to a 2 cc syringe filled with saline and then introduced through the inferior punctum via the inferior canaliculus into the lacrimal sac to ascertain patency.

The cannula is removed and then passed in a similar manner through the superior canaliculus into the lacrimal sac, and saline is injected to wash out any mucopurulent material. With gentle pressure over the sac, the procedure is repeated until the fluid clears.

Finally with the cannula left in the sac, the syringe is gently detached from the cannula filled with air and reattached to the cannula. To ease the cannula toward the superior opening of the nasolacrimal duct at the inferior medial aspect of the orbital rim, the thumb of the opposite hand is placed over the opening of the superior part of the nasolacrimal duct.

The anesthesiologist removes the mask and 0.5 to 2 cc of air is injected into the lacrimal sac (Fig. 62.2). With thumb of the opposite hand compressing the everted inferior canaliculus against the inferior orbital rim to prevent air from escaping through the lower punctum, a distinct "plop" may be heard as the obstruction is cleared.

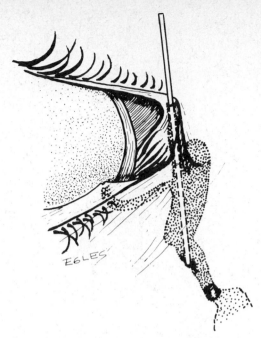

Figure 62.1 Standard probe can damage NLD mucosa.

The opening of the nasolacrimal duct can be performed by placing a drop of surgical soap on the nares and observing for bubbles as the air escapes into the nasal cavity.

The insufflation technique allows a bolus of air to follow the preformed lumen of the nasolacrimal duct forcing debris downward and rupturing fine membranes without damage to the mucosa itself. This technique avoids damage or tearing of the mucosa, which might occur by passing a probe down the nasolacrimal duct where the inferior portion enters the vestibule of the nose at approximately a 20-degree angle to the general direction of the boney canal.

BIBLIOGRAPHY

Sevel D: Insufflation treatment of occluded nasolacrimal apparatus in the child. *Ophthalmology* 89:329, 1982.

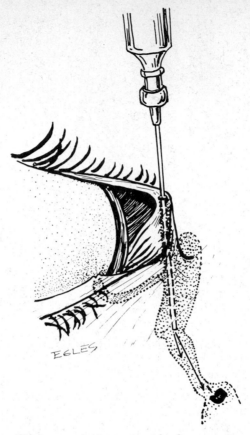

Figure 62.2 Insufflation technique avoids damage to mucosa.

63

Dacryocystography

Michael J. Hawes

INTRODUCTION

Radiographic technique of dacryocystography can be useful in lacrimal evaluation such as canalicular obstruction, tumors in the region of the sac and duct, diverticula and fistulas, dacryoliths, foreign bodies, failed dacryocystorhinostomy, and nasolacrimal duct obstruction. Conventional cannulation (1) of a single canaliculus with a metal cannula usually does not allow for visualization of the canaliculi or even the entire sac or duct. The physician's hand must be close to the x-ray beam if fluoroscopy is performed.

These problems can be avoided with the method below.

TECHNIQUE

Catheterization of both canaliculi with Teflon catheters* tapered to 0.5 mm outside diameter (1.5 French) allows complete opacification and visualization of the drainage system and permits fluoroscopy and patient head movements without risk of radiation exposure to the physician (2). Simultaneous bilateral dacryocystograms can be performed if desired. Acqueous contrast medium, such as iothalamate meglumine,† is preferred because of its lower viscosity.

A contrast medium is injected through the catheters to eliminate air from the system. The punctum and the initial portion of the canaliculus are intubated (Fig. 63.1). With both catheters in place (Fig. 63.2), contrast medium is injected (Fig. 63.3) under fluoroscopy with exposures taken as desired. Posteroanterior and oblique views are usually sufficient.

---

* Available from Cook, Inc. Box 489, Bloomington, Indiana, 47402 (# T 3.0 15 30 P NS O). Three-way Y manifold (TWY-1FLL-2MLL) also available.

† Conray-60, MallincKrondt, Inc. St. Louis, Mo., 63134.

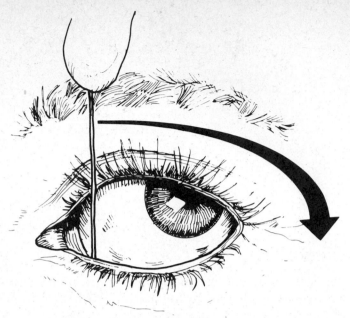

Figure 63.1 Catheter in lower punctum.

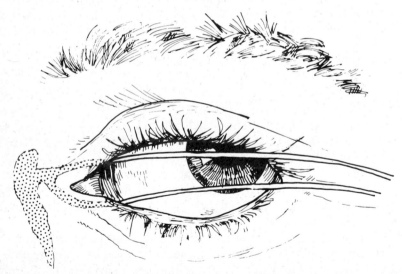

Figure 63.2 Catheter intubation of both canaliculi.

REFERENCES

1. Milder B: Dacryocystography, in Milder B (ed): *The Lacrimal System*. Norwalk, Appleton–Century–Crafts, 1983.
2. Gullotta U, v Denffer H: *Dacryocystography: An Atlas and Textbook*. New York, Thieve–Stratton, 1980.

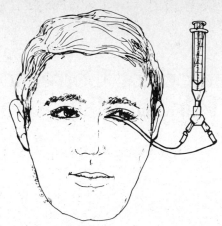

Figure 63.3   Injection of contrast medium for dacryocystography.

64

Method for Correction of Punctal Malposition

Hampson A. Sisler

INTRODUCTION

Epiphora can arise from malpositioning of the punctum, whether caused by trauma, inflammation, or an aging process. With the punctum located too far nasally, the caruncle or semilunar fold may occlude the punctum. With a position too far temporally, the corneal bulge may be a problem. With the punctum rotated inwardly against the eye, pressure by the eyeball may occlude the punctum.

Punctal malpositioning from trauma or inflammation can be corrected by releasing the proximal or vertical part of the canaliculus and punctum, excising tissues located in the direction of the desired relocation, and resuturing the freed proximal canaliculus to the newly created tissue defect.

TECHNIQUE

An operating microscope is used to perform the procedure ten minutes after injecting 1% lidocaine or bupivacaine with 1:200,000 epinephrine containing hyaluronidase below the nasal end of the inferior tarsus and the placement of 4% lidocaine hydrochloride solution topically to the punctum. A medium-sized Bowman probe is passed to define the vertical portion of the canaliculus. A small, straight-tipped blade is used to circumscribe the peripunctal mucosa and to make cuts about 1.5 mm outside and around the canaliculus (Fig. 64.1A,B,C,D, and E).

With the operating microscope, care can be exercised to avoid cutting into the canaliculus and to simply free its proximal extent down to the region of the ampulla. The vertical canaliculus is mobilized to facilitate its placement in the desired direction. A 1.5-mm trephine can be used to excise adjacent tissue, either medially or laterally in the direction of desired replacement of the punctum and proximal canaliculus (Fig. 64.1F,G, and H).

194

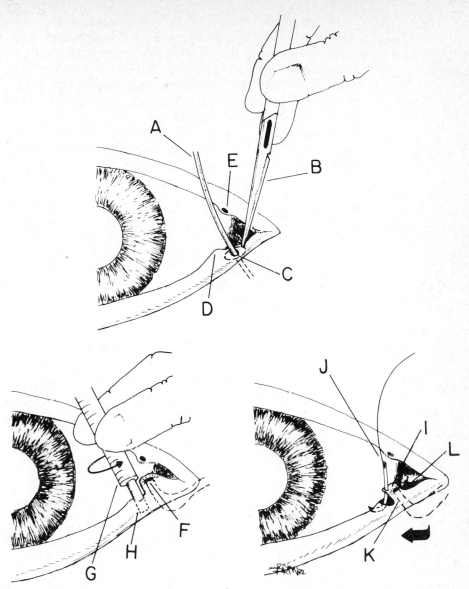

Figure 64.1 Medium Bowman probe (A) in inferior punctum (C). Straight blade (B) used to incise 1.5 mm around the punctum, which is displaced nasally from lower lacrimal papilla (D). Normal superior punctum (E). 1.5 mm trephine (G) used to create defect (H) for repositioning of punctum (F). Using operating microscope, 10-0 nylon (J) passed through wall of punctum (I) pulling freed canaliculus (K) into proper position. Tissue gap (L) left unsutured.

A very fine suture is passed through the peripunctal mucosa and submucosa tissue on the side toward the defect created by the trephine, with the needle passed across the gap of the excision at a corresponding depth to emerge from the surface (Fig. 64.1I,J,K, and L). The suture is secured tightly, thereby rotating the punctum and the proximal canaliculus in the desired direction. With the patient blinking slowly, the newly positioned punctum can be evaluated in its new position.

This technique allows for repositioning the punctum with the simple technique under local anesthesia to correct the malposition of the punctum, whether internal, lateral, or medial.

65

Finding a Lost Proximal End of a Canalicular Laceration

Craig E. Berris

INTRODUCTION

The proximal end of a severed canaliculus after medial canthal trauma can be difficult to locate if the cut has been tangential or if significant tissue swelling has occurred. The search for the lost proximal end can be a prolonged, frustrating experience for any surgeon.

Traditional methods to find the lost proximal end of the canalicular laceration are frequently unsatisfactory. Milk or penicillin can be irrigated through the opposite punctum of the canalicular system and the proximal end of the canalicular laceration identified. However, no reflux will occur unless there is an obstruction of the nasolacrimal duct below the injection site. The irrigation of milk or penicillin passes into the nose without reflux through the involved canalicular system.

A pigtail probe may be passed through the noninvolved canalicular system to exit out the severed canaliculus. Frequently, passage of the probe through the inferior system is impossible, and the surgeon may create a false passage. Surgical repair with a pigtail probe has a poorer patency rate and a high instance of damage to the uninvolved canalicular system.

Another technique injects air through the uninvolved canalicular system while the surgical site is under a puddle of water. A tampon is placed to close off the valve of Hasner at the distal end of the nasolacrimal duct. Visualization of the exit of the air bubbles is difficult as is placement of the tampon at the distal ostium of the nasolacrimal duct.

The canaliculus can be located at the site of refluxed fluid with a 2.5 French double-lumen balloon-tipped catheter with a port 2-mm proximal to the balloon. The balloon can be passed through the normal canaliculus into the NLD, the balloon inflated, and fluorescein injected (Fig. 65.1). This technique works well, but the catheters are not stocked in every operating room.

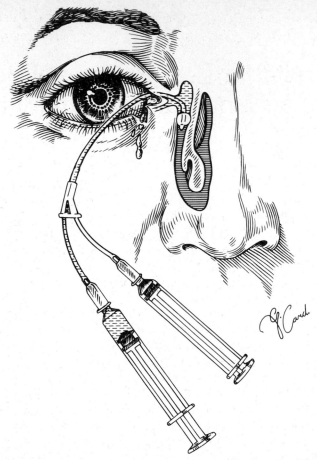

Figure 65.1 *Method of locating severed canaliculus by blocking NLD with French 2.5 double-lumen catheter.*

Using readily available materials, the technique below can be used to identify the lost proximal end of a canalicular laceration through an unobstructed view of refluxed fluid.

TECHNIQUE

This method uses a temporary obstruction of the nasolacrimal duct distal to the common canaliculus. Silastic tubing, 0.037 inches in outside diameter and 0.020 inches in inside diameter is inserted onto a size 0 Quickert rod. The inside diameter of the Silastic tube will accommodate the standard nasolacrimal cannula. After passage of the Quickert rod and Silastic tubing through the uninvolved canalicular system and out through the nose, a "fly" is tied around the tube with two pieces of Silastic tubing, creating a knot approximately 2 to 3 mm in diameter. Proximal to this knot, the surgeon makes multiple passes of a 27-gauge needle through the

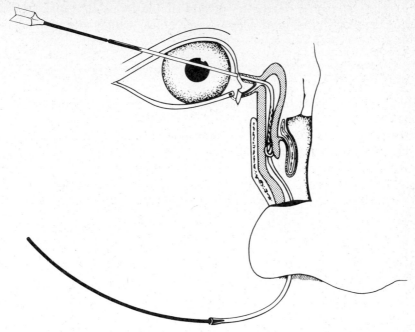

Figure 65.2 *Readily available Silastic "fly" method to create fluid reflux through cut canaliculus.*

Silastic tubing. The tubing, with knot attached, is then pulled back through the nasolacrimal system so the knot rests in or proximal to the valve of Hasner to create an effective obstruction of the nasolacrimal system.

Next, a nasolacrimal cannula is inserted in the free end of the Silastic tubing. A syringe containing either dye or other solutions may be used to inject forcibly through the Silastic tubing. The fluid exits through the perforations made with the 27-gauge needle in a manner similar to sprinkler hoses seen in any garden shop (Fig. 65.2).

The fluid preferentially passes retrograde through the common canaliculus and out the proximal end of the lacerated canaliculus, because the distal nasolacrimal system is obstructed with the fly. After location of the proximal end of the lacerated canaliculus, the nasolacrimal cannula is removed from the Silastic tubing and a Quickert rod is attached to this end as well. The Quickert rod is placed through the distal end of the lacerated canaliculus, through the now-localized proximal end, and out the nose. The Silastic tubing is then tied on itself in a standard fashion.

The surgeon should avoid making excessively large openings in the Silastic tubing with the needle or putting over-zealous traction to bring the fly back into the nasolacrimal system, which could break the weakened Silastic tubing. The knot should be small enough to pass under the inferior turbinate so that it does indeed obstruct the valve of Hasner.

The 27-gauge needle or smaller needle should be used to make multiple puncture sites rather than a few larger holes, which might weaken the tubing.

BIBLIOGRAPHY

Morrison F: An aid to repair of lacerated tear ducts. *Arch Ophthalmol* 72:341, 1964.

Quickert M, Dryden R: Probes for intubation of lacrimal in lacrimal drainage. *Trans Am Acad Ophthalmol Otolaryngol* 74:431, 1970

Saunders D, Shannon G, Flanagan J: The effectiveness of the pigtail probe method of repairing canalicular lacerations. *Ophthalmic Surg* 9:33, 1978.

Wurst J: Method for reconstructing torn canaliculus. *Am J Ophthalmol* 53:520, 1962.

66

Use of Neurosurgical Canal Elevator to Separate Nasal Mucosa from Rhinostomy

James R. Boynton

INTRODUCTION

During dacryocystorhinostomy the nasal mucosa should be preserved to facilitate an anastomosis with the lacrimal sac for successful lacrimal drainage procedure. Even with careful exposure of the mucosa, stripping mucosa from the bone may be difficult.

TECHNIQUE

The use of a neurosurgical canal elevator (Storz N-1704-6 Jordan Round Sharp) allows the surgeon (Fig. 66.1) to strip nasal mucosa from the internal boney surface of the nose. This facilitates separation of the nasal mucosa so that a Kerrison or other rongeur may be introduced with the usual technique to enlarge the rhinostomy before incising the nasal mucosal flaps for dacryocystorhinostomy.

This instrument can be used to create enough space for the Kerrison punch without trauma to the nasal mucosa.

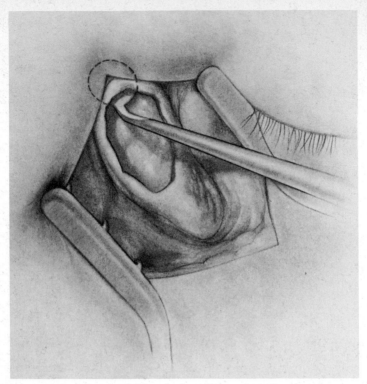

Figure 66.1 Neurosurgical canal elevator separates nasal mucosa.

67

Identification of Lacrimal Sac in Dacryocystorhinostomy

Robert M. Dryden
T. David I. Wilkes

INTRODUCTION

Opening a relatively normal lacrimal sac during dacryocystorhinostomy (DCR) by cutting down on a lacrimal probe passed into the sac through a canaliculus surgery usually presents no problems. Opening the sac can be difficult when the mucosa has scarred or the internal punctum remains imperforate. This essential step in DCR surgery can be simplified using the technique described below.

TECHNIQUE

After standard DCR technique has been used to incise the skin, identify the lacrimal fossa, and create the bony ostium, the nasolacrimal duct can be identified in the nasolacrimal canal suspended as a tubular structure (Fig. 67.1). A blunt probe or small tenotomy hook inserted into the nasolacrimal canal verifies the position of the nasolacrimal duct.

With a number 12 Bard–Parker blade, the medial wall of the nasolacrimal duct is opened superiorly exposing the nasolacrimal mucosa (Fig. 67.2).

To avoid confusion in opening the nasolacrimal duct, a small tenotomy hook is then passed through the incision into the collapsed sac and used to suspend the sac open (Fig. 67.3). An incision into the sac can be performed with scissors or a number 12 blade in a controlled manner with the sac elevated with the tenotomy hook without fear of transecting both walls of the sac.

The remainder of the sac can be opened with the number 12 blade (Fig. 67.4), as the nasolacrimal duct remains suspended by the bony canal

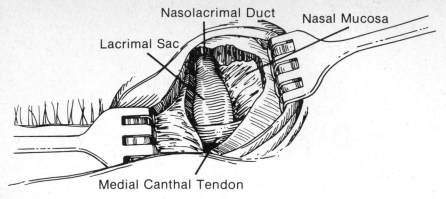

Figure 67.1 *Nasolacrimal duct, forehead view.*

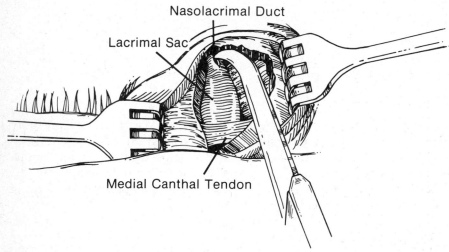

Figure 67.2 *Medial wall of nasal lacrimal duct opened with number 12 blade.*

despite a collapsed lacrimal sac. This technique may be used on routine cases, but this method helps to avoid the complications of opening only the periosteal sac, incising too deeply cutting both the medial and lateral walls of the sac with common punctum damage, orbital fat collapse, and disorientation with regard to anatomic landmarks.

BIBLIOGRAPHY

Dryden RM, Wilkes TDI: Lacrimal sac identification in dacryocystorhinostomy surgery. *Ophthalmic Surg* 14:661, 1983.

Jones LT, Wobig JL: Surgery of the tear sac, in *Surgery of the Eyelids and Lacrimal System*. Birmingham, Aesculapius, 1976, pp 198–208.

Quickert MH: Lacrimal drainage surgery, in Soll DB (ed): *Management of Complications in Ophthalmic Plastic Surgery*. Birmingham, Aesculapius, 1976, p 105.

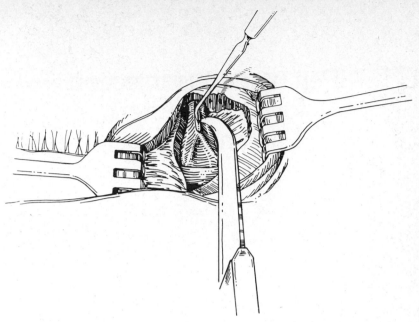

Figure 67.3 *A small tenotomy hook suspends collapsed sac allowing controlled opening of the sac.*

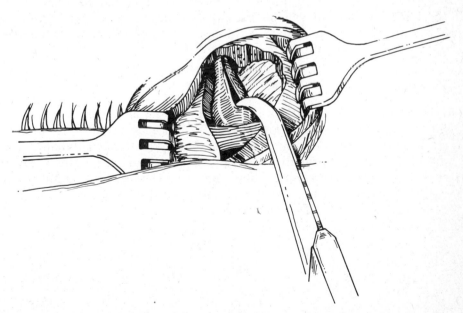

Figure 67.4 *Remainder of the sac incision easily performed with either number 12 blade or scissors. (Reprinted with permission. Ophthalmic Surgery 14:661–662, 1983.)*

68

Percutaneous Injection for Occult Atretic Lacrimal Puncta

Francis G. LaPiana

INTRODUCTION

Patients with apparent congenital absence of the superior and inferior punctum may, in fact, have atresia of the lacrimal puncta. If the atretic puncta can be opened, a functional lacrimal system may be established. Incisions into the lid can be fraught with difficulty in identifying an atretic lacrimal system. This technique shows a simple method to identify occult atretic lacrimal puncta.

TECHNIQUE

To find the probable locus of an atretic punctum, methylene blue can be injected percutaneously through a 27- or 30-gauge needle into the lacrimal sac while pressure is exerted over the inferior portion of the sac and the surgeon observes whether or not dye fills the canaliculus. If dye can be seen in the eyelids (Fig. 68.1), then a punctum can be created at the point where the dye ends and patency maintained with silicone intubation thus creating a functioning lacrimal system.

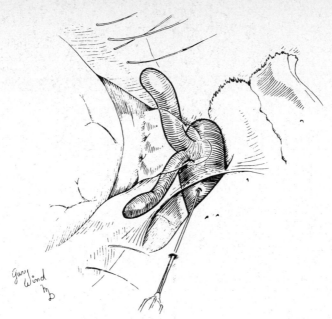

Figure 68.1 Atretic lacrimal system distended with methylene blue to identify site laterally to form punctum.

69

Separation of Nasal Mucosa from Rhinostomy During Dacryocystorhinostomy

James R. Boynton

INTRODUCTION

Separation of the nasal mucosa from the overlying bone during dacryocystorhinostomy allows the nasal mucosa to be kept intact for anastomosis with the lacrimal sac. Conventional trephines and punches may damage the nasal mucosa.

TECHNIQUE

With use of a diamond burr (Striker No. 1608693), the bone over the desired rhinostomy site can be cut away in a controlled manner without cutting the underlying nasal mucosa (Fig. 69.1). Once the mucosa is identified, a Kerrison punch can be introduced to push the nasal mucosa inward and remove the desired bone for the rhinostomy site.

The nasal mucosa is left intact until incised to form flaps for the dacryocystorhinostomy.

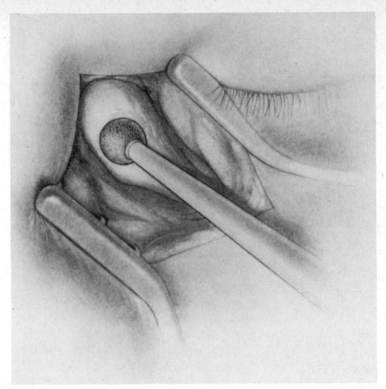

Figure 69.1 Diamond burr for dacryocystorhinostomy leaves nasal mucosa intact.

70

Use of a Silicone Sponge for Retention of Canalicular Silicone Intubation

Russell W. Neuhaus
Norman Shorr

INTRODUCTION

Silicone intubation of the lacrimal system can be used as an effective stent in canalicular lacerations, canalicular stenosis, medial canthal trauma, nasolacrimal duct obstructions, and dacryocystorhinostomy surgery. Problems can arise from the method of securing the ends of the tube in the nose.

With tube secured too tightly, erosion of the upper and lower punctum occurs. If inadequately secured in the nose, the ends of the tube may retract up the nasolacrimal duct, particularly if the loop between the upper and lower lid is grasped by a child.

Even when numerous knots are tied in the ends of the silicone tubes within the nose, the tube can still be retracted up the nasolacrimal duct. Suturing the ends to the side of the nose may provide only temporary fixation. Fixation of the ends of the tube with a retinal band attached to the knots can prevent loop retraction, but may cause punctal erosion.

With the method below, tubes remain in the end of the nose without undue tension on the canalicular system.

TECHNIQUE

The silicone tubing should be inserted into the lacrimal system using the surgeon's preferred technique such that silicone tubing is placed through the upper and lower canalicular system, down the nasolacrimal duct, and two free ends brought out the nose. Castroviejo forceps (0.5 mm) are

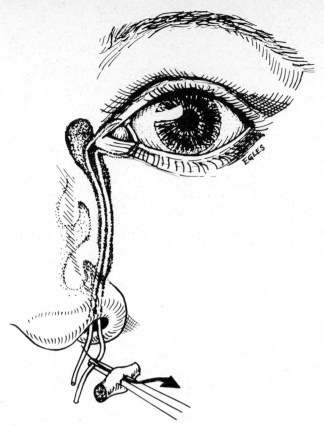

Figure 70.1 Forceps pull tube back through sponge.

pushed through a silicone retinal sponge 3 mm in diameter and approximately 10 mm in length in order to grasp the silicone tubing (Fig. 70.1). The forceps are then used to pull the silicone tubing through the sponge (Fig. 70.2). The other free end of the silicone tubing is pulled through the sponge approximately 3 mm away from the first in a similar manner. The silicone loop should then be adjusted for the appropriate loop tension.

The silicone tubing should be stabilized with a hemostat and brought out the external nares while multiple knots are placed in the silicone 1 cm sponge (Fig. 70.3). Then, 4-0 silk can be used to secure the final throw of the silicone knot to prevent unraveling. The sponge is then positioned in the inferior meatus with the ends of the silicone tubing left on the floor of the nose (Fig. 70.4).

Friction between the silicone tubing and sponge will maintain the correct tension of the loop. Should excessive tension develop, the silicone tubing can slip through the sponge until the correct tension is obtained, preventing punctal erosion.

Loop retraction at the medial canthus is prevented by the knots and the silicone sponge lying at the right angles to the nasolacrimal duct. The

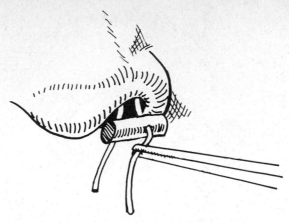

Figure 70.2 First silicone loop pulled through retinal sponge.

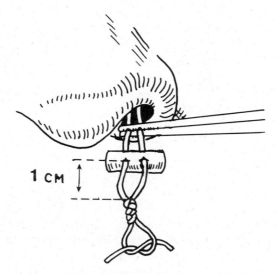

1 CM

Figure 70.3 Hemostat fixes tubing as knots are tied 1 cm from sponge.

excess silicone tubing allows for inadvertent loop retraction postoperatively as the loop can be easily repositioned in the nose by identifying the silicone sponge, which is fixated as the silicone tubing pulled back through the sponge for correction of the proper tension.

At the time of silicone tube removal, the silicone sponge facilitates finding the exposed tubing in the nose. The silicone loop between the upper and lower punctum can be cut, and the silicone sponge and attached sponging can be easily removed from the nose.

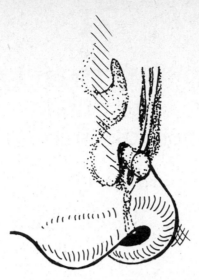

Figure 70.4 Tension on tubing adjusted to prevent punctal erosion. (Reprinted with permission. Ophthalmic Surgery 14:1026–1028, 1983.)

BIBLIOGRAPHY

Anderson RL, Edwards JJ: Indications, complications, and results with silicone stents. *Ophthalmology* 86:1474, 1979.

Neuhaus RW, Shorr N: Modified lacrimal system intubation. *Ophthalmic Surg* 14:1026, 1983.

Quickert MH: Probes for intubation and lacrimal drainage. *Trans Am Acad Ophthalmol Otolaryngol* 74:431, 1970.

71

Technique to Open Lacrimal Sac during Dacryocystorhinostomy

James R. Boynton

INTRODUCTION

A large anterior flap of lacrimal sac is desirable for most dacryocystorhinostomy procedures. Exposure can be troublesome if this sac is small or scarred. To incise posteriorly as far as desired may be very difficult. This step in dacryocystorhinostomy can be facilitated by using the technique listed below.

TECHNIQUE

A Bard–Parker number 11 blade is heated, preoperatively, over a Bunson burner and the tip bent to an angle between 60 degrees and 90 degrees. The length and angle of the tip can be varied. Once the lacrimal sac is exposed, the incision can be easily performed (Fig. 71.1) with such a blade. Blades should be bent in both directions to be able to cut up or down or to incise a right or left lacrimal sac.

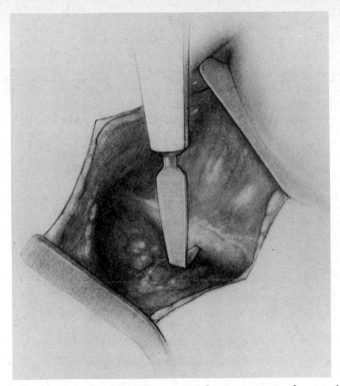

Figure 71.1 Number 11 blade prepared preoperatively used to open lacrimal sac.

72

Mucous Membrane Graft and Conjunctivodacryocystorhinostomy (Jones Tube Placement)

Charles B. Campbell III
Joseph C. Flanagan

INTRODUCTION

Patients with an obliterated canaliculus require a CDCR (conjunctivodacryocystorhinostomy) with a Jones glass tube placement to obtain satisfactory lacrimal function. Traditionally these tubes, which are left in place for a lifetime, have a high instance of local complications such as infection, tube extrusion, obstruction, or local irritation, which makes many surgeons use these only as a last resort.

The technique of lining the tract with a full-thickness mucous membrane graft obtained from the lip virtually eliminates the local tube complications and allows for removal of the tube 6 months after surgery. With reduced complications and the possibility of removing the glass tube, the surgeon can become much more aggressive in offering relief to patients with intractable epiphora from canalicular stenosis.

TECHNIQUE

CDCR is performed by opening an osteotomy in the lacrimal bone, often already performed with a previous dacryocystorhinostomy, resecting the caruncle, and opening a track between the caruncle and the nasal cavity with an oblique orientation to facilitate the flow of tears (Fig. 72.1).

The lower lip is ballooned with saline or local anesthetic (Fig. 72.2), and a mucotome or dermatome is used to harvest the full-thickness mucous membrane graft (Fig. 72.3). The graft is wrapped around the tube with the epithelial surface toward the lumen and sutured with 7-0 Vicryl to create a tube graft (Fig. 72.4).

The tube and graft are then inserted into the previously constructed

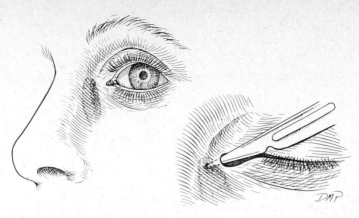

Figure 72.1 CDCR prepared.

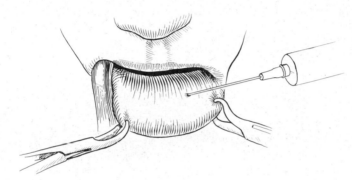

Figure 72.2 Lower lip ballooned with anesthetic.

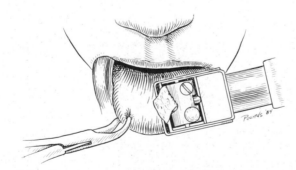

Figure 72.3 Full-thickness mucous membrane graft taken with muco-tome.

CDCR tract (Fig. 72.5). Tubes should be secured to the medial canthus with a nonabsorbable suture (Fig. 72.6).

The surgeon does not need to trim excess graft within the nose, as that portion not supported by nutritive connective tissue will spontaneously slough. Postoperative care consists of antibiotics, daily cleansing of the

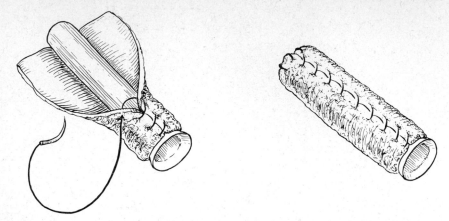

Figure 72.4 Graft sewed with epithelium against glass Jones tube.

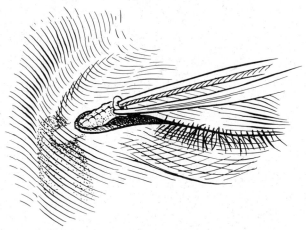

Figure 72.5 Insertion of Jones tube with mucous membrane graft.

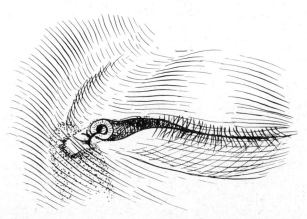

Figure 72.6 Tube and graft secured with nonabsorbable suture.

opening of the tube, and clearing the tube with negative intranasal pressure. After 6 months, the tube can be removed the conduit lined with epithelium functioned for lacrimal drainage.

Use of mucous membrane graft around the tube in CDCR has significantly reduced the instance of infection, tube extrusion, and granulation tissue. The option of removing the tube at 6 months allows the surgeon to be much more aggressive in correcting epiphora from canalicular obstruction.

BIBLIOGRAPHY

Campbell CB III, Shannon GM, Flanagan JC: Conjunctivodacryocystorhinostomy with mucous membrane graft. *Ophthalmic Surg* 14:647, 1983.

Jones LT: Conjunctivodacryocystorhinostomy. *Am J Ophthalmol* 59:773, 1965.

73

Use of Skin Biopsy Punch to Form Conjunctivodacryocystorhinostomy Tract in Placement of Jones Tubes

Ralph E. Wesley
Marcia Egles

INTRODUCTION

The placement of a Jones tube through a CDCR (conjunctivodacryo-cystorhinostomy) is required to bypass the entire lacrimal system to reestablish tear drainage in upper system problems such as canalicular stenosis.

   The use of a dermatology punch makes forming the track easier. Removal of a plug establishes a permanent drainage fistulae.

TECHNIQUE

The CDCR is performed with the usual technique in which an incision is carried out through the skin down to the anterior lacrimal crest. The lacrimal sac is elevated out of the fossa and a generous rhinostomy anteriorly and inferiorly performed into the nose, and the lacrimal sac is opened.

   The inferior portion of the caruncle should be excised and then a CDCR track formed at a 45-degree angle down through the sac into the nose.

   Using a disposable 3 mm dermatology punch (Fig. 73.1) directed with appropriate orientation, the punch can be twisted and slowly advanced into the lacrimal sac, and a plug can be removed from the track.

   The tube can be easily inserted (Fig. 73.2) into the track to ensure the appropriate length tube. We recommend fixation of the tube for 4 weeks with a 4-0 Vicryl suture passed through the tube and tied with a knot at the edge; then a bite of the suture is passed through the upper lid and tied to prevent the tube slipping into the nose postoperatively.

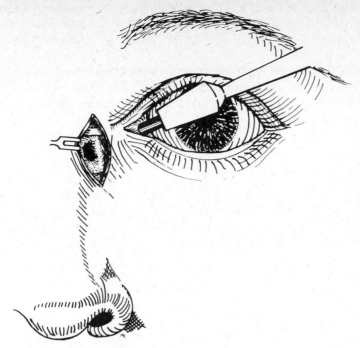

Figure 73.1 A 3-mm skin pouch to make CDCR tract.

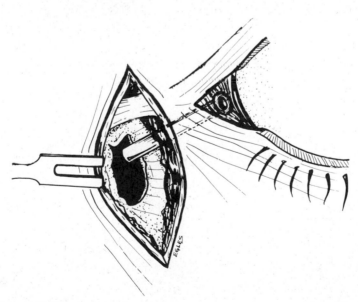

Figure 73.2 Jones tube in place.

Removing a plug instead of simply making an incision with a long keratotomy knife not only makes the insertion of the tube easier, but also allows for better preservation of the track if the tube is removed or manipulated.

With this technique, we have observed tubes seat better without migration of the tubes or irritation to the patient's eye. This technique can be combined with the placement of mucous membrane graft (see Chapter 72).

74

Removal of Middle Turbinate in Lacrimal Surgery

Ralph E. Wesley

INTRODUCTION

Even when a DCR is properly performed, a large anteriorly developed middle turbinate can occlude the rhinostomy and spoil the result.

Removing the anterior portion of the middle turbinate in appropriate cases provides adequate room in the nose for lacrimal drainage, especially when the patient has a deviation of the nasal septum.

TECHNIQUE

At the time of DCR, an assessment should be made of the middle turbinate from an intranasal examination as well as through the rhinostomy. Vasoconstriction of the mucosa may deceive the surgeon into thinking adequate space is available. When the middle turbinate appears next to the rhinostomy, the DCR may fail to function after surgery. After the vasoconstrictor on the mucosa has worn off, the middle turbinate swells and plugs off the DCR site (Fig. 74.1).

For hemostasis, the middle turbinate should be injected with 2% lidocaine with epinephrine (1:100,000). After a few minutes a Jantzen–Middleton forceps can be used from the nares or from the rhinostomy site to bite off the middle turbinate. The turbinate should not be twisted, as this can rip off the nose, causing a CSF leak.

Once an adequate amount of turbinate has been removed, Gelfoam soaked in thrombin should be packed onto the raw site to prevent late hemorrhage.

With the anterior portion of the middle turbinate removed, the rhinostomy has a clearer opening into the anterior nose (Fig. 74.2). Electrocautery should be avoided as a method of removing the turbinate due to the proximity of the frontal nasal duct, which can become inflamed from the electrocautery and result in frontal sinusitis.

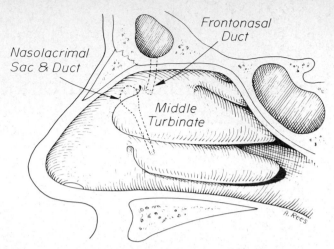

Figure 74.1 Prominent, anteriorly developed middle turbinate overlying nasolacrimal duct and lacrimal sac.

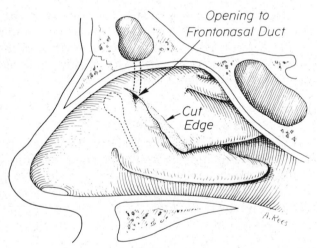

Figure 74.2 Removal of a part of middle turbinate for adequate clearance.

This technique can also be used on failed DCRs in which a middle turbinate occludes the rhinostomy site. In that instance, the middle turbinate can be removed from an intranasal approach or by making a secondary incision at the previous rhinostomy site through the skin at the anterior lacrimal crest.

75

Vein Grafting
and Nasolacrimal Reconstruction

David B. Soll

INTRODUCTION

The CDCR (conjunctivodacryocystostomy) with placement of a Jones Pyrex tube (1), the procedure of choice for establishing tear drainage with an irreparably damaged canalicular system, can fail due to obliteration of the track should the tube accidentally come out early in the postoperative period or even while servicing the Pyrex tube.

Placement of a saphenous vein graft around the tube during the initial procedure provides an immediate lining and safeguards the CDCR track during manipulation or inadvertent extrusion.

TECHNIQUE

A standard CDCR is performed with an anastomosis of the anterior and posterior flaps of the lacrimal sac (2) (Fig. 75.1A–L). Frequently, the anterior portion of the middle turbinate must be removed when obstructing the internal nasal osteum created during rhinostomy surgery.

To establish an immediate lining for the CDCR tract of the Jones tube, a 2-inch segment of the long saphenous vein should be obtained from the lower leg just above the ankle. After outlining the vein on the skin surface, a cutdown can be made directly over the length of the vein to be excised.

Both the proximal and distal ends of the vein are double ligated with 4-0 Dacron sutures. Then, 5-0 Vicryl sutures are used for subcutaneous closure, and the skin is closed with 6-0 chromic or silk sutures. Elastic bandage and pressure are kept against the donor site for several days (a venous pressure of 9 mm Hg with the patient standing can break double ligatures causing hematoma in patients without pressure bandage).

The vein graft is passed over a Pyrex tube of appropriate length (2) with the Callahan measuring set. The veins of the valve should be in the same direction that blood flows when a Pyrex tube is passed (Fig. 75.1E–H).

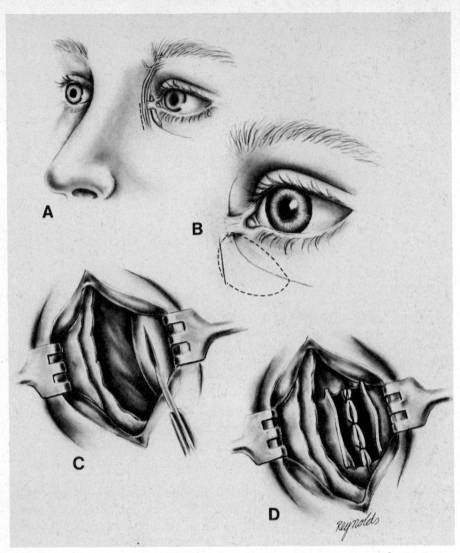

Figure 75.1 (A and B) DCR incision. (C) Lacrimal sac opened. (D) Anastamosis. (E and F) Tube placement. (G and H) Vein graft placement. (I and J) Tube position. (K) Nasal appearance. (L) Closure. (Reprinted with permission. Ophthalmic Surgery 14:656–660, 1983.)

After lower end of the vein graft is ligated at the inferior end of the tube, the tube and vein graft complex are passed through the CDCR tract.

With the tube in proper position, the exposed excess of the vein graft should be trimmed and sutured to adjacent conjunctiva with interrupted 9-0 nylon sutures, which will eventually slough out and do not have to be removed. The vein graft covering the end of the Pyrex tube in the nose should be trimmed so a free lumen exists between the conjunctival side of the tube and the inside of the nose.

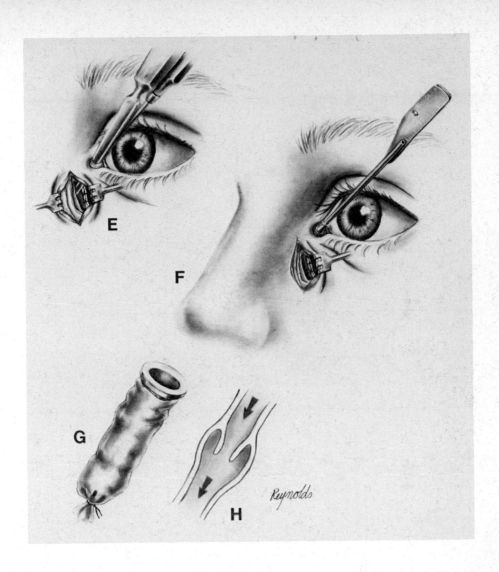

E

F

G

H

Reynolds

On nasal examination, the distal end of the tube should be covered with the vein graft extending several millimeters into the nasal cavity and lying anterior to the tip or severed end of the middle turbinate (Fig. 75.1I–L). The distal vein graft covering the exposed portion of the Pyrex tube seen in the nose will slough within several weeks. After 2 or 3 weeks, the Pyrex tube may be removed and replaced without difficulty in finding the lumen of the tract.

This procedure allows for the tract to be maintained with inadvertent extrusion of the tube or during replacement. If the Pyrex tube is removed, the walls of the vein graft tend to become opposed preventing drainage of tears (3).

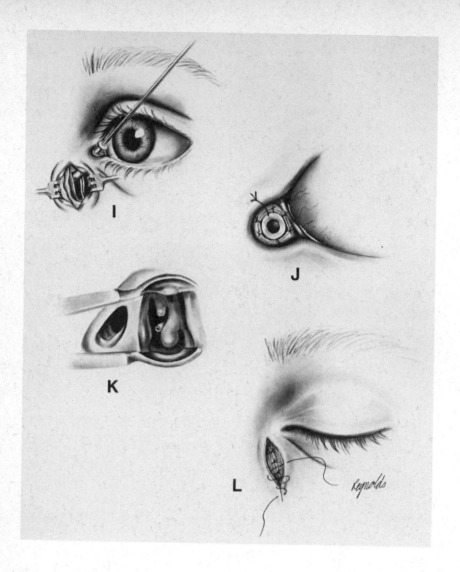

REFERENCES

1. Jones LT: Conjunctivo-dacryocystorhinostomy. *Am J Ophthalmol* 59:773, 1965.
2. Callahan A, Callahan MA: Ophthalmic Plastic and Orbital Surgery. Birmingham, *Aesculapius*, 1979, p 120.
3. Soll DB: Vein grafting and nasolacrimal system reconstruction. *Ophthalmic Surg* 14:656, 1983.

76

Canaliculodacryocystorhinostomy

Timothy W. Doucet and Jeffrey J. Hurwitz

INTRODUCTION

Canalicular obstruction and failed lacrimal surgery (DCR) have been treated with bypass procedures, such as the Jones tube regardless of the site of obstruction. The Jones tube requires placement of a permanent prosthesis and long-term follow up. With the technique described below, these patients may have successful microsurgery reconstruction of the canaliculus to avoid the problems of Jones tube conjunctivocystorhinostomy.

TECHNIQUE

Accurate localization of the obstruction is a requirement that can best be determined with dacryocystography (DCG) combined with probing. The surgical technique varies according to the location of the obstruction.

Probes are passed into the canaliculi until the obstruction is met. A combination of blunt and sharp dissection separates the anterior limb of the medial canthal tendon and subcutaneous tissue. The probe inside the common canaliculus can be identified as well as the obstruction. The obstruction is then excised proceeding toward and including the lacrimal sac, if involved. A rhinostomy is performed and the remaining patent, common canaliculus is then anastomosed to the lateral aspect of the lacrimal sac (Fig. 76.1) or directly to the nasomucosa (Fig. 76.2) if the sac has been involved. Silicone intubation is used for 3 months postoperatively.

With lateral obstruction in the lower canaliculus, the procedure is then modified so the canalicular obstruction is excised and the anastomosis created between the individual canaliculus and the lacrimal sac or nasomucosa. This anastomosis is technically no more difficult than repairing a lacerated canaliculus. The difficulty is in dissecting the obstruction without losing anatomic orientation.

With previously failed lacrimal surgery (DCR), a repeat DCR with a larger rhinostomy may be curative. However, many patients with failed surgery have no recognizable lacrimal sac. These patients benefit from a common canalicular-nasal mucosa anastomosis. An estimated 75% of

229

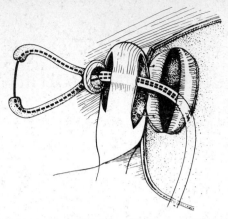

Figure 76.1 Anastomosis of the posterior canaliculus to existing lacrimal sac.

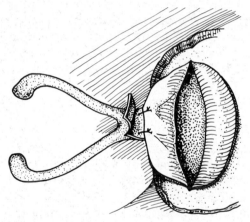

Figure 76.2 With scarred lacrimal sac removed, anastomosis made directly to nasomucosa flaps.

previous Jones tube candidates have had successful reconstructive surgery. Failures are most often associated with short canalicular remnant of less than 8 mm.

BIBLIOGRAPHY

Doucet TW, Hurwitz JJ: Caniculo-dacryocystorhinostomy and the treatment of canalicular obstruction. *Arch Ophthalmol* 100:306, 1982.

Doucet TW, Hurwitz JJ: Canaliculo-dacryocystorhinostomy in the management of unsuccessful lacrimal surgery. *Arch Ophthalmol* 100:619, 1982.

Jones LT: The cure of epiphora due to canalicular obstruction of trauma and surgical procedures of the lacrimal passage. *Trans Am Acad Ophthalmol Otolaryngol* 66:506, 1962.

77

Gelfoam Stent
in Dacryocystorhinostomy

Ralph E. Wesley

Traditionally a red rubber catheter has been used to stent the flaps of nasal mucosa and lacrimal sac in dacryocystorhinostomy surgery. The catheters cause significant discomfort to the patient. They have an odor. The catheter requires a fixation stitch, and the patient must return for removal.

Using Gelfoam soaked in thrombin for the stent provides an effective stent for the flaps, improves hemostasis, eliminates discomfort, and requires no removal.

TECHNIQUE

During surgery the lacrimal sac should be retracted away from the lacrimal canal. An anterior-inferior rhinostomy is performed with an air drill (Fig. 77.1) or by forcing a Kerrison punch through the posterior lacrimal crest into the nasal cavity.

After opening the nasal mucosa and the lacrimal sac, the posterior flaps of nasal mucosa and lacrimal sac are sewed together (Fig. 77.2).

To stent the rhinostomy, small pieces of Gelfoam are compressed with a toothless forceps, soaked in thrombin briefly, and placed into the rhinostomy (Fig. 77.3) to maintain separation of the anterior and posterior flaps.

A cotton-tipped applicator can be used to force the Gelfoam into the rhinostomy, or a toothless bayonette forceps can be used to place the material in the proper position. If posterior flaps cannot be sutured, the Gelfoam should be packed to keep the posterior lacrimal flap directed posteriorly.

In cases in which the anterior portion of the middle turbinate must be removed to provide adequate lacrimal drainage (see Chapter 74), the Gelfoam with thrombin can be packed onto the cut turbinate before packing the rhinostomy. The Gelfoam provides lasting hemostasis avoiding the trauma and possible nosebleed associated with traditional gauze packing.

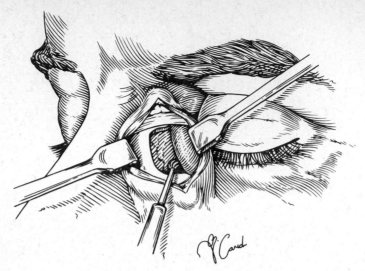

Figure 77.1 Rhinostomy formed with air drill.

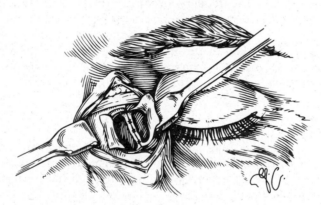

Figure 77.2 Posterior lacrimal flaps sutured. Anterior flaps of nasal mucosa and lacrimal sac retracted open.

BIBLIOGRAPHY

Leone CR Jr: Gelfoam-thrombin dacryocystorhinostomy stent. *Am J Ophthalmol* 94:412, 1982.

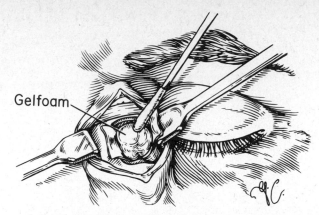

Gelfoam

Figure 77.3 Q-tip packs Gelfoam soaked in thrombin into rhinostomy before closing anterior flaps.

ANOPHTHALMOS

PART VI

78

Conjunctival Marking Sutures in Enucleation

Christine L. Zolli

INTRODUCTION

Accurate closure of the cut edges of the conjunctiva after enucleation promotes rapid healing of the socket, reduces the chance of tissue foreshortening, and establishes a smooth surface for ocular prosthetic fitting.

Difficulty can arise trying to find the conjunctival edges after enucleation because the tissue edema distorts the incisional planes, especially if the orbital tissues are congested or inflamed.

This problem can be solved with two running 4-0 black silk marking sutures passed through the conjunctival edges during enucleation when the freshly cut edges of the conjunctiva are easily discernible. The sutures serve as a guide for easily recognition of the conjunctival borders later in the procedure when the conjunctival borders must be closed.

TECHNIQUE

After completing the peritomy (Fig. 78.1) and undermining the conjunctiva widely to expose the muscle insertions during enucleation, two 4-0 silk sutures are woven horizontally into the cut edges of the conjunctiva (Fig. 78.2), one to mark the inferior border (Fig. 78.3) and one to mark the superior border (Fig. 78.4). These sutures are kept long and left in position during the remainder of the enucleation surgery.

When the surgeon is ready to close the conjunctiva, no time is lost as the marking sutures identify the conjunctival edges. The 4-0 silk sutures are pulled out as the closure of the conjunctival edges proceeds (Fig. 78.5 and 78.6).

The technique helps simplify the enucleation procedure with more accurate conjunctival approximation to conserve conjunctiva and possibly reduce the incidence of epithelial inclusion cysts in these sockets.

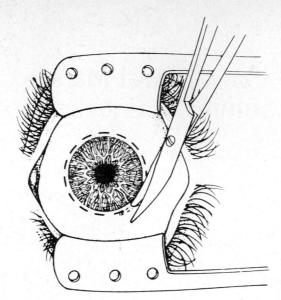

Figure 78.1 Performing peritomy.

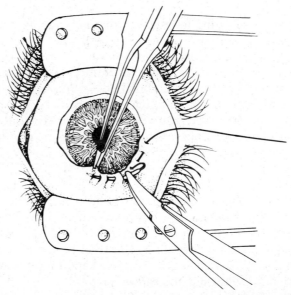

Figure 78.2 Some 4-0 silk sutures woven into cut edge of conjunctiva.

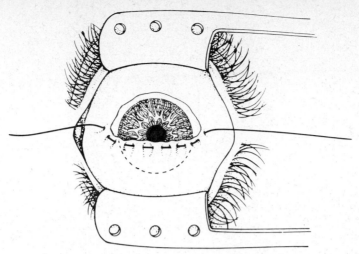

Figure 78.3 Conjunctiva border marked with silk suture.

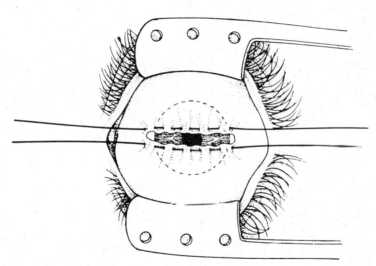

Figure 78.4 Marking sutures in place.

Note, the marking sutures should be left long or tied together to avoid pulling them out prematurely during the procedure.

BIBLIOGRAPHY

Fox SA: *Ophthalmic Plastic Surgery.* New York, Grune & Stratton, 1970, p 475.
Illif CE: *Oculoplastic Surgery.* Philadelphia, Saunders, 1979, p 204.
Zolli CL: Conjunctival-marking suture in enucleation procedure. *Ann Ophthalmol* 14:679, 1982.

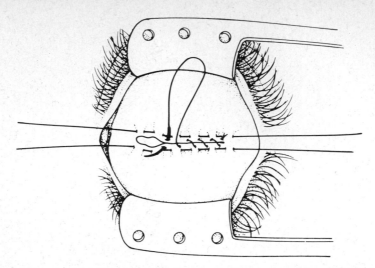

Figure 78.5 A 4-0 silk suture pulled out as conjunctiva closed.

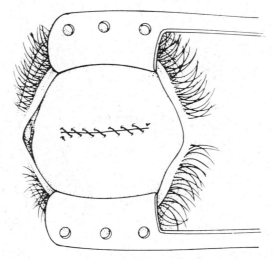

Figure 78.6 Final conjunctival closure. (Zolli C: Conjunctival marking suture in enucleation procedure. Ann Ophthalmol 14:679–680, 1982.)

79

Optic Nerve Clipping for Hemostasis During Enucleation

Ralph E. Wesley

INTRODUCTION

Postoperative hemorrhage from enucleation can result in infection, pain, and extrusion of the implant. The snare device, commonly used to cut the optic nerve during enucleation surgery, does not identify and ligate the vessels within and around the optic nerve. A tamponade may be required to stop the bleeding. Postoperatively, the bleeding may recur, particularly with increasing blood pressure, coughing, or straining. The technique below uses readily available material to provide permanent hemostasis of the optic nerve.

TECHNIQUE

A Weck right-angled, medium-large, applicator (Fig. 79.1, top) can be used to place a permanent, nonreactive tantalum ligaclip around the optic nerve before cutting the optice nerve (Fig. 79.1, middle) during enuclea-tion surgery (Fig. 79.1, bottom). These clips have been used for years with vasucular surgery to facilitate ligating vessels to minimize blood loss.

Conn (1) has modified this instrument by mounting a pair of knife blades on its jaws to allow for cutting and clipping in the same motion. With the technique described above, the surgeon must first clip poste-riorly and then cut the nerve anterior to the ligaclip.

REFERENCES

1. Conn H: Optic nerve clipping for hemostasis during enucleation. *Ophthalmic Surg* 12:352, 1981.

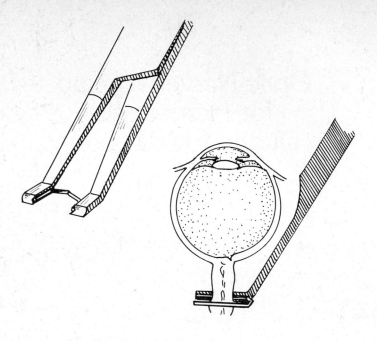

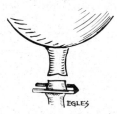

Figure 79.1 Improved hemostasis during enucleation by placing liga-clip before transecting the optic nerve.

80

Use of Absolute Alcohol to Destroy Cysts After Enucleation

Albert Hornblass

INTRODUCTION

Orbital cysts after enucleation can cause such pain and socket distortion that the patients cannot wear a prosthesis. Aspiration and injection by steriods are ineffective. The cysts frequently recur after surgical removal.

The injection of absolute alcohol provides a simple, effective method to eliminate cysts after enucleation.

TECHNIQUE

One drop proparacaine hydrochloride is applied to the involved socket every 2 minutes for 10 minutes. A 25-gauge needle on a 3 cc syringe should be inserted to the center of the cyst. All fluid is then aspirated. The needle is left in the cyst, being careful not to penetrate the cyst wall. The syringe is removed, and a second 2 cc syringe of absolute alcohol is attached to the needle. The alcohol is injected (Fig. 80.1) and topical antibiotics applied.

This technique provides an effective alternative to surgery.

BIBLIOGRAPHY

Hornblass A, Bosniak S: Orbital cysts following enucleation: The use of absolute alcohol. *Ophthalmic Surg* 12:123, 1981.

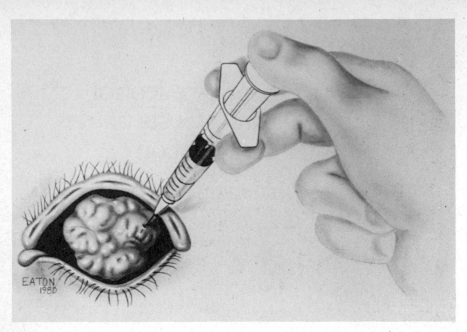

Figure 80.1 Absolute alcohol injected to eliminate cyst after enuclea-tion. (Reprinted with permission. Ophthalmic Surgery 12:125–126, 1981.)

81

Double-Sphere Implantation Technique for Enucleation

Albert Hornblass

INTRODUCTION

An ideal enucleation technique should replace enough orbital volume to prevent enophthalmos and provide good prosthetic motility without increasing implant extrusion. The double-sphere implantation technique allows the surgeon to replace lost volume and enhance prosthetic motility without increased risk of implant migration or extrusion.

TECHNIQUE

In enucleation, one sphere is implanted in the muscle cone, and another sphere is placed within tenon's capsule to replace the globe. With evisceration, the first sphere is placed in the muscle cone and the second enclosed within the scleral shell.

In patients who are submitting to enucleation, a 16-mm glass implant in an introducer is placed through the rent in tenon's capsule lateral to the optic nerve. The sphere is positioned posteriorly into the orbital apex within the muscle cone (Fig. 81.1). A 14-mm glass sphere is placed within the capsule anterior to the first sphere in line with the anterior-posterior axis. A continuous purse string suture of 4-0 Mersilene is used to close tenon's capsule anteriorly, incorporating a fibromuscular bundle (Fig. 81.2).

If undue pressure seems to develop on the suture, a smaller sphere can be placed. Three additional interrupted 5-0 Mersilene sutures are used to close the anterior tenon's capsule. The conjunctiva is closed with continuous suture of 5-0 chromic. A fenestrated conformer should be placed under the lids; a tarsorrhaphy and pressure patch are used for the first 24 hours.

In patients submitting to evisceration, meticulous removal of uveal tissue should be performed and then posterior and tenon's capsule in-

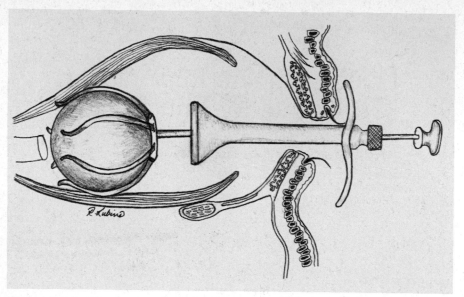

Figure 81.1 A 16-mm glass sphere posterior to Tenon's capsule.

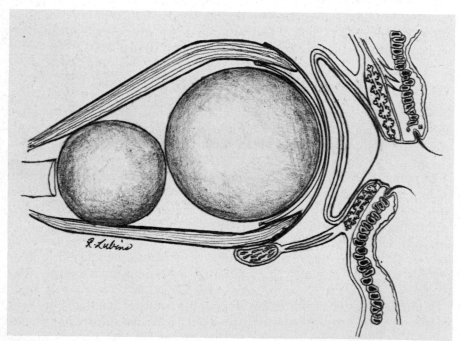

Figure 81.2 Anterior 14-mm glass sphere within Tenon's capsule. (Hornblass A: Double-sphere implantation technique. Ophthalmic Plast Reconstr Surg, 1985.)

cised in a vertical direction for 10 mm. The rent is spread by blunt dissection to facilitate introduction of the 16-mm hollow glass sphere, as described during enucleation (Fig. 81.1). Posterior tenon's capsule should be closed with interrupted 5-0 chromic suture. The rent in the posterior wall of the scleral shell may be closed with 4-0 Dexon suture.

Next, a 12-mm hollow glass sphere is placed within the scleral shell. The anterior scleral incision should be sutured continuously with a 4-0 Dexon suture. Tenon's capsule should be closed with a purse string of 5-0 chromic. The conjunctiva is sutured with a continuous 6-0 chromic suture. A fenestrated plastic conformer is placed under the lids, and a tarsorrhaphy is maintained for 24 hours.

In cases of enophthalmitis, the orbital implantation should be performed as a secondary procedure 6 weeks later. The volume of the scleral shell can be maintained between surgeries with gauze packing.

The volume replacement to the orbit after enucleation or evisceration by this procedure maintains symmetry between the orbits and prevents postoperative enophthalmos and superior sulcus depression. The larger implant wedged posteriorly supports the muscle tone, which would otherwise collapse with time. The smaller implants within tenon's capsule reduces the risk of extrusion.

The hollow implants reduce the burden of weight to which the orbital structures are subjected. The two spheres appear to enhance prosthetic motility via a translation of movement of orbital contents and fornices generated by the extraocular muscles as the anterior sphere functionally pivots on the fiberoptic surface of the posterior sphere.

This method provide a simple technique to enhance motility, reduce loss of orbital volume, and prevent implant migration or extrusion.

82

The Dermis-Fat Graft in Orbital Soft Tissue Reconstruction

Richard L. Petrelli

INTRODUCTION

Enucleation is the most common cause of soft tissue defects within the orbit. Classically, the eye is removed and a light acrylic sphere is placed within or behind tenon space. With deficient orbital volume, a typical flattened, superior sulcus may develop with pseudoptosis. The plastic sphere may migrate with the implant and distort the socket. Socket contraction may occur with foreshortened fornices.

The technique of dermis-fat graft, which has been used for over 10 years as a solution to the problems of exposed or migrating implant, superior sulcus deformity, contracted socket, can be used as the primary procedure at the time of enucleation to avoid these problems.

TECHNIQUE

The exposed implant can be removed through a 25-mm midline incision over the area of the exposed implant (Fig. 82-1 and 2). Tenon's cavity is identified. If the rectus muscle stumps can be identified; the insertions are tagged (Fig. 82.3), and the posterior capsule of tenon's cavity is removed to create a raw recipient surface for vascularization of the dermis-fat graft.

The dermis-fat graft is obtained from the lateral aspect of the thigh in the vicinity of the buttock, which is rich in subcutaneous fat. A circle 20 mm in diameter is marked with a number 15 blade and infiltrated with 1% xylocaine. The blade is introduced at one edge of the circle (Fig. 82.4) and tunneled to either side by massaging the blade forward and backward until the entire epidermis of the outlined circle has been removed.

A number 10 blade is then used to complete the 20 mm circular incision to obtain the cylindrical plug of dermis-fat with a depth of about 20

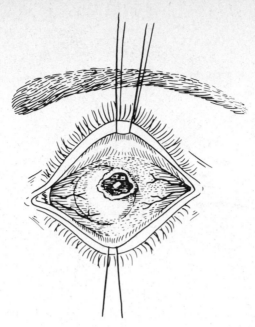

Figure 82.1 Migrated and extruding implant.

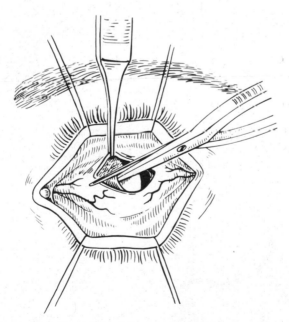

Figure 82.2 A 25-mm midline incision made directly over extruded implant.

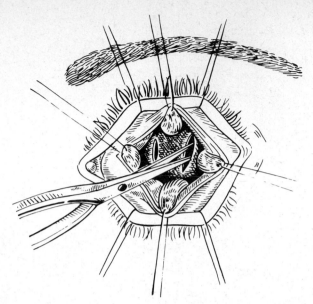

Figure 82.3 Rectus muscle stumps identified and tagged and posterior Tenon's cavity removed to create recipient raw surface for dermis-fat graft.

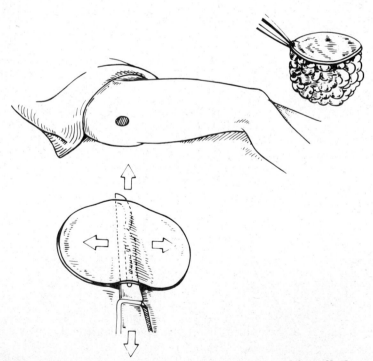

Figure 82.4 Dermis fat taken from lateral thigh and handled carefully; below shows a number 15 blade tunneling under the epithelium to separate the surface from the dermal edge.

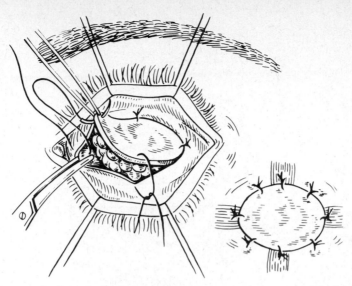

Figure 82.5 *A dermis-fat graft sutured to the conjunctival-Tenon edge with 4-0 chromic catgut.*

mm. After removal of the graft, the donor site is closed with 4-0 chromic and 4-0 black silk vertical mattress sutures.

The graft is transported gently to the recipient bed and sutured to the adjacent tenon-conjunctival edge with interruped 4-0 chromic gut sutures. The rectus muscle stumps, if they have been identified, can be sutured as the needle passes from the dermis edge of the graft to the adjacent tenon's conjunctival edge (Fig. 82.5). Attachment of the rectus muscles enhances the motility of the graft. Excess fat from the graft is trimmed as the graft is sutured into each quadrant. A doughnut conformer is placed in the socket at the end of the procedure, and a light dressing is applied (Fig. 82.6). A prosthesis may be fitted after 4 weeks.

Potential complications of the procedure are central pitting of the graft, suture granulomas, and fat atrophy. Central graft necrosis is avoided by harvesting grafts with diameters less than 25 mm. Fat atrophy can be avoided by gentle manipulation of the graft, preparation of the host bed, and selection of patients with healthy, vascular sockets. The chemically burned avascular socket is a poor recipient bed and should not be used with this technique in dermis-fat grafting.

This technique can be used for both primary enucleation as well as for replacement of a migrated implant.

BIBLIOGRAPHY

Guberina C, Hornblass A, Meltzer M, et al: Autogenous dermis-fat orbital implantation. *Arch Ophthalmol* 101:1586, 1983.
Petrelli RL: Management of the contracted eye socket. *Ophthalmol* 5:33, 1982.

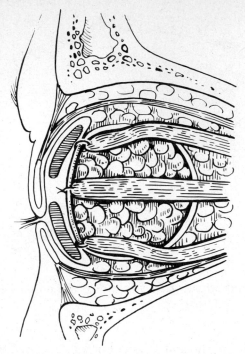

Figure 82.6 Doughnut conformer used to maintain fornices after place-ment of dermis-fat graft.

Smith B, Petrelli R: Dermis-fat graft as a movable implant within in the muscle cone. *Am J Ophthalmol* 85:62, 1978.

Smith B, Bosniak S, Lisman R: An autogenous kinetic dermis-fat orbital implant. *Ophthalmology* 89:1067, 1982.

83

Reversed Split-Skin/Dermis-Fat Composite Graft for Severely Contracted Sockets

Ralph E. Wesley
Marcia Egles

INTRODUCTION

Patients whose eyes are removed for conditions such as acid or lye burns, cicatricial conjunctiva diseases such as pemphigoid, or severe trauma can develop such a severe contraction of the socket that it makes the wearing of an artificial eye impossible.

Socket reconstruction with full-thickness mucous membrane grafts provide initially gratifying results, but late contraction occurs that requires a smaller and smaller prosthesis to be worn. Patients can have considerable pain around the graft donor site.

Split-thickness skin grafts are considerably more durable, but late contraction can occur. Split-thickness skin graft donor sites involve considerable morbidity, taking up to 6 weeks for healing.

With the technique below, a one-stage procedure can be used to reconstruct even completely contracted sockets. The minimal donor site morbidity allows for much quicker rehabilitation of the patient.

TECHNIQUE

The socket is lined with a dermis-fat graft for the central portion, and the epithelium overlying the dermis-fat graft is used to line the fornices, as shown in Figure 83.1. The epithelium from the split-thickness graft eventually covers the raw dermis as the socket heals. Most grafted substances, such as split-thickness skin or full-thickness mucous membrane, tend to contract with time.

A large dermis-fat graft is marked on the abdomen to allow for immediate contraction, which occurs on harvesting (Fig. 83.2A). The epithelium of approximately 3.5 × 3.0 cm is harvested first making an incision with a number 15 blade and then undermining with scissors. Next, an incision is carried through the dermis into the fat so that the

253

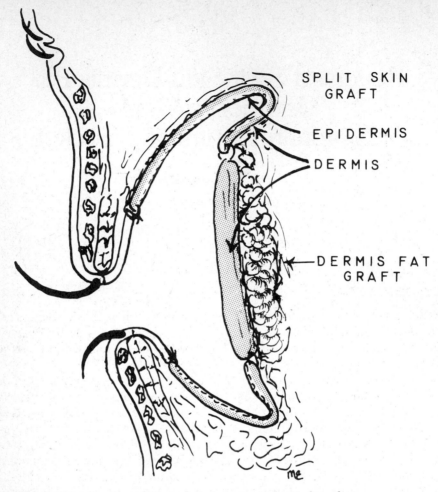

SPLIT SKIN GRAFT

EPIDERMIS

DERMIS

DERMIS FAT GRAFT

Figure 83.1 *Source of lining of the reconstructed socket.*

underlying dermis-fat graft can be harvested (Fig. 83.2B). In sockets that are sunken as well as contracted, a considerable amount of fat may need to be implanted. If little enophthalmos exists, virtually no fat is required on the graft.

Figure 83.2C shows the split-thickness skin graft being placed onto the dermal graft, but in a reversed position so that epithelium faces the raw dermal service. Running or interrupted 5-0 Vicryl sutures hold this snugly in place. Next, an aperture is made for the conformer to fit into this composite graft using a number 15 Bard–Parker blade or scissors (Fig. 83.2D and E).

To prepare the recipient site of the contracted socket, an incision is made in the central portion, and any remnants of mucous membrane are freed to fold up onto the upper and lower eyelids. Frequently, virtually no mucous membrane remains after the dissection has been performed (Fig. 83.3).

254

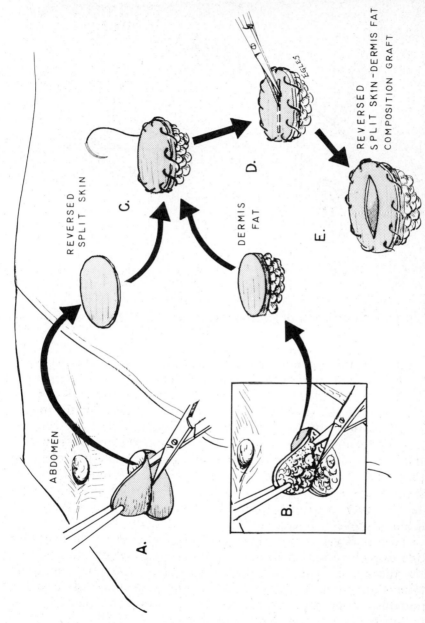

ABDOMEN

A.

B.

REVERSED SPLIT SKIN

C.

DERMIS FAT

D.

EGLES

REVERSED SPLIT SKIN - DERMIS FAT COMPOSITION GRAFT

E.

Figure 83.2 Skin surface reversed onto dermis-fat for composition graft.

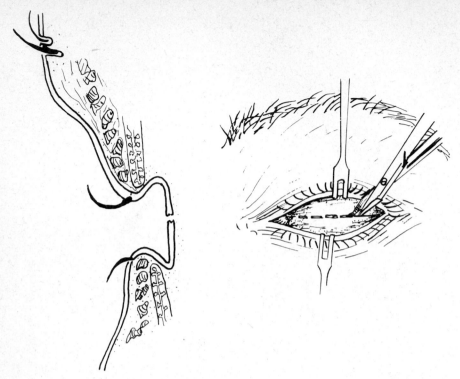

Figure 83.3 *Preparation of recipient site.*

The composite split-skin/dermis-fat graft can be placed into the socket (Fig. 83.4). The graft will be somewhat unwieldly. To stent the graft, a silicone conformer is placed into the socket. First, sutures such as double-armed 4-0 prolene are passed through the conformer, and then the needle is passed into the split-thickness graft at the point where the surgeon desires to stretch down to make the inferior fornix. The needle should be passed down to grasp the inferior periosteum and brought out through the skin (Fig. 83.5). Once these sutures are in place, the upper and lower eyelid should be sewn together, which will place the upper fornix on stretch. The traction sutures from the lower fornix are tied through a dental roll to prevent sloughing of the skin externally.

On suture removal 10 days later, the socket should be cleaned with peroxide to remove any desquamated epithelium that occurs from the split-thickness skin. This procedure produces a socket with minimal long-term contraction. As with any socket graft with skin, daily cleaning is required for proper hygiene. The patient with a properly closed donor site on the abdomen has virtually no morbidity compared to split thickness skin graft sites or buccal mucous membrane donor sites.

The eyelids should be sewn together no longer than 10 days as the desquamated epithelium can cause a superficial infection. The patient can usually have an artificial eye custom fabricated in 4 to 6 weeks.

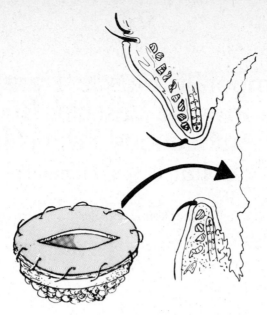

Figure 83.4 Composite graft placed into recipient site.

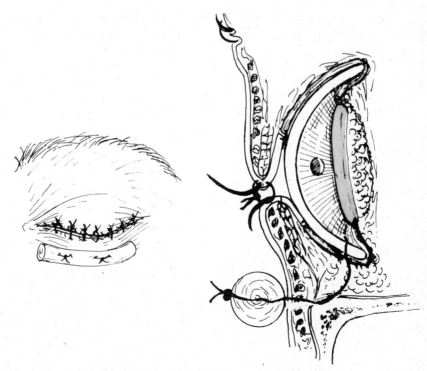

Figure 83.5 Graft stinted with silicone conformer.

84

Temporalis Muscle Transfer to Provide Vascular Bed for Autogenous Dermis-Fat Orbital Implantation

Stephen L. Bosniak

INTRODUCTION

Insults to the orbit such as thermal burns, radiation therapy, chemical burns, and multiple surgical procedures leave a relatively avascular socket that defies standard reconstructive procedures designed to permit the patient to wear an artificial eye.

Though conventional dermis-fat grafts do not survive satisfactorily due to a poor blood supply, these sockets can be reconstructed by transposing temporalis muscle into the depths of the orbit through a window in the lateral orbital wall providing a blood supply to implant an autogenous dermis-fat graft within Tenon's capsule.

TECHNIQUE

An incision begins 2 mm lateral to the lateral canthus continuing horizontally to the preauricular area where the incision sweeps superiorly in the hairline for approximately 4 cm. A skin flap should be retracted temporarily. The superficial muscular aponeurotic system (SMAS) containing branches of the facial nerve should be dissected from the anterior temporalis fascia and retracted laterally.

The temporalis muscle is separated from the temporal bone with a Freer elevator. With the temporalis muscle retracted, the exterior of the lateral orbital is exposed. With an air drill, a 3.0 × 2.0 cm window in the lateral orbital wall is created (Fig. 84.1).

Now the conjunctiva, submucosal cicatrix, and Tenon's capsule are opened centrally. The rectus muscle stumps should be identified and tagged with a locking 5-0 Vicryl suture. If muscle stumps cannot be

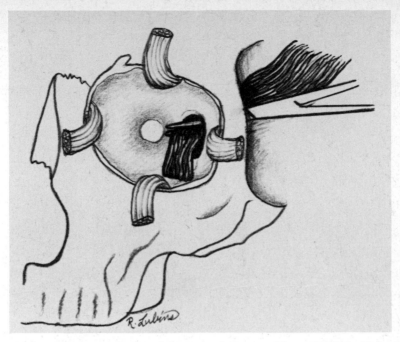

Figure 84.1 *Temporalis muscle provides vascular pedicle for dermis-fat graft in avascular sockets.*

identified, double-armed 5-0 Vicryl sutures can be passed through the anterior edge of Tenon's capsule and the edge of the conjunctiva at positions of 3, 6, 9, and 12 o'clock meridians. A lateral defect in Tenon's capsule should be made to overlie the previously created bony window in the lateral orbital wall.

Outlined with methylene blue, a 1.5 × 5.0 cm pedicle of temporalis muscle flap is incised and transposed though the defect in the lateral orbital wall (Fig. 84.1) to be sutured into the orbit at the medial periosteum and Tenon's capsule.

A dermis-fat graft is taken from the midpoint of a line joining the anterior iliac crest and the greater trochanter in an area that has healthy subcutaneous tissue, but without hair. The diameter of the graft should be no larger than 2.0 cm or 75% of the horizontal palpebral aperture.

The graft can be demarcated freehand, with a cutting compass, or with a trephine. Sterile saline injected intradermally facilitates lamellar dissection of the keratinized epithelium with a number 15 blade or razor fragment (Fig. 84.2). A number 10 blade or graft trephine incises the donor site to a depth of 2.5 cm. Enucleation scissors are used to transect the base of the dermis-fat graft.

The cylindrical graft is placed within Tenon's capsule in the orbit, and the rectus muscle stumps are attached to the dermal edges at positions of 3, 6, 9 and 12 o'clock. The sutures are passed through the adjacent Ten-

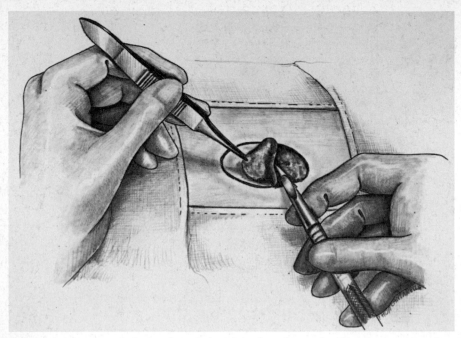

Figure 84.2 *Intradermal injection of saline facilitates separating epithelium from dermis-fat graft.*

on's capsule and conjunctiva drawing these tissues to the margin of the graft (Fig. 84.3).

Interrupted 5-0 Vicryl sutures approximate the remaining graft and conjunctival margins. A donut conformer is placed behind the eyelids to maintain the fornix.

At the temporalis muscle donor site, the SMAS layer can be closed with 4-0 chromic sutures and the skin with 5-0 nylon sutures. Intravenous tubing left in the temporalis defect and attached externally to a vacutainer tube can be left in place 2 to 3 days as a vacuum drain. A headroll dressing can be used for pressure; the socket and eyelids are covered with one loosely applied eyepad. The sutures are removed in 7 days.

The dermis-fat donor site can be closed with 3-0 black silk vertical mattress sutures and a running, locking 7-0 silk suture. Pressure is applied to the wound with Telfa, fluffs, and elastoplast. The running suture can be removed in 2 weeks, and the mattress sutures can be removed in 3 to 4 weeks.

The temporalis muscle flap provides a vascular supply for survival of the dermis-fat graft. Once the bare surface of the dermis has been covered with epithelium and orbital edema subsided, the patient should have an adequate socket to wear a prosthetic eye.

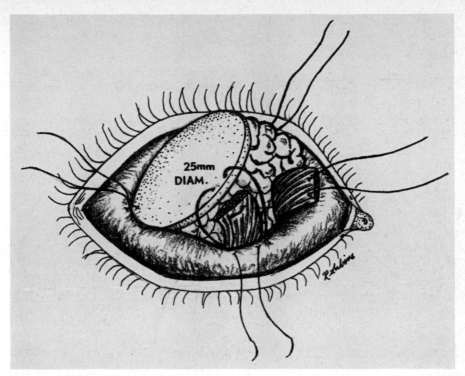

Figure 84.3 Fixation of dermis-fat graft to pedicle of temporalis muscle.

85

Enucleation with Myoconjunctival Attachment to Improve Prosthetic Motility

William P. Chen

INTRODUCTION

Enucleation can be complicated by orbital hemorrhage, migration of the orbital implant, lack of movement, obliteration of inferior forniceal space, and poor retention of the ocular prosthesis. Integrated implants experience a high incidence of erosion, exposure, infection, and ultimate extrusion. Techniques that insert a spherical orbital implant with the muscles criss-crossed or allowed to retract are technically easy to perform but may result in an immobile prosthesis with a poor functional appearance.

The technique described below helps to avoid these problems by providing a physiologic myoconjunctival attachment to improve motility.

TECHNIQUE

A retrobulbar injection with 3 cc of 1% xylocaine with 1:100,000 epinephrine and hyaluronidase is performed for anesthesia and hemostasis. After making 360-degree peritomy, the Tenon's space is exposed. Each of the four rectus muscles is isolated with a double armed 6-0 Dexon suture and detached from the globe.

Then, 4-0 silk sutures are placed over the insertional stump of the medial and lateral recti for traction (Fig. 85.1). The superior oblique muscle is severed. The inferior oblique muscle, however, is hooked and isolated with a 6-0 Vicryl suture and disinserted using a cutting bovie cautery.

A curved clamp is placed around the optic nerve from the medial side, and the steel wire loop of an enucleation snare is positioned around the optic nerve anterior to the clamp from the lateral side (Fig. 85.2). The

262

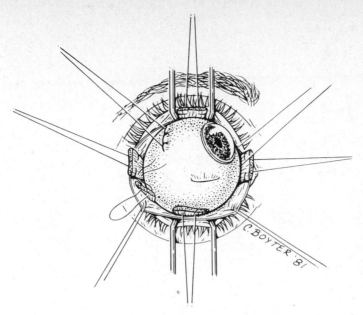

Figure 85.1 Four rectus muscles with traction sutures.

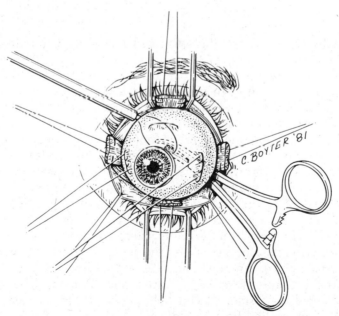

Figure 85.2 Snare around optic nerve just anterior to enucleation clamp.

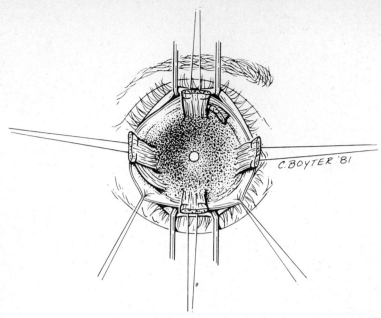

Figure 85.3 *Optic nerve and vessels cauterized before releasing muscles.*

snare is tightened, severing the optic nerve, such that the globe can be removed intact.

After applying electrocautery to the nerve stump, the clamp is removed to provide visualization of the socket (Fig. 85.3). The inferior oblique is attached to the inferior edge of the lateral rectus 8 mm from the cut end of the lateral rectus to serve as an inferior hammock.

An 18-mm soft, silicone spherical implant is inserted into the sub-Tenon's space with the four recti tunneling forward toward the conjunctival surface (Fig. 85.4). Smaller sized implants are used for children. Anterior Tenon's capsule from opposite and adjacent quadrants is closed using 5-0 Dexon interrupted sutures (Fig. 85.5).

Each rectus muscle is then anchored to the back surface of its respective conjunctival fornix with the knots exteriorized so the superior rectus is 25 mm from the inferior rectus, and the medial rectus is 25 mm from the lateral rectus. The conjunctival edges are closed horizontally using running absorbable sutures (Fig. 85.6). Antiobiotic ointment is instilled, and a medium-sized conformer placed behind the eyelids. A semipressure dressing is then applied for 2 to 3 days.

The technique of myoconjunctival attachment transfers contractile forces of the extraocular muscles to the forniceal space (Fig. 85.7). The extraocular muscles are maintained within their approximate physiologic state on their length-tension curve thus improving movement of the artificial eye. Use of the curved clamp and cauterization of the optic nerve minimizes any orbital hemorrhage. Avoiding excessive manipulation of

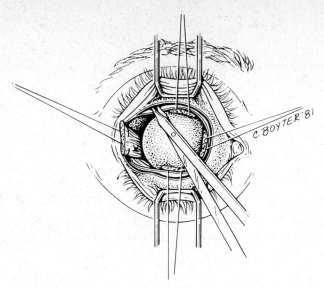

Figure 85.4   Spherical implant inserted with anterior Tenon's layer dissected from conjunctiva.

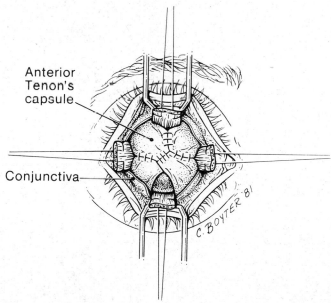

Figure 85.5   Method of closure of Tenon's from opposite quadrants.

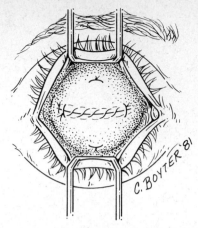

Figure 85.6 *Myoconjunctival suture illustrated after closure of conjunctiva.*

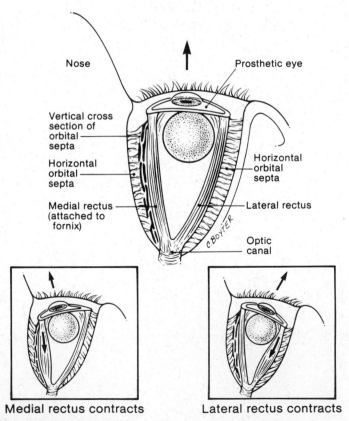

Figure 85.7 *Transmission of muscle forces to fornices.*

the sub-Tenon's tissue preserves the orbital musculofibrous tissue, check ligaments, and intermuscular septa.

Postoperative ptosis and loss of forniceal space are minimized. Excellent prosthetic movement occurs on lateral gaze, upgaze, and downgaze. The most limited movement is on medial gaze, which can be judged to be fair to acceptable.

BIBLIOGRAPHY

Breinin G: The electrophysiology of extraocular muscles. Toronto, University of Toronto Press, 1962.

Chen WP: Biomechanics of socket and prosthetic motility: A proposed enucleation technique to improve motility. Thesis for Fellowship Candidacy, read before the 12th Annual Meeting of the American Society of Ophthalmic Plastic and Reconstructive Surgery, Atlanta, November 1981.

Kennedy RE: The effect of early enucleation on the orbit: In animals and humans. *Am J Ophthalmol* 60:277, 1965.

Kornneef L.: Spatial aspects of orbital musclo-fibrous tissue in man. Amsterdam and Lisse, Swets and Zeitlinger, 1977, p 103.

Soll DB: Enucleation surgery. *Arch Ophthalmol* 84:196, 1972.

PTOSIS

PART **VII**

86

Pull-Out Stitch
for Adjustment
of Fasanella–Servat Procedure

Charles M. Stephenson

INTRODUCTION

Even with very careful clamp placement, the Fasanella–Servat procedure may result in over correction of ptosis, or a poor contour may develop from a segmental overcorrection (Fig. 86.1A). A simple postoperative correction of these problems is possible if a pull-out suture has been used for closure.

TECHNIQUE

A running 6-0 prolene suture is used to approximate the cut edges of tarsus and Müller's muscle with each end anchored to the pretarsal skin with an adhesive strip or a loop in the suture (Fig. 86.1B). Prolene can be readily removed avoiding the pain and difficulty encountered with nylon sutures.

The lid position and contour is evaluated 2 days postoperatively. If the lid has segmental overcorrection (Fig. 86.1A), topical anesthetic is applied and traction placed on the opposite end of the suture until pulled half-way (Fig. 86.1C).

A gentle downward pull on the lid margin is then applied until a slight wound separation is felt. A drop or two of blood may appear. Figure 86.1D illustrates the wound separation that can be produced. However, massage or pulling the lid is used rather than averting the lid over Desmarres retractor, which might cause excessive wound separation. Figure 86.1E shows the final correction of lid contour.

A bandage soft contact lens should be inserted to prevent eye irritation by the loose end of the suture. The entire suture is pulled out 1 week after surgery.

271

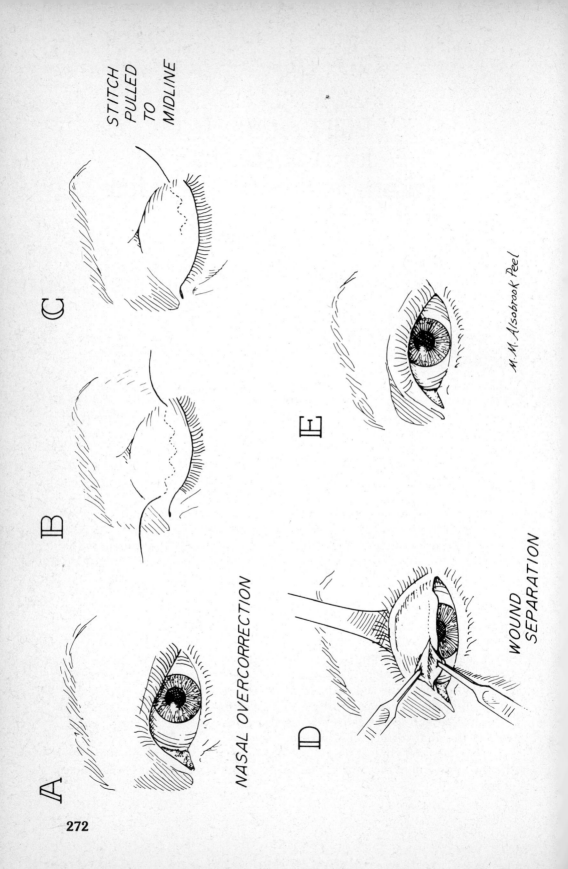

A

B

C

STITCH
PULLED
TO
MIDLINE

NASAL OVERCORRECTION

D

WOUND
SEPARATION

E

M. M. Alsobrook Peel

If the entire eyelid should be excessively elevated by the ptosis repair, the pull-out suture is completely removed 2 or 3 days postoperatively and the wound separated slightly by gentle downward traction on the lid margin as previously described. With removal of the entire suture, separation of the wound margins must be accomplished with great care to avoid recreating the ptosis.

Figure 86.1 *With nasal over correction after Fasanella–Servat procedure (A), the running pullout suture (B) should be pulled out the opposite side (C) so the wound can be separated when the lid is massaged or pulled downward, but not evererted as in (D), to produce a normal contour (E).*

87

Prevention of Corneal Irritation in Fasanella–Servat Ptosis Procedure

Richard Carroll

INTRODUCTION

The Fasanella-Servat procedure is a reliable, technically simple operation to correct up to 4 mm of acquired ptosis. Patients may experience severe irritation when the involved eye comes in contact with the exposed running sutures used to close the wound edges inside the upper lid.

The suture technique below eliminates the problem of ocular irritation or corneal abrasion from the Fasanella–Servat procedure.

TECHNIQUE

The Fasanella–Servat procedure is performed according to standard techniques, with the upper eyelid everted and curved hemosats placed so that the width of the tarsal resection is the same across the central two-thirds of the eyelid (Fig. 87.1).

After the resection of the tissues included in the clamp has been accomplished, the wound should be sutured together using a buried plain catgut suture with each end passed out the skin. As the running 5-0 plain catgut is used to close the wound, the sutures are placed obliquely joining the Müller's muscle and tarsus so all suture loops are buried beneath the conjunctiva. No suture is left exposed, as shown in the two upper methods in Fig. 87.2.

The suture can be tightened and tied over bolsters, as shown in Fig. 87.3. One week later, the suture can be pulled out if it has not absorbed.

This method avoids any immediate irritation of the cornea or conjunctiva.

274

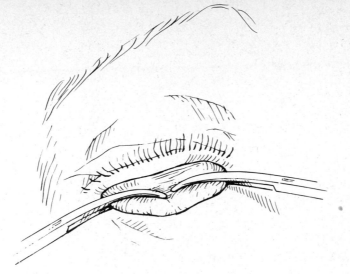

Figure 87.1   Correction application of hemostats.

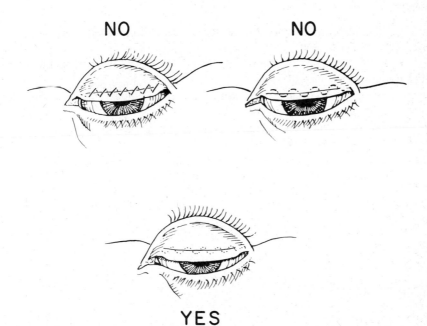

Figure 87.2   Burried pull-out suture.

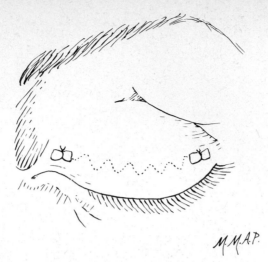

Figure 87.3 External appearance of pull-out suture.

BIBLIOGRAPHY

Beard C: Blepharoptosis repair by modified Fasanella–Servat operation. *Am J Ophthalmol* 69:850, 1970.

Carroll RP: Preventable problems following the Fasanella–Servat procedure. *Ophthalmic Surg* 11:44, 1980.

Fasanella RM, Servat J: Levator resection for minimal ptosis: Another simplified operation. *Arch Ophthalmol* 65:494, 1961.

Putterman AM: A clamp for strengthening Müller's muscle in the treatment of ptosis. *Arch Ophthalmol* 87:665, 1972.

Wiggs EO: The Fasanella–Servat operation. *Ophthalmic Surg* 9:48, 1978.

88

Technique for Threading Fascia Latae Strips

Don Liu
Orkan G. Stasior

INTRODUCTION

Manipulating a fascia strip can be a delicate and time-consuming procedure. Special instruments to facilitate the threading of fascia may not always be readily available.

Passing large instruments through a fascia stripper can macerate the fascia and damage the Crawford fascia stripper. Passing the fascia through the eye of a needle can be even more difficult due to the small size of the opening.

With the technique below, readily available instruments can be used to pull fascia through the eye of a needle or the fascia stripper without damaging the material.

TECHNIQUE

A 2-inch 22-gauge needle should be bent near its hub at approximately a 120-degree angle. The tip of the needle is bent a full 180-degrees to form a small hook at the end in a plane perpendicular to the first bend (Fig. 88.1). The needle can be held by hemostat and passed through the stripper, the fascia hooked and pulled into the stripper (Fig. 88.1). To thread the fascia through the eye of a needle, the 27-gauge needle can be passed through the eye and the fascia hooked and pulled back through the needle and released (Fig. 88.2).

This simple technique eliminates the frustration of passing fascia through the stripper or the eye of a needle and prevents damage to the fascia.

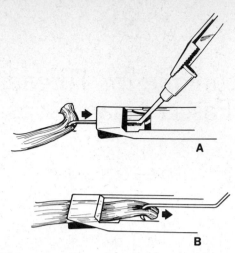

Figure 88.1 Bent 27-gauge needle used to introduce fascia into Crawford fascia stripper.

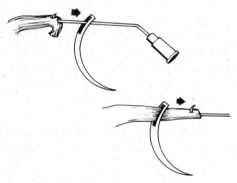

Figure 88.2 Bent needle facilitates passage of fascia through eye of needle. (Reprinted with permission. Ophthalmic Surgery 14:511–512, 1983.)

BIBLIOGRAPHY

Liu D, Safran TM, Stasior OG: A new technique of threading fascia lota strip. Ophthalmic Surg 14:511, 1983.

89

Lasso Technique with Upper Eyelid Fascia Latae Frontalis Suspension for Blephoptosis

Sanford D. Hecht

INTRODUCTION

During ptosis surgery using frontalis suspension, the surgeon may have difficulty passing the fascia through the small tunnels under the orbicularis muscle and skin. The passage is especially difficult through the levator aponeurosis/skin connection at the lid fold and across the orbital septum.

An easier passage can be obtained using extra large tunnels, but that method involves more trauma, which is especially undesirable in small children. With the lasso technique, the bulk of the leading edge of the fascia can be reduced as it passes through the tissue, allowing for ease in securing the fascia from one incision to the other.

TECHNIQUE

This technique uses a thin suture at the leading edge of the fascia, rather than a bulky, nonyielding instrument. Any of the usual instruments can be used with this technique to pass fascia through the lid. With the lasso technique, a 1-0 suture is passed through the eye of the right needle and tied on itself to form the loop, or lasso.

The lasso is dragged through the tunnel as the needle is passed. Then the fascia is lassoed (Fig. 89.1, left) and pulled back through the tunnel by pulling on the suture and right fascia needle simultaneously (Fig. 89.1, right). The fascia needle and then the fascioletta are brought up to the incision without difficulty.

The surgeon can pass the fascia atraumatically for more comfortable, pleasing postoperative course and cosmetic result.

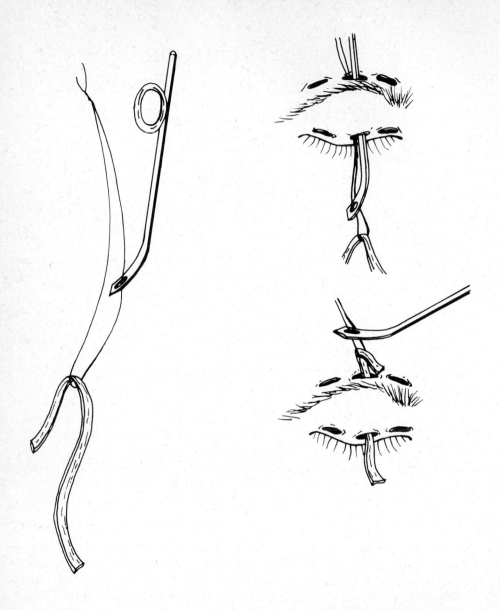

Figure 89.1 *Lasso technique for passing fascia. (Reprinted with permission. Ophthalmic Surgery 9:78–79, 1978.)*

BIBLIOGRAPHY

Hecht SD: Lasso technique in upper lid fascia lata frontalis fixation for ptosis. *Ophthalmic Surg* 9:78, 1978.

90

4-0 Silk Traction Sutures for Upper Eyelid Eversion

Richard K. Dortzbach

INTRODUCTION

The upper eyelid must be everted for surgery, such as ptosis repair from the internal approach, chalazion surgery, biopsies, and for reconstructive procedures using free tarsal grafts or tarsal-conjunctiva flaps. Everting the upper eyelid over a Desmarres retractor pushes the eyelid tissues posteriorly and makes dissection in the proper plane difficult.

Upper eyelid traction sutures described below provide easy access underneath the upper lid for surgery on the tarsoconjunctival surface or for a more involved techinque such as ptosis repair.

TECHNIQUE

This technique was originally described as part of a ptosis procedure using an internal approach to resect the superior tarsal muscle through an incision just above the superior tarsus with the lid everted (a 12-mm resection of the superior tarsal, or Müller's muscle, will very closely approximate the preoperative elevation by phenylephrine eyedrops) (1).

With the upper eyelid everted, two 4-0 silk traction sutures are placed in the posterior surface of the eyelid medially and laterally through the tarsus near the superior tarsal border (Fig. 90.1). Placing the sutures horizontally through the tarsus just below the superior tarsal border decreases the chance of piercing the superior internal arcade lying at, or just above, the superior tarsal border.

The 4-0 silks may be tied separately to the upper tarsal plate and then draped up over the operative field to be held with hemostats or clamped as needed for constant eversion of the upper eyelid.

This simple technique eliminates the frustration of trying to keep the upper eyelid everted.

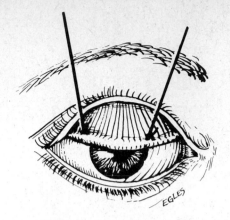

Figure 90.1 Upper eyelid eversion with 4-0 silk sutures.

REFERENCES

1. Dortzbach RK: Superior tarsal muscle resection to correct blepharoptosis. *Trans Am Acad Ophthalmol Otolaryngol* 86:1883, 1979.

91

Conjunctival Advancement Flap for Inferior Exposure Keratitis

David F. Kamin

INTRODUCTION

Keratitis from lagophthalmos after ptosis surgery nearly always resolves shortly after surgery. In some problem cases, the inferior keratitis persists, despite treatment with lubricants or artificial tears.

In patients needing ptosis surgery or revision of previous ptosis surgery, inferior keratitis would be a contraindication to further ptosis surgery.

The technique below provides an advancement flap of conjunctiva over the lower portion of the cornea to alleviate existing keratitis or to allow for additional ptosis surgery.

TECHNIQUE

The eye with inferior keratitis will show staining of the inferior cornea (Fig. 91.1). A 180-degree inferior peritomy is performed to develop a conjunctival flap. Using the operating microscope, the conjunctival flap is freed from Tenon's for advancement on the inferior third of the cornea.

A superficial lamellar keratectomy on the inferior cornea, below the lower pupillary border, should be performed. The conjunctiva is advanced in a "bridge flap" fashion and tacked to the corneal bed with a running number 10 nylon pull-out suture (Fig. 91.2).

Two or 3 weeks later, the pull-out suture can be removed leaving the inferior cornea protected by conjunctival epithelium (Fig. 91.3). Symptomatic keratits does not occur on the conjunctival epithelium.

This procedure is appropriate for patients with longstanding, medically resistant, symptomatic, inferior keratitis or patients with inferior keratitis needing further ptosis surgery.

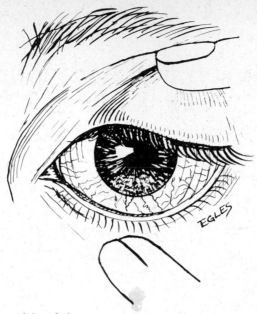

Figure 91.1   Keratitis of the inferior cornea due to lagophthalmos.

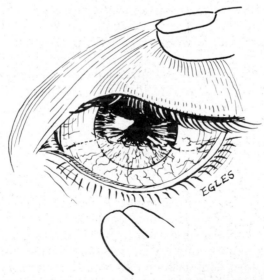

Figure 91.2   After lamellar keratectomy, conjunctival flap is attached to the cornea.

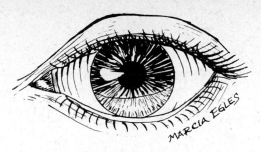

Figure 91.3 Conjunctival epithelium prevents inferior keratitis.

92

Elongation of a Short Fascia Strip

Mark R. Levine
Ido Sternberg

INTRODUCTION

Frontalis muscle should be used to elevate a ptotic lid when levator function is 4 mm or less. Despite the simplicity and availability of nonabsorbable and homogenous material, the complications of infection (1) and absorption still favor autogenous fascia for frontalis suspension.

The advantages of fascia are substantial: relative technical ease, excellent tensile strength, and no absorption (2).

Problems arise in children less than 2 years of age with insufficient amounts of fascia or when a dull fascia stripper makes the fascia difficult to harvest. In either case, an adequate length of fascia may be difficult to obtain.

The technique below describes a simple method to use effectively a short strip of fascia.

TECHNIQUE

If a short piece of fascia is obtained, the surgeon proceeds in the following manner. The fascia strip obtained is freed of any subcutaneous tissue and placed flat on a skin graft board. An incision 2 to 3 mm wide and parallel to one of the borders is made the entire length of the strip, stopping approximately 2 to 3 mm from the end (Fig. 92.1). The second incision, 2 to 3 mm wide and parallel to the first incision, is then made in an opposite direction, stopping 2 to 3 mm from the end. Additional strips as needed may be accomplished by making the incision as marked (Fig. 92.1, top).

The fascia is unfolded and placed on tension. The areas at the end of the strips are reinforced with 6-0 Vicryl suture (Fig. 92.1, midsection) and some remnant redundant fascia excised giving a uniform linear strip (Fig.

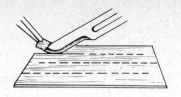

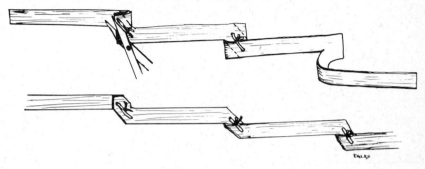

Figure 92.1 A short piece of fascia can be lengthened and strengthened with reinforcing sutures.

92.1, bottom). The fascia lata strip is then woven from the eyelid to the frontalis muscle using any of the conventional procedures of the surgeon's choice.

The tensile strength is more than adequate. Placing the fascia on stretch once the piece has been lengthened allows for easier placement of the reinforcing sutures at each of the corners.

BIBLIOGRAPHY

Beard C: *Ptosis*. St. Louis, Mosby, 1969, p 71.

Fox SA: *Ophthalmic Plastic Surgery*. New York, Grune & Stratton, 1970, p 373.

Quickert AE, Beard C: Studies of autogenous and homogenous fascia lata. *Eye Ear Nose Throat Monthly* 50:18, 1971.

93

Right-Angle Technique to Elongate Fascia

Marcia Egles

INTRODUCTION

Autogeneous fascia is the material with the least complication and best long-term results when used in frontalis suspension. The technique described below shows a method to elongate fascia with increased stability.

TECHNIQUE

Once the fascia has been obtained, the strips should be marked and cut with the incisions including alternate ends (Fig. 93.1). If the strips are then folded at right angles (much like one folds paper dolls), the strips will be folded into a single line and appropriate reinforcement sutures of 6-0 Dexon or a permanent suture placed at each junction.

This technique provides elongation of the fascia and eliminates any shearing forces by suturing the fascia totally at right angles (Fig. 93.1).

REFERENCES

1. Levine MR: Short fascia strip—What next? *Arch Ophthalmol* 95:1621, 1977.

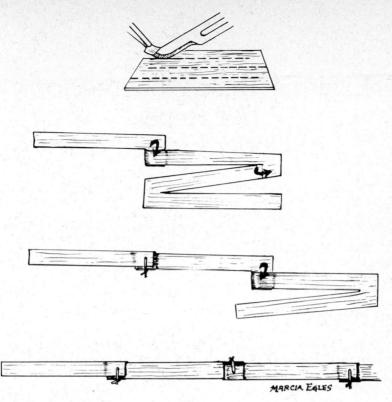

Figure 93.1 Folding fascia at right angles reduces shearing forces on fascia.

94

External Tarsoaponeurectomy for Repair of Upper Eyelid Ptosis

William R. Nunery

INTRODUCTION

The Fasanella–Servat procedure has been a simple, predictable way to correct minimal ptosis. The procedure must be limited to patients with only 2 to 3 mm of ptosis and those with greater than 12 mm of levator function.

The Fasanella–Servat procedure cannot be used in patients that require repositioning of the lid fold externally. The procedure requires everting the upper lid, which can be extremely difficult in cases involving conjunctival scarring. The procedure cannot be applied to patients with a high lid fold from dehiscence of the levator aponeurosis, which requires an external incision. Another procedure must be applied to patients with greater than 3 mm ptosis.

The external tarsoaponeurectomy can overcome these difficulties with predictable results.

TECHNIQUE

The Fasanella–Servat procedure consists of everting the tarsus, clamping and excising 4 to 6 mm of superior tarsal and levator tissue from the conjunctival surface, and then closing the defect with absorbable sutures. With the tarsoaponeurectomy, a similar resection can be accomplished through an external lid crease incision.

For the tarsoaponeurectomy, patients should have at least 12 mm of levator function. Then, 2% lidocaine with epinephrine and hyaluronidase are injected in to the external and conjunctival aspects of the upper eyelid before marking the lid crease 10 mm above the lash margin in the desired lid crease line. A blepharoplasty incision is outlined above the lid crease if the patient has dermatochalasis (Fig. 94.1).

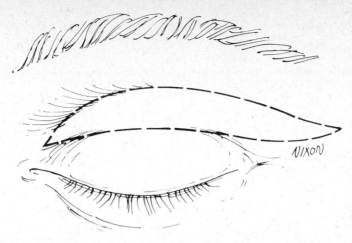

BLEPHAROPLASTY INCISION FOR TARSO-APONEURECTOMY

Figure 94.1 *Blepharoplasty and lid crease procedures can be performed with tarsoaponeurectomy.*

Cutaneous tissue can be excised with a Bard–Parker blade and Wescott scissors. Sharp dissection is carried down to the superior border of the tarsal plate. The tarsus is undermined anteriorly for visualization and identification of the entire superior half of the tarsus and adjoining levator aponeurosis (Fig. 94.2). After hemostasis is achieved, an Ehrhart clamp is placed on the tarsal plate. An ellipse of tissue straddling the superior border of the tarsal plate and extending across the entire horizontal aspect of the eyelid is then outlined with methylene blue marking.

The vertical extent of the ellipse generally measures 3 mm plus the amount of the ptosis. If levator function exceeds 14 mm, this measurement is reduced by 1 to 2 mm. For example, a patient with 3 mm of ptosis and 16 mm of levator function would require 6 mm of vertical excision. A patient with 3 mm of ptosis and 16 mm of levator function would only require 4 to 5 mm of vertical excision.

The elliptical incision includes the tarsal strip, conjunctiva, levator aponeurosis, and Müller's muscle (Fig. 94.3). The cut edge of the tarsal plate is then resutured to the cut edge of levator aponeurosis with three interrupted 7-0 silk sutures. These sutures are placed in the midpupillary line, the medial limbus line, and approximately 3 mm lateral to the lateral limbus line. Care is taken to avoid suturing the tarsus to the septum (Fig. 94.4).

The lid crease is then created in the desired position by placing at least three 7-0 silk sutures from the lower skin edge through the cut edge of the levator aponeurosis to the upper skin edge. The skin incision is closed with running 7-0 silk suture or other appropriate suture (Fig. 94.5).

Conservative amounts of excision are employed to prevent overcorrection. Overcorrection will be less acceptable to patients than slight undercorrection. If an overcorrection is observed on the day following surgery,

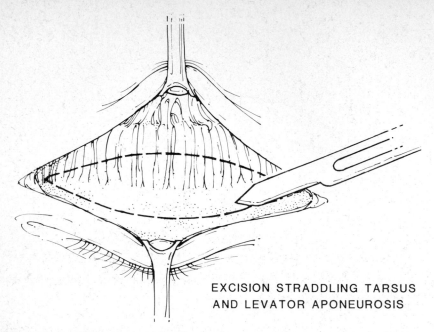

EXCISION STRADDLING TARSUS
AND LEVATOR APONEUROSIS

Figure 94.2 Excision marked at tarsoconjunctival border.

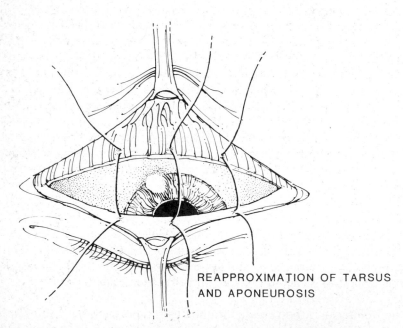

REAPPROXIMATION OF TARSUS
AND APONEUROSIS

Figure 94.3 Placement of sutures after excision of ellipse of tarsus, conjunctiva, levator aponeurosis, and Müller's muscle.

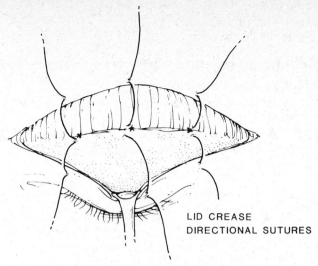

LID CREASE
DIRECTIONAL SUTURES

Figure 94.4   *Upper tarsus sutured to cut edge of levator aponeurosis.*

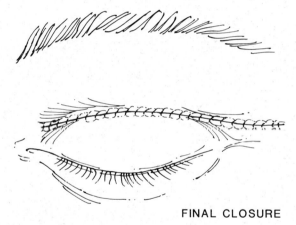

FINAL CLOSURE

Figure 94.5   *Running 7-0 silk skin closure.*

the midpupillary levator fixation suture can be removed from the conjunctival surface, allowing the lid position to relax 1 to 2 millimeters.

The advantages of the tarsoaponeurectomy procedure over the Fasanella–Servat procedure include application of the procedure to patients in whom the upper eyelid cannot be everted, or everted only with difficulty, improved cosmesis through blepharoplasty incision, redirection of the normal lid crease line, and elimination of superior sulcus deformity defect. Also, the amount of ptosis that can be corrected through this procedure has a much wider range since the procedure can be graded and applied to patients with severe ptosis, provided the levator function exceeds 12 mm. Finally, contouring of the lid margin can be accomplished with greater ease through this incision than through the traditional Fasanella–Servat incision.

BIBLIOGRAPHY

Beard, C: Ptosis. St. Louis, Mosby, 1969.

Fasanella RM, Servat J: Levator resection for minimal ptosis: Another simplified operation. *Arch Ophthalmol* 65:493, 1961.

McCord CD Jr: An external minimal ptosis procedure: external tarsoaponeurectomy. *Trans Am Acad Ophthalmol Otolaryngol* 683, 79:683, 1975.

95

Phenylephrine Test in Ptosis

Gil A. Epstein

INTRODUCTION

When should one use the Fasanella–Servat and when should the more complicated repair of the levator aponeurosis procedure be used? The phenylephrine test can distinguish the optimal surgical approach for ptosis surgery.

TECHNIQUE

A drop of 10% phenylephrine hydrochloride is instilled into the superior fornix with the patient leaning backward and looking downward. With the upper lid manually lifted upward the superior fornix can be easily seen. Two instillations of the drop are performed 1 minute apart. The patient can be evaluated 5 minutes later. With hypertension or cardiovascular disease, 2.25% phenylephrine has worked well.

The fissure width is not measured but rather the margin reflex distance (MRD)—the distance from a light reflex to the superior lid in primary gaze. This test is more accurate than measuring fissure width which reflects stimulation by phenylephrine of the Müller's muscle in both the upper and lower eyelids.

If the upper eyelid elevates to an acceptable level, the test is considered positive (Fig. 95.1). Poor elevation is considered negative.

With a positive response to the phenylephrine test, a Müllers muscle-conjunctiva resection (Fasanella type) surgical procedure can be expected to duplicate the appearance after the eyedrops in 95% of cases. If the test is negative, an external levator repair, advancement, and/or tuck is indicated.

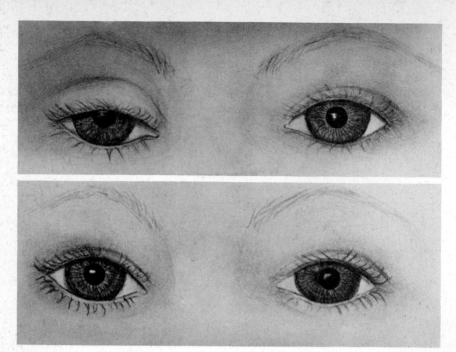

Figure 95.1 Phenylephrine instilled into right eye with ptosis (top). Good response (bottom) indicates Fasanella–Servat procedure will be effective. The distance from light reflex to the upper lid should be measured rather than the fissure width, which reflects stimulation of both upper and lower eyelids.

96

Finding the Levator Muscle

Gil A. Epstein

INTRODUCTION

Isolating the levator muscle constitutes the key step in ptosis surgery. This technique provides ready access to the levator muscle during external ptosis repair.

TECHNIQUE

A skin incision is made at the proposed horizontal lid crease (Fig. 96.1). The inferior skin is retracted downward over the eye; the superior skin wound is lifted up toward the sky. The orbicularis muscle adheres to the skin and the levator follows posteriorly adjacent to the superior rectus muscle. Separating the wound edges as described above reveals a space between the levator and orbicularis.

The orbicularis can be buttonholed and this space extended across the entire aspect of the wound while lifting the scissors skyward (Fig. 96.2). After the orbicularis incision is completed, two forceps can grasp the orbital septum, which eminates from the superior orbital rim.

To confirm the orbital septum, one can palpate under the superior orbital rim and notice the tenseness of the orbital septum. If the orbital septum is intact, it can be buttonholed with Westcott scissors and then opened across the entire wound up on the orbital septum to avoid injury to the levator muscle. A wet cotton-tipped applicator can be employed for blunt dissection (Fig. 96.3).

After the orbital septum has been opened, the orbital fat can be easily identified. Just under the orbital fat lies the levator muscle.

Under local anesthesia, the levator can be confirmed by tagging with a suture and directing the patient to look upward.

Careful identification of the anatomic structure of the eyelid, particularly the levator muscle complex, greatly simplifies ptosis surgery, blepharoplasty, and upper eyelid reconstruction.

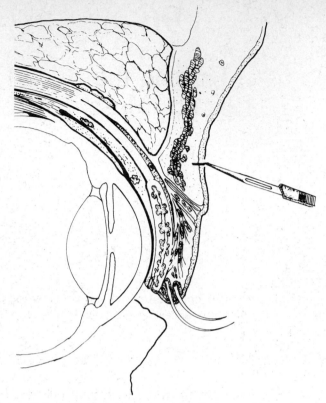

Figure 96.1 Skin incision at proposed lid crease.

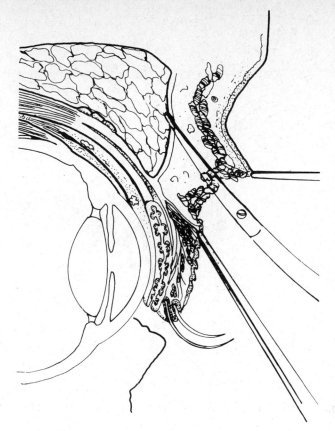

Figure 96.2   Buttonhole made through orbicularis muscle.

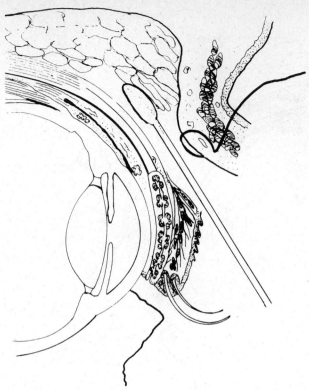

Figure 96.3 Cotton-tipped applicator for blunt dissection to expose the levator.

97

Adjustable Silicone Rod Frontalis Sling for the Correction of Blepharoptosis

Charles R. Leone, Jr.
John W. Shore
John V. Van Germet

INTRODUCTION

Autogenous fascia is generally considered to be the material of choice in frontalis suspension in congenital ptosis. In special cases in which poor corneal protective mechanisms coexist with severe ptosis, as in third nerve palsies or chronic progressive external ophthalmoplegia, a technique that allows for easy adjustment of the sling must be used.

This technique uses a readily available silicone rod for frontalis suspension due to the case of postoperative adjustment to alleviate exposure or to place the lid in a more desireable position.

TECHNIQUE

An incision is carried through the proposed lid crease 7 to 9 mm above the lash line (Fig. 97.1A). The orbicularis is separated from the anterior tarsus. Four sutures of 5-0 Dacron are placed vertically through the midportion of the tarsus, and the 1-mm solid silicone rod is placed over the sutures to be tied securely to the tarsus.

Brow incisions medially, centrally, and laterally are carred to the deep frontalis fascia. A Wright fascia needle is passed through the medial and lateral brow incisions along the curve of the superior orbital rim deep to the orbital septum in the plane of the levator aponeurosis exiting at the superior tarsal border. The silicone rod, placed through the eye of the needle, can be pulled back through the tunnel and externalized at the medial and lateral brow incisions.

Through each of the brow incisions, a 4-0 Dacron suture is placed through the deep frontalis fascia. A number 0 lacrimal probe is placed

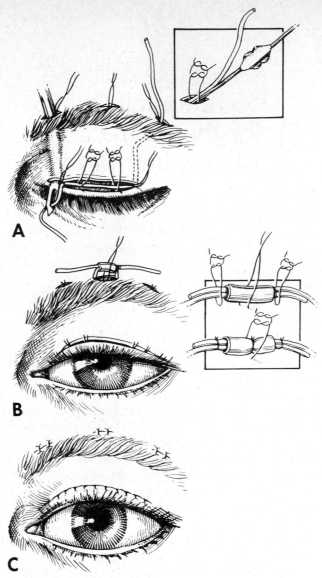

A

B

C

Figure 97.1 Fixation of adjustable silicone rod frontalis suspension. (Reprinted with permission. Ophthalmic Surgery 12:881–887, 1981.)

alongside the silicone rod in the medial and lateral brow incisions, and the Dacron suture is tied around both structures. When the probe is removed, a small suture pulley will remain through which the rod can easily slide. The two ends of the rod are brought out through the central brow incision with the Wright fascia needle.

The two ends of the rod are passed through a 1.5 mm inside diameter silicone tube (Watzke sleeve) measuring 5 mm in length. A Watzke forceps is placed within the tube to stretch it open to allow the two rods to pass through the lumen. The two ends are pulled tight within the silicone sleeve to adjust the lid margin to the desired height.

With congenital ptosis, the lid is placed at the superior limbus. In chronic progressive ophthalmoplegia, the lid is placed between the pupil and superior limbus. The lid margin should be forcefully pulled down to remove any kinks of loops in the rod. The sleeve is placed within the central incision to obtain as true an evaluation of the upper eyelid position as possible

The sleeve is then pulled out of the central incision and the overlapped rods on each side of the sleeve tied together with a 4-0 Dacron suture. The 5 mm of excess rod on each side of the sleeve allows for later adjustment. A third Dacron suture is tied around the sleeve, and the preplaced deep Dacron suture is tied over the sleeve to secure it within the depth of the incision (Fig. 97.1B).

In adults, the upper eyelid incision is closed with 6-0 silk, catching the tarsus at the superior border to fixate the skin. In children, double-armed 6-0 plain catgut suture are brought through the superior fornix at the superior tarsal border then through the upper and lower skin edges to be tied to invaginate the skin edges. Brow incisions are closed with either interrupted 6-0 prolene in adults or 6-0 plain catgut in children (Fig. 97.1C). A Frost suture of 6-0 silk through a number 40 silicone band peg is placed through the lower eyelid pulling the lower lid over the cornea on taping the sutured ends to the brow.

A liberal amount of antibiotic ointment is placed over the eye and incision areas, and then a wet eye pad is applied. The next day, the Frost suture can be loosened to observe how the patient tolerates the open fissure during the day. It is retaped to the brow at night. If the patient can tolerate 2 days of an open fissure, the Frost suture is completely removed. Lubricating ointment is liberally applied each night along with saline-soaked eye pads.

For overcorrection or undercorrection, the central brown incision is opened; the sleeve is located and lifted out of the incision. The sutures are removed around the rods, and the lid is either raised or lowered to the desired level and resutured as previously described.

The adjustment can be made early in the postoperative period or years later. The elasticity allows for good eyelid approximation with minimal effort reducing postoperative corneal problems. The nonbiodegradeable silicone rod becomes encased in a fibrous connective tissue through which it can slide for late readjustment of eyelid position. With the fixation directly to the tarsus, a satisfactory eyelid crease is created.

BIBLIOGRAPHY

Leone CR, Shore JW, Van Gemert JV: Silicone rod frontalis sling for the correction of blepharoptosis. *Ophthalmic Surg* 12:881, 1981.

Leone CR, Rylander G: A modified silicone frontalis sling for the correction of blepharoptosis. *Am J Ophthalmol* 85:802, 1978.

98

Adjustable Eyelid and Eyebrow Suspension for Blepharoptosis

Arthur J. Jampolsky

INTRODUCTION

When the results of a surgical procedure are variable, as with frontalis suspension, a technique that allows for postoperative adjustment should be used. The technique below allows for postoperative adjustment of both eyelid height and contour after brow suspension.

TECHNIQUE

This technique uses two separate rhomboid suspension slings with removable loop sutures at points where suspension material bends to permit postoperative adjustment of the height and contour.

Skin markings are made 3 to 4 mm above the lid margin (Fig. 98.1) centrally, medially, and laterally. Some of the markings are made above the brow separated by approximately 15 mm. The eyelid incisions are carried out to the depth of the tarsus and the brow incisions to the depth of the periosteum of the frontal bone. The surgeon's choice of suspension material may be used.

A Wright fascia needle or large, curved needle is used to pass one end of the suspension material from the center eyebrow incision to exit the lateral eyebrow incision. A loop of 5-0 nonabsorbable suture is tied around the suspension material (Fig. 98.1, right) to allow manipulation of the eyelid position either during the operation or for postoperative adjustment. The rhomboid is continued as the suspension material is passed from the lateral eyebrow incision to the lateral upper eyelid incision beneath the orbicularis muscle and brought out through that incision.

A similar 5-0 nonabsorbable suture is passed around the suspension at this point, and the material is then passed beneath the orbicularis muscle in front of the tarsal plate to the central eyelid incision. No loop is used at

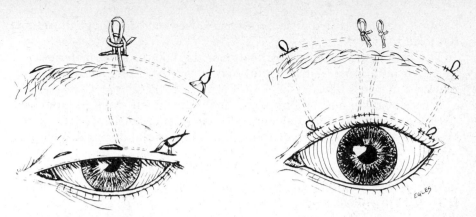

Figure 98.1 Adjustable frontalis suspension technique. (Carlson MR, Jampolsky A: Adjustable eyelid and eyebrow suspension for blepharoptosis. Am J Ophthalmol 88:109–112, 1979. Published by The American Journal of Ophthalmology. Copyright by The Ophthalmic Publishing Company.)

this point, but the suspension material is then passed up to the upper eyelid and allowed to exit at the central eyebrow incision where the rhomboid was initiated (Fig. 98.1). A similar rhomboid is performed medially with adjustment sutures passed around the suspension material at the medial eyebrow and medial eyelid incision.

Now the suspension can be adjusted. The end of the suspension material from the central eyelid incision is grasped at the central brow incision with gentle traction to elevate the lid to the desired level in the central portion. A small hemostat at the skin can be used to hold the suspension at this level. Eyelid contour is now elevated, and the tension of the sling material at the medial and lateral incisions can be locally adjusted with the loop sutures.

For more elevation, the corresponding suture in the eyebrow can be pulled to increase tension on the suspension. To lower the lid, the loop in the eyelid margin should be pulled to loosen the suspension material. At the final adjustment, there should be no slack in the suspension material. The hemostats can be removed and the suspension material tied in a bow knot (Fig. 98.1, right). Skind incisions are sutured in an interrupted fashion allowing the loops to remain exposed. Antibiotic ointment is applied, and the lower eyelid is elevated with a Frost suture.

Four to 12 hours after surgery, with the patient alert, the material can be adjusted with the patient sitting and looking directly ahead. Adjustment, under sterile conditions, can be made by loosening the bow knot and retying it after the adjustment of a higher eyelid had been made. This can be repeated until optimal eyelid position has been achieved.

Eyelid contour can be altered by pulling the appropriate loop sutures to adjust the extreme medial and lateral contour. When completed, the suspension material is tied. The excess is excised, and the loop sutures are removed.

The skin can be allowed to heal over the knot of sling material centrally, or additional skin closures can be added. Frost sutures can be removed in 2 to 3 days.

If considerable edema exists, the final adjustment should be delayed until the edema has subsided, and a sterile dressing can be placed over the eye and eyebrow to avoid contamination of the wound during this waiting period.

Previous techniques have described adjustable frontalis suspension, but none have included the postoperative adjustment of contour, as described in this technique.

BIBLIOGRAPHY

Carlson MR, Jampolsky AJ: Adjustable eyelid and eyebrow suspension for blepharoptosis. *Am J Ophthalmol* 88:109, 1979.

Crawford JS: Repair of ptosis using frontalis muscle and fascia lata. *Trans Am Acad Ophthalmol Otolaryngol* 60:672, 1956.

99

Repair of Ptosis in Blepharophimosis

David F. Kamin

INTRODUCTION

Blepharophimosis consists of telecanthus (wide intercanthal distances), epicanthus inversus, ectropion, and ptosis (Fig. 99.1). Due to poor levator function, correction of the ptosis has required obtaining fascia to perform frontalis suspension.

A simpler procedure, which does not require a separate incision either to obtain fascia lata or for the placement of foreign material, can be used to provide excellent lid fold, contour, and height.

The technique of anterior levator and tarsal resection can correct ptosis in blepharophimosis while avoiding the problems with lid crease, contour height, and asymmetry frequently seen with frontalis suspension.

TECHNIQUE

The skin incision is carried through the lid crease, and the tarsal plate is exposed with dissection. The levator aponeurosis is isolated and dissected free (Fig. 99.2). A 5-mm full-thickness contoured excision of the tarsus and conjunctiva is performed (Fig. 99.3). The excised piece of tarsus should be a elliptical and approximate the shape of the upper eyelid. This resection essentially shortens the tarsus in the vertical dimension while allowing the upper lid to retain its original shape.

After the tarsal plate is excised and a maximum resection performed, the levator aponeurosis is reattached to the distal end of the tarsus. This creates both an advancement of the levator and a resection of the tarsus (Fig. 99.4). The levator is resected and secured to the tarsal border, and the lid incision is closed (Fig. 99.5). Figures 99.6 and 99.7 show the preoperative and postoperative positions that typify elevation of the lid with this procedure.

This procedure provides an effective alternative to frontalis suspension and uses a single operative site.

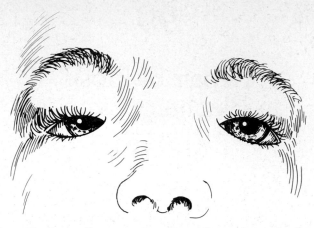

Figure 99.1 Blepharophimosis patient with ptosis and telecanthus.

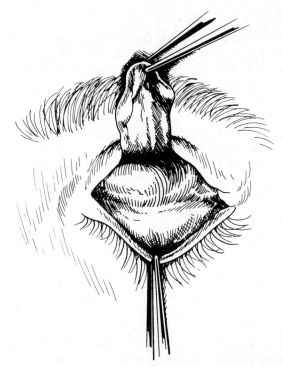

Figure 99.2 Levator resection: superior forceps holding levator aponeurosis.

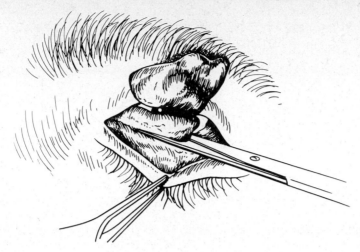

Figure 99.3 Elliptical spindle of tarsus and conjunctiva excised.

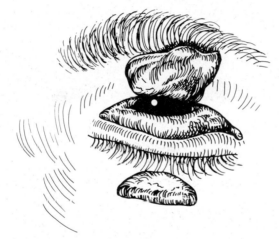

Figure 99.4 Excised tarsus (below). Levator, aponeurosis (above).

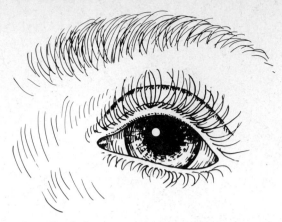

Figure 99.5 View after closure with deep stitches to create lid fold.

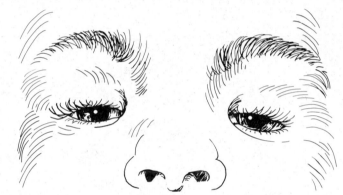

Figure 99.6 Blepharophimosis patient preoperatively.

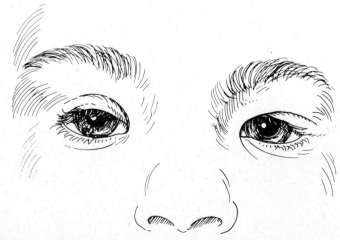

Figure 99.7 Expected appearance postoperatively.

100

Clothesline Operation for Ptosis

R. Bruce Ramsey
Martin L. Leib

INTRODUCTION

The Fasanella–Servat procedure has served as a simple, quick, effective means for minimal ptosis that is particularly effective in disorders involving Müller's sympathetically inervatived muscle such as Horner's syndrome. The Fasanella–Servat procedure will not correct ptosis from underacting levator superiorus muscle from attenuation or dehiscence of the levator aponeurosis.

The clothesline operation is a simple, effective procedure for ptosis, whether myogenic, neurogenic, or aponeurogenic.

TECHNIQUE

Satisfactory anesthesia can be accomplished with a regional frontal nerve block. The lid is doubly everted over a Desmarres retractor (Figure 100.1A), and a 3-0 silk clothesline suture is placed in the upper lid from the conjunctival surface in the following manner: At the lateral one-fifth approximately 3 to 4 mm above the tarsus, depending on the amount of correction required, the suture is introduced to traverse the middle three-fifths of the lid at a depth to include conjunctiva, Müller's muscle, as well as levator aponeurosis (Fig. 100.2).

The suture is passed in a curve parallel to the superior tarsal border to exit at a juncture at the medial one-fifth of the eyelid. The Desmarres retractor should be removed and the anterior lid inspected to determine if the skin and orbicularis muscle have been included in the suture. If traction on the suture produces dimpling of the skin, the suture should be withdrawn and reintroduced with a more shallow bite.

The clothesline suture should be pulled tight and the upper lid everted with a hook as two hemostats are applied to the lid (Fig. 100.1B). The

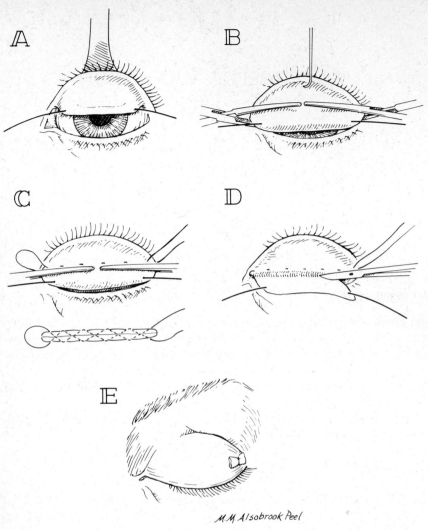

Figure 100.1 (A) Clothesline suture to incorporate levator aponeurosis. (B) Retraction by clothesline. Placement of clamps approximately 4 mm onto tarsus. (C) Diagonal suture technique to protect corneal. (D) Excision of clamp tissue. (E) Externalized suture to be tied over bolster.

level of the clamp application is variable and depends on the degree of ptosis. An average distance is 4 mm to 5 mm. The skin hook retracting upward helps to stabilize the lid during placement of the clamps.

Beginning nasally and immediately posterior to the clamps, one end of a double-armed 6-0 Dexon or Vicryl suture should be woven through the full thickness of these tissues in a continuous, diagonal mattress fashion (Fig. 100.1C). To prevent postoperative corneal irritation, the minimum amount of sutures should be exposed on the conjunctival surface; as each

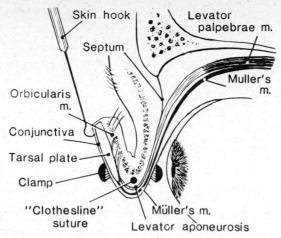

Figure 100.2 *Sagittal section: clothesline suture incorporating levator aponeurosis.*

bite exits, the next bite should be taken right at that exit site so that the suture can sink slightly into the tarsoconjunctival substance.

The clamps can be removed and the clothesline suture tightened while a full-thickness scissor cut is made along the crush tracks left by the clamps (Fig. 100.1D). The ends of the double-armed suture are now passed to the skin surface temporally to be tied over a bolster of Telfa or cotton (Fig. 100.1E).

Any technique other than the diagonal suturing technique that buries the Vicryl or Dexon within the lid substance will cause the corneal irritation. Antibiotic ointment should be instilled three times a day for the first postoperative week. The suture can be cut flush with the skin and the bolsters discarded.

This operation, while similar to the Fasanella–Servat, uses the principle of resecting levator aponeurosis as well as the Müller's conjunctival complex. The surgeon can better understand this technique by noting the anatomy in Figure 100.2 and 100.3. The clothesline suture, pulled tight, incorporates the levator aponeurosis into the resection (Figs. 100.4 and 100.5), making this procedure effective in cases of levator aponeurosis disorders, which will not be corrected by the Fasanella–Servat operation.

Furthermore, the traction and countertraction provided by the clothesline suture and the hook retractor allow much better control in placement of the clamps as compared to the Fasanella–Servat operation. Long-term follow-up has shown the results to be predictable and persistent.

313

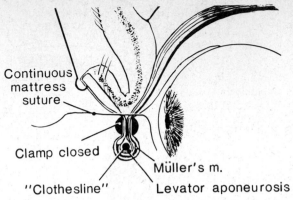

Figure 100.3 *Relation of clamps, levator aponeurosis, and clothesline* suture.

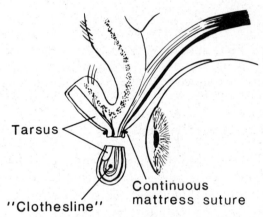

Figure 100.4 Tissue excised in clothesline procedure.

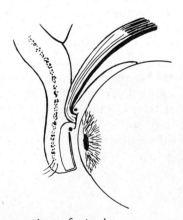

Figure 100.5 After correction of ptosis.

101

Full-Thickness Eyelid Resection for the Treatment of Undercorrected Blepharoptosis and Eyelid Contour Defects

Henry I. Baylis
Kevin I. Perman

INTRODUCTION

The most frequent complications of ptosis surgery are undercorrection and lid contour defects. The scarring and altered anatomy can make these complications difficult to correct.

This technique repairs under corrected eyelid ptosis and contour deformities after a blepharoptosis procedure.

TECHNIQUE

With either local infiltration or general anesthesia, a marking pen is used to delineate an ellipse of skin representing the amount of desired correction on a millimeter-for-millimeter basis (Fig. 101.1A). The vertical dimension of the ellipse is equal to the amount of ptosis correction desired (Fig. 101.1B). The ellipse may be skewed to compensate for eyelid contour abnormalities. The closer to the eyelid margin the full-thickness resection can be performed, the more predictable will be the amount of correction.

The full-thickness resection should be performed in the lower 10 mm of the eyelid. The vascular supply of the eyelid margin is not compromised because of the complex of vessels present on the tarsal conjunctiva as well as the marginal vessels of the lid.

A number 15 Bard–Parker blade can be used to make an incision through the skin and orbicularis muscle. Next, a lid plate should be placed between the globe and the lid and the full-thickness blepharop-

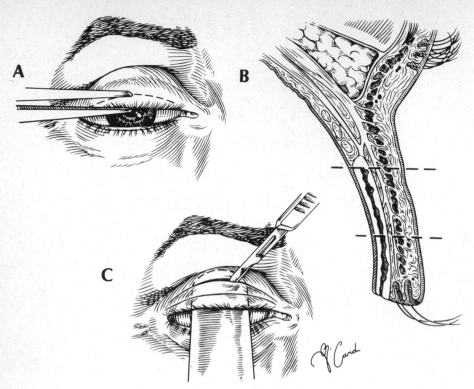

Figure 101.1 (A) Amount of ptosis measured to determine quantity of lid resection. (B) Sagittal section: lower incision at least 4 mm above lid margin. (C) Incision through skin and orbicularis.

tomy completed (Fig. 101.1C). Scissors can be introduced through the full-thickness incisions in both the upper and lower portions to remove the entire ellipse en block (Fig. 101.2A). Once the full-thickness incision has been completed, 6.0 Dexon sutures on a half-curved needle are carefully used to close the posterior layers in an interrupted fashion (Fig. 101.2B) with care, making sure the needle does not penetrate the conjunctiva to avoid ocular irritation.

The eyelid contour and lid level can be inspected and adjusted by excising additional full-thickness eyelid tissue or loosening the Dexon sutures. The suture used for skin closure should incorporate the levator aponeurosis to enhance the eyelid crease (Fig. 101.2C,D).

The tissue excised in this procedure is illustrated in Figure 101.1B. The inferior incision should not be lower than 4 mm above the lid margin, and the superior incision should not penetrate the orbital septum. This procedure provides a simple, effective, one-stage correction of eyelid height and contour abnormalities.

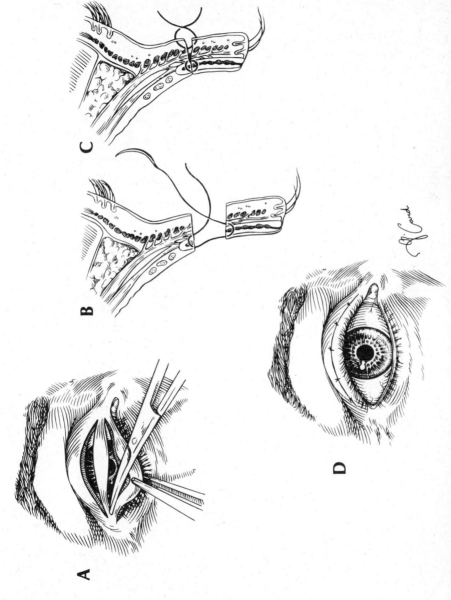

Figure 101.2 (A) Scissors complete full-thickness excision. (B and C) Layered closure. (D) Closure after ptosis correction.

BIBLIOGRAPHY

Baylis HI, Axelrod RN, Rosen N: Full thickness eyelid resection for the treatment of undercorrected blepharoptosis and eyelid coutour defects, in Bosniak SL (ed): *Advances in Ophthalmic Plastic and Reconstructive Surgery*. New York, Pergammon Press, 1982, vol 1, p 212.

Baylis HI, Shorr N: Anterior tarsectomy reoperation for upper eyelid blepharoptosis or contour abnormalities. *Am J Ophthalmol* 84:67, 1977.

McCord CD Jr: External minimal ptosis procedure/external tarsoaponeurectomy. *Trans Am Acad Ophthalmol Otolaryngol* 79:683, 1975.

Mustarde JC: Problems and possibilities in ptosis surgery. *Plast Reconstruct Surg* 56:381, 1975.

102

The A-Frame
Ptosis Operation

Robert G. Small

INTRODUCTION

Acquired blepharoptosis can frequently be repaired by suturing the edge of the disinserted levator aponeurosis to the upper tarsus. In many instances, the levator aponeurosis is merely thinned. In such cases, aponeurosis repair is really the old tuck operation.

With the A-frame technique, acquired ptosis from thinning, but not disinsertion, of the levator aponeurosis, is performed rapidly and predictably by resecting the levator aponeurosis and Müller's muscle.

TECHNIQUE

An incision is marked in the lid crease of the upper eyelid and carried through skin and orbicularis muscle. A white oval will be visible as the orbicularis muscle is opened. Scissors complete the incision with one blade inserted beneath the orbicularis muscle. The attachment of the septum to the levator aponeurosis is identified, and the orbital septum is opened the full length of the eyelid. Preaponeurotic fat prolapses through the opening in the septum.

The preaponeurotic fat is retracted with a Desmarres retractor to reveal Whitnall's ligament. If disinsertion of the levator aponeurosis is found, the repair can be accomplished by attaching the levator aponeurosis to the upper tarsal plate. If the aponeurosis is simply thinned, the surgeon continues with the A-frame modification.

A muscle hook is passed under the upper eyelid (Fig. 102.1) approximately 4 mm from the upper tarsal border. The tip of the muscle hook is pressed up against the conjunctiva, Müller's muscle, and thinned levator aponeurosis, which is then grasped with a forceps (Fig. 102.2). With the forceps holding the levator tissue in an A-frame configuration (Fig. 102.3) a clamp is placed across the tissue (Fig. 102.4).

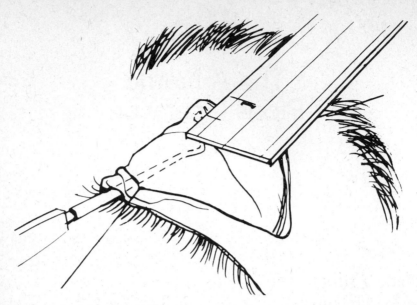

Figure 102.1 Muscle hook tip under lid, 4 mm above tarsus.

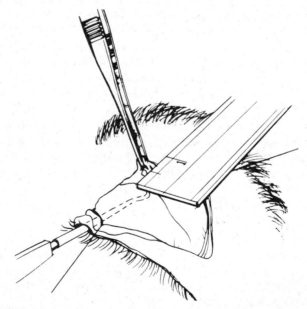

Figure 102.2 Forceps grasps Müller's muscle, conjunctiva, and levator aponeurosis.

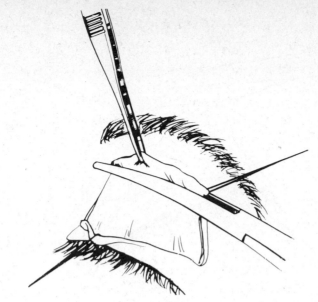

Figure 102.3 Elevation of A-frame to be clamped.

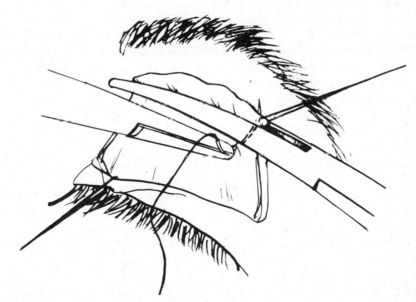

Figure 102.4 Running suture beneath clamp.

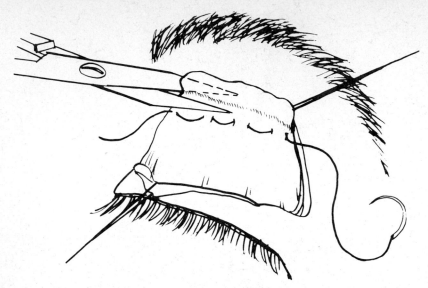

Figure 102.5 *Cutting along serration marks left by clamp.*

Note that the forcep is placed medial to the center of the eyelid so that the curve of the resected tissue will correspond to the normal upper eyelid curvature with the highest point just medial to the center of the eyelid. The assistant may need to hold the tissue with a second forcep while the clamp is applied. If 4 mm of tissue is pulled into the clamp, an 8 mm resection will be accomplished.

A 5-0 braided polyester running mattress suture is placed beneath the clamp (Fig. 102.5). The clamp can be removed and the tissue excised along the serration marks left by the clamp. The sutures are brought back as a running suture either above the running mattress suture (Fig. 102.6) or below the mattress suture and then tied to complete the A-frame resection.

Eversion of the upper eyelid shows the running suture is covered by conjunctiva avoiding the danger of corneal abrasion. The height and contour of the upper eyelid are inspected. If necessary, the suture is removed, and cut edges are reapproximated for proper eyelid curvature and height. The skin is closed with a running suture of 6-0 mild chromic catgut or subcuticular suture of 6-0 nylon.

The procedure is designed for acquired adult ptosis, but can be used in moderate congenital ptosis with good levator function.

BIBLIOGRAPHY

Small RG: The A-frame operation for acquired blepharoptosis. *Arch Ophthalmol* 98:516–519, 1980.

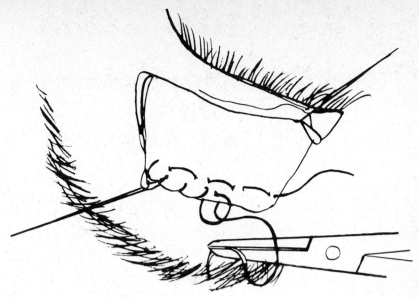

Figure 102.6 Repair of thinned levator aponeurosis with running closure.

103

Suture Tarsorrhaphy System for Keratopathy After Ptosis Surgery

Allen M. Putterman

INTRODUCTION

Patients with ptosis from external ophthalmoplegia, third nerve palsy, or myasthenia gravis are vulnerable to severe keratitis from lagophthalmos produced by ptosis surgery due to abnormal ocular motility or poor Bell's phenomenon. The tarsorrhaphy suture system prevents serious postoperative exposure keratopathy in these patients while the cornea adapts gradually to the lagophthalmos (difficulty in closing the eyelids) that follows ptosis surgery.

This technique keeps eyelids partially closed in the early postoperative weeks in patients who have difficulty lowering their eyebrow and closing their eyelids from postoperative forehead pain and edema after frontalis sling surgery.

TECHNIQUE

At the completion of ptosis surgery, a 4-0 black silk double-armed Frost tarsorrhaphy suture is passed through the central lower eyelid and forehead. The suture should pass through skin and orbicularis muscle at the center of the lower eyelid 2 mm below the eyelashes (Fig. 103.1A and B). One arm is passed through the skin and frontalis muscle just above the central eyebrow and above the frontalis sling suture. Two other double-armed sutures are passed through the temporal and nasal lower eyelid and forehead (Fig. 103.1A). Cotton pledgets are placed beneath the nasal and temporal loops of suture in the lower eyelid skin to prevent cheese wiring through the eyelid.

A fourth 4-0 black silk double-armed suture is passed through the skin, orbicularis muscle, and superficial tarsus and into the central lower eyelid just under the central Frost suture (Fig. 103.1A). The ends of the suture

324

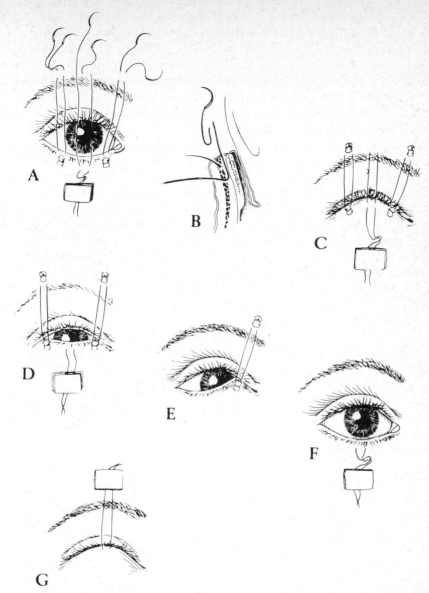

Figure 103.1 Suture tarsorrhaphy system to manage keratitis after ptosis surgery.

are knotted about 6 mm from the eyelid and taped to the lower eyelid at the inferior rim region.

Tha nasal forehead tarsorrhaphy suture ends are tightened. When the nasal lower eyelid margin meets the upper eyelid margin, each arm is tied over a cotton pledget. The temporal tarsorrhaphy suture is tied similarly. When the central Frost suture is tied, the entire cornea is covered by eyelids (Fig. 103.1C). A light pressure dressing is applied.

On the first day postoperatively, the dressing and central Frost suture are removed (Fig. 103.1D). Lacrilube ophthalmic ointment is applied to each eye every 2 to 3 hours during the day and once in the middle of the night for 2 to 3 days. If the cornea shows only minimal staining with fluorescein, the treatment can be reduced to four applications of ointment each day, and the nighttime instillation ceased. If the cornea remains stable, the ointment is further reduced to two applications each day, beginning 5 to 6 days postoperatively.

If the cornea is stable by the seventh postoperative day, the temporal tarsorrhaphy suture can be removed (Fig. 103.1E), and the application of ointment can be increased to the same frequency as when the first suture had been removed 1 week previously. The ointment is tapered in a similar manner, and if only minimal corneal staining remains, the nasal tarsorrhaphy suture can be released at the end of the second week (Fig. 103.1F). At night, the central suture previously taped to the cheek should be taped to the forehead so the lower eyelid covers the cornea during sleep (Fig. 103.1G). Ointment instillation is again tapered. After 3 days, taping of the central lid suture to the forehead is discontinued. When the cornea has adapted to the lagophthalmos, the lower eyelid suture can be removed.

As long as keratitis appears to be a potential problem, the lower lid suture can be taped to the forehead. After removal of the lid suture, the patient can be maintained on a regimen of artificial tears and ointment as needed to control any lingering keratopathy.

BIBLIOGRAPHY

Putterman AM: Suture tarsorrhaphy system to control keratopathy after ptosis surgery. *Ophthalmic Surg* 11:577, 1980.

104

Prevention of Vertical Tarsal Buckling in Repair of Levator Aponeurosis Defects in Acquired Blepharoptosis

Michael Patipa
Robert B. Wilkins

INTRODUCTION

Acquired blepharoptosis from defects in the levator aponeurosis can be corrected through a lid crease incision to expose the disinserted edge of the levator aponeurosis, which can be reattached to the anterior tarsal plate. The amount of advancement of the levator aponeurosis can cause overcorrection or undercorrection. Reattachment of the levator aponeurosis below the vertical center of the tarsal plate can cause vertical buckling of the tarsal plate (Fig. 104.1) with upper eyelid entropion and a deformed upper eyelid.

Late correction of this deformity can require reoperation to adjust the sutures, a symblepharon ring, placement of 4-0 silk mattress sutures from the fornix, or even a Weis procedure to correct entropion. This complication can be avoided by reattaching the levator aponeurosis to the upper tarsus as described below.

TECHNIQUE

The levator aponeurosis can be isolated in the affected upper eyelid through a lid crease incision and separated from preaponeurotic orbital fat according to usual methods. The levator aponeurosis can be repaired or advanced onto the anterior tarsal plate the desired amount, and tempo-

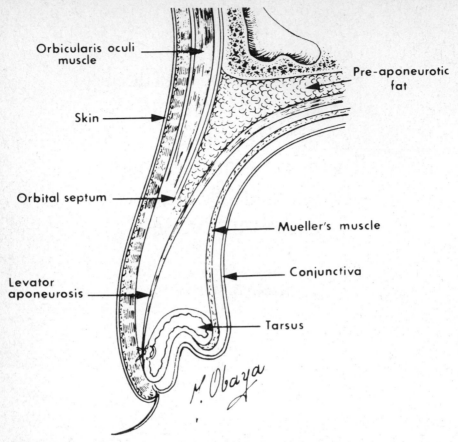

Orbicularis oculi muscle

Pre-aponeurotic fat

Skin

Orbital septum

Mueller's muscle

Conjunctiva

Levator aponeurosis

Tarsus

M. Obaya

Figure 104.1 *Tarsus buckles when levator aponeurosis is attached below vertical center of tarsus.*

rary sutures can be placed in the upper tarsus, approximately 2 mm below the upper edge. If additional elevation is required, the levator aponeurosis should not be advanced further down the tarsal plate (Fig. 104.2).

Instead, the temporary sutures should be removed from the levator aponeurosis. Additional correction, or elevation of the eyelid, should be accomplished by placing the sutures higher in the levator aponeurosis, not by attaching the aponeurosis further down onto the tarsal plate. Fig. 104.3 shows the correction incision and reattachment of the levator aponeurosis to the tarsal plate to avoid vertical tarsal buckling.

BIBLIOGRAPHY

Anderson RL, Dixon RS: Aponeurotic ptosis surgery. *Arch Ophthalmol* 97:1123, 1979.
Anderson RL, Beard C: The levator aponeurosis: Attachments and their clinical significance. *Arch Ophthalmol* 95:1437, 1979.

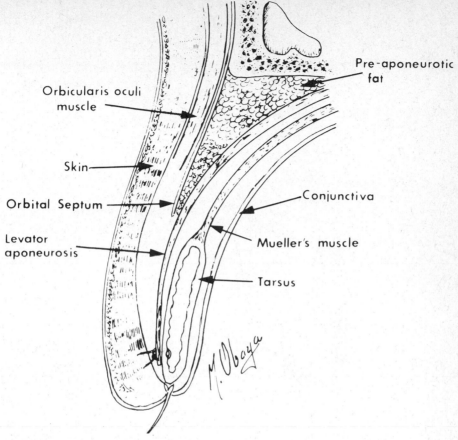

Orbicularis oculi muscle

Skin

Orbital Septum

Levator aponeurosis

Pre-aponeurotic fat

Conjunctiva

Mueller's muscle

Tarsus

M. Obaya

Figure 104.2 *Levator improperly attached to inferior tarsus to provide additional elevation.*

Patipa M, Wilkins RB: Vertical tarsal buckling as a complication of levator aponeurosis repair for acquired blepharoptosis. *Am J Ophthalmol* 97:93, 1984.

Weiss IS, Shorr N: Tarsal buckling after sutureless Fasanella–Servat procedure. *Am J Ophthalmol* 90:377, 1980.

Wilkins RB, Patipa M: The recognition of acquired ptosis in patients considered for upper eyelid blepharoplasty. *Plast Reconstr Surg* 70:431, 1982.

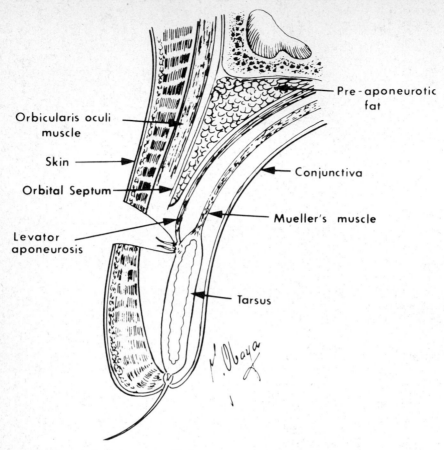

Orbicularis oculi
muscle

Skin

Orbital Septum

Levator
aponeurosis

Pre-aponeurotic
fat

Conjunctiva

Mueller's muscle

Tarsus

Figure 104.3 Levator attached to superior tarsus. If additional elevation is needed, levator aponeurosis should be resected rather than pulling the aponeurosis further down onto the tarsal plate. (Patipa M, Wilkins RB: Vertical tarsal buckling as a complication of levator aponeurosis repair for acquired blepharoptosis. Am J Ophthalmol 97:93–99, 1984. Published with permission from The American Journal of Ophthalmology. Copyright by The Ophthalmic Publishing Company.)

EYELID
RETRACTION

PART VIII

105

Controlled Recession
of Upper Eyelid

Robert G. Small

INTRODUCTION

Several methods have been described to reduce eyelid retraction, but the results are variable and may be asymmetric.

With this technique, the surgeon can adjust the height of the upper eyelid postoperatively.

TECHNIQUE

The upper eyelid is doubly everted over a Desmarres retractor, and the conjunctiva is ballooned with an injection of saline (Fig. 105.1). The conjunctiva is dissected from Müller's muscle down to the upper fornix (Fig. 105.2). Figure 105.3 shows excision of Müller's muscle with the previously freed conjunctiva lying over the cornea. The levator aponeurosis is then freed from the tarsus across the entire extent, as well as medially and laterally from all eyelid attachments (Fig. 105.4).

Two 5-0 nylon mattress sutures are symmetrically placed through the cut edge of the levator and brought through the eyelid at the level of the superior tarsus and out the skin at the superior lid crease (Fig. 105.5). The sutures are passed through a cylindrical segment of rubber cut from the edge of a surgeon's glove. The friction of the rubber against the sutures permits adjustment by drawing the sutures through the bolster until the eyelid is at the desired height (Fig. 105.6).

The dissected conjunctiva is replaced to its normal position at the conclusion of the operation to heal without sutures.

The upper lid can be observed on the operating table and sutures adjusted accordingly. After surgery, when the local anesthetic effect has subsided, the sutures are again adjusted. The medial or lateral eyelid can be raised or lowered by adjusting one suture, or the entire eyelid level can be adjusted.

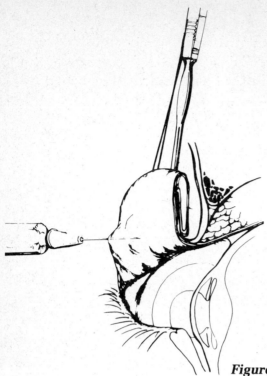

Figure 105.1 Upper eyelid doubled everted

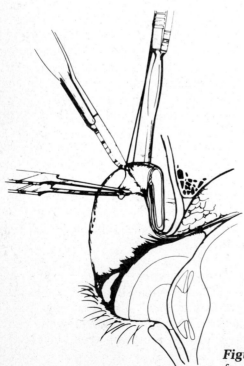

Figure 105.2 Conjunctiva separated from Müller's muscle to fornix.

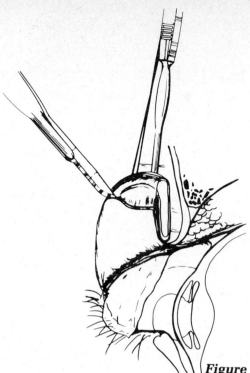

Figure 105.3 Müller's muscle excised.

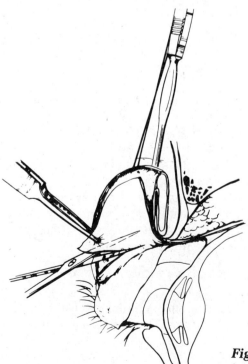

Figure 105.4 Levator aponeurosis
freed from upper tarsus.

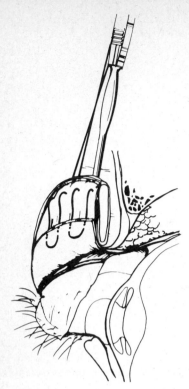

Figure 105.5 *Sutures through edge of levator and out skin crease.*

The best adjustment can be done right after the operation. Postoperative swelling, particularly in patients with thyroid disease, may make later adjustment less satisfactory. Some adjustment can be made one or more days after surgery.

The sutures are removed between the second and third postoperative week. The 4-0 traction suture in the edge of the eyelid to provide downward traction on the lid can be removed after the initial adjustment.

If further adjustment is contemplated, the nylon sutures should be left long and taped to the forehead. If the surgeon is satisfied with the eyelid position, the nylon sutures are tied and cut short.

As with any eyelid procedure, reoperation may be necessary occasionally, but this procedure allows effective postoperative adjustment in eyelid retraction and occasionally for primary ptosis procedures. The author frequently uses the external incision for this procedure.

BIBLIOGRAPHY

Small RG: Controlled recession of the upper eyelid, in Bosniak SL (ed): *Advances in Ophthalmic Plastic and Reconstructive Surgery.* New York, Pergammon Press, 1982, vol. 1, pp 263–274.

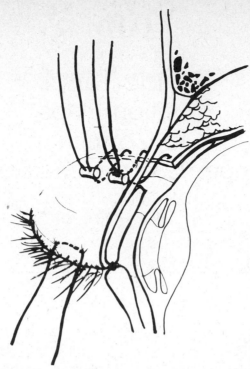

Figure 105.6 Sutures through bolsters for friction. (Reprinted with permission. Small RG: Controlled recession of the upper eyelid. Adv Ophthalmic Plast Reconstr Surg 1:263–274, 1982. Copyright by Pergamon Press, Ltd.)

106

Pedicle Tarsal Rotation Flaps to Correct Upper Eyelid Retraction

Roger Kohn

INTRODUCTION

With the technique described below, the surgeon can correct upper eyelid retraction with two pedicle tarsal rotation flaps that allow the levator aponeurosis to be attached to the tarus directly in a normal anatomic insertion, avoiding the placement of additional foreign or grafted material. This procedure can also be used to correct lower eyelid retraction or overcorrected ptosis.

TECHNIQUE

In cases of upper eyelid retraction (Fig. 106.1) the incision at the desired lid fold is marked with methylene blue and local anesthesia administered at the injection site to provide analgesia without akinesia. The incision is carried through the skin and orbicularis muscle to the anterior tarsal surface (Fig. 106.2). The preseptal orbicularis muscle is separated from the orbital septum. The septum should be opened along its entirety to expose the levator aponeurosis below the preaponeurotic orbital fat.

The levator aponeurosis and underlying Müller's muscle and conjunctiva should be dissected free as one complex. Next, two pedicle flaps are fashioned from the upper border of the tarsus with the bases medially and laterally (Fig. 106.3). The pedicles should be 2 mm wide and curved somewhat centrally for easier rotation. The width between the flaps should be equal to the width of the levator aponeurosis that has been recessed. Conjunctival tissue beneath the tarsal flaps should be removed by sharp dissection.

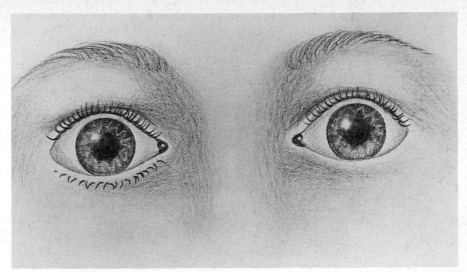

Figure 106.1 Retraction of upper eyelids.

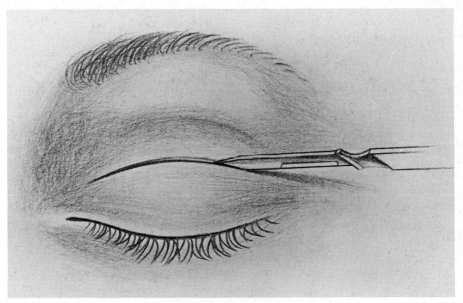

Figure 106.2 Incision at desired lid crease.

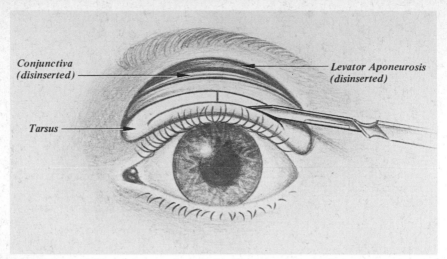

Figure 106.3 Dissection of pedicle flaps and recession of retractors.

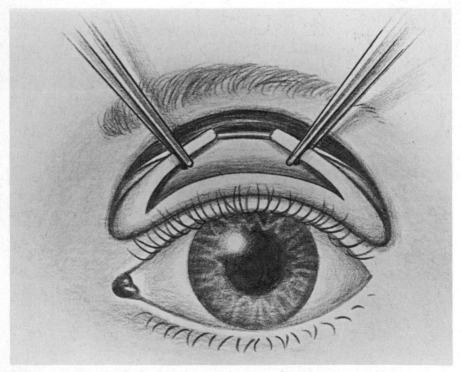

Figure 106.4 Pedicle flaps rotated upward.

340

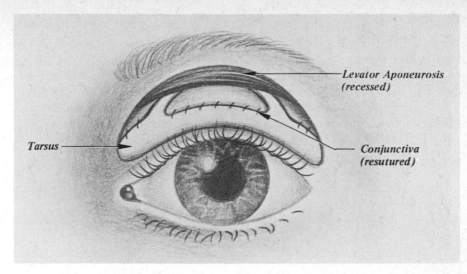

Figure 106.5 Pedicle flaps attached to recessed levator aponeurosis.

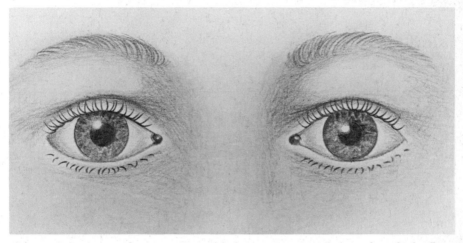

Figure 106.6 Final correction of lid retraction with tarsal pedicle flap. (Kohn R: Pedicle tarsal rotation flaps to correct upper eyelid retraction. Am J Ophthalmol 95:539–544, 1983. Published by The American Journal of Ophthalmology. Copyright by The Ophthalmic Publishing Company.)

In cases of overcorrected ptosis, the conjunctiva should be resutured to the superior tarsal border and the levator aponeurosis should be recessed. In patients with Graves' disease or who have had previous motility surgery, the entire levator aponeurosis and underlying Müller's muscle and conjunctiva are recessed as one complex.

The tarsal pedicles are rotated superiorly (Fig. 106.4) and sutured to each end of the levator aponeurosis or the levator aponeurosis complex with a 6-0 Vicryl mattress suture (Fig. 106.5). Tying temporary knots

341

allows for observation and adjustment of eyelid position. Directing the surgical lights off the patient's eyes allows for more accurate adjustment. The eyelid should be 1 to 2 mm below the recommended position to compensate for mild postoperative contracture. Once the corrected position has been reached, the sutures should be tied permanently and cut. The incision is closed with 7-0 silk running sutures, taking deep bites of the distal levator aponeurosis if an eyelid fold is desired (Fig. 106.6).

BIBLIOGRAPHY

Grove AS: Levator lengthening by marginal myotomy. *Arch Ophthalmol* 98:1433, 1980.

Hamako C, Baylis HI: Lower eyelid retraction after blepharoplasty. *Am J Ophthalmol* 89:517, 1980.

Kohn R: Treatment of eyelid retraction with two pedicle tarsal rotation flaps. *Am J Ophthalmol* 95:539, 1983.

107

Marginal Myotomy of the Levator for Correction of Eyelid Retraction

Arthur S. Grove, Jr.

INTRODUCTION

Upper eyelid retraction, a common feature of ophthalmic Graves' disease, can produce a severe cosmetic deformity and possible ocular injury from corneal exposure. Various surgical procedures have been used to correct upper eyelid retraction (1–4), but the proper amount of division or replacement of the levator, Müller's muscle, or tarsus can be difficult to determine. Frequently, foreign materials or donor sclera must be implanted to recess or lengthen the retractors of the eyelid, which can produce inflammation or damage to the eye. None of the traditional operations correct subcutaneous inflammatory adhesions that form anterior to the levator and contribute to upper eyelid retraction.

The technique below corrects upper eyelid retraction through a skin excision using marginal myotomies similar to strabismus surgery to lengthen the levator aponeurosis and the separation of adhesions between the levator and overlying tissues to correct upper eyelid retraction (5).

TECHNIQUE

The patient should be observed for 6 months or more after treatment of a thyroid disorder before surgical correction of the upper eyelid deformity (Fig. 107.1, upper left) to allow for any variation in upper eyelid position with treatment. The levator marginal myotomy can be performed with local anesthesia. The amount of eyelid lowering should be estimated before surgery.

To correct the eyelid position (Fig. 107.1), a horizontal incision should be made through the skin and orbicularis muscle in the position of the upper eyelid crease. Adhesions between the levator aponeurosis and overlying orbicularis muscle should be divided. With the lid everted,

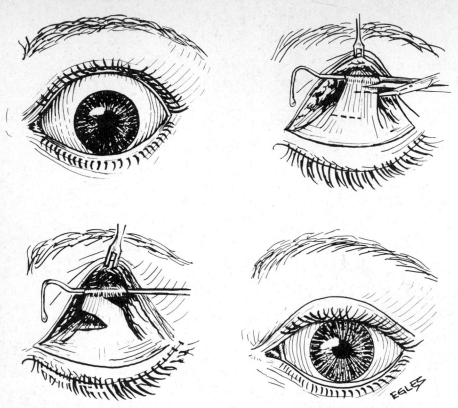

Figure 107.1 *Correction of lid retraction with marginal myotomies.*

local anesthetic with epinephrine can be injected to elevate the conjunctiva from the underlying tissue with good hemostasis. Scissors are passed through a perforation in the mucosa, and a palpebral conjunctiva is dissected from Müller's muscle on the levator aponeurosis. The conjunctival dissection should be carried superiorly for at least 15 mm above the upper tarsal margin. Then the conjunctival perforation can be closed with an absorbable suture with the knot tied away from the eye.

A muscle hook can be passed between the levator muscle/levator aponeurosis and Müller's muscle—palpebral conjunctiva. The levator and Müller's muscle can be pulled downward for additional dissection of the structures free from the orbicularis muscle and orbital septum.

With scissors, a marginal myotomy extending over half the width of the levator aponeurosis and Müller's muscle should be performed in opposite directions at two locations (Fig. 107.1, upper right). The first cut should be placed in one margin several millimeters above the upper edge of the tarsus. The second cut in the opposite direction should be approximately 5 to 10 mm above the first. These incisions must cross the central area of the levator for adequate lengthening to be achieved. The lid is then placed on a stretch downward, and the cuts are extended, if necessary, so that the measured lengthening of the levator is approximately one and a half times the desired amount of lid lowering (Fig. 107.1, lower left). The skin incision can be closed and the upper lid held downward for 1 to 2 days by suture, taped, or sewn to the lower lid or cheek. In the early postoperative period, the upper lid can be expected to be ptotic, after which it will rise to a stable position (Fig. 107.1, lower right).

This procedure allows for correction of upper eyelid retraction with a one-stage graded procedure that does not require the insertion of any foreign material.

REFERENCES

1. Putterman AM, Urist M: Surgical treatment of upper eyelid retraction. *Arch Ophthalmol* 87:401, 1972.
2. Chalfin J, Putterman AM: Müller's muscle excision and levator recession in retracted upper lid: Treatment of thyroid-related retraction. *Arch Ophthalmol* 97:1487, 1979.
3. Baylis HI, Cies WA, Kamin DF: Correction of upper eyelid retraction. *Am J Ophthalmol* 82:790, 1976.
4. Flanagan JC: Eyebank sclera in oculoplastic surgery. *Ophthalmic Surg* 5:45, 1974.
5. Grove AS Jr: Eyelid retraction treated by levator marginal myotomy. *Ophthalmology* 10:1013, 1980.

RECONSTRUCTION

PART IX

108

Cilia Transplantation to Reconstruct Eyelashes

Thomas C. Naugle, Jr.
Delmar R. Caldwell

INTRODUCTION

When eyelashes are lost as a result of injury, infection, tumor removal or inadvertently from ptosis surgery, traditional methods correct the defect are frequently unsatisfactory. False eyelashes can cover a defect, but most men will not use them, and many women find false eyelashes cumbersome. A full-thickness lid resection with primary closure can eliminate smaller gaps in eyelashes (1–4), but more extensive defects require transplantation of hair from the brow, or other areas. Such grafts do not match well, and the hair frequently is misdirected on the eyelid margin.

With the technique below, the surgeon can transplant either a strip of lashes or individual lashes from the lateral aspect to the patient's upper and lower eyelids to fill the defective area with transplanted lashes that have a pleasing appearance with the lash growing in the proper direction.

TECHNIQUE

Each patient must be evaluated to determine whether individual follicles, segments of follicles, or a combination should be used to fill the particular defect. This procedure transfers cilia from relatively plentiful inconspicious area to the prime areas of cosmetic defect.

When a strip of lashes is to be transplanted, methylene blue is used to outline approximately 3 to 4 mm of lashes in the lateral canthal areas to be transplanted to the central defect (Fig. 108.1). The strips can be taken from the lateral areas of all four lids. A local anesthetic with epinephrine should be injected for hemostasis. Using the microscope, a number 75 Beaver blade is used to carry an incision around the lashes to be transplanted, leaving a margin of approximately 0.5 mm to allow for suturing of the segment or the individual cilia (Fig. 108.2). Disection is carried

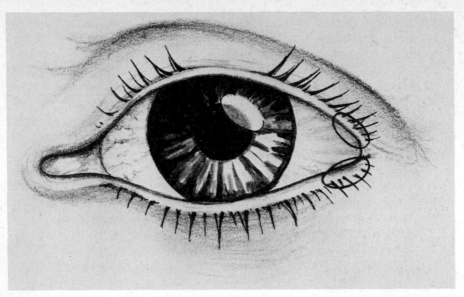

Figure 108.1 Central lash defect to be reconstructed with grafts from the lateral lids.

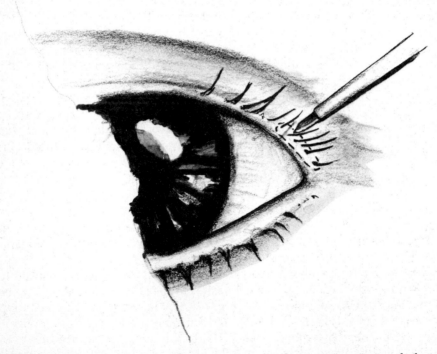

Figure 108.2 Number 75 blade used to make incision around donor lashes.

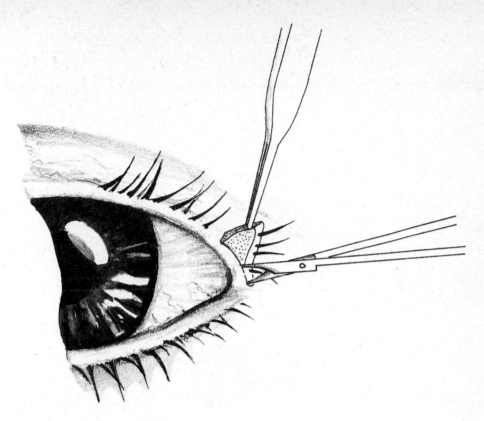

Figure 108.3 *Scissors dissecting lash segment without injury to bulb roots.*

beneath the root bulbs using Westcott scissors with meticulous care to avoid injury to the follicle (Fig. 108.3).

The segment of follicles (Fig. 108.4A) is transferred to balanced salt solution in the Petri dish. The donor site can be allowed to heal by secondary intention.

The recipient area should be marked with methylene blue (Fig. 108.4B) before injecting local anesthetic with epinephrine. If the strip is to be implanted, a plug of lid margin approximately the same size as the graft should be excised with the number 15 blade and Westcott scissors. The segment of lashes can then be placed into the defect (Fig. 108.4C) and secured with 9-0 monofilament nylon (Fig. 108.4D). To avoid injuring vessels necessary to support the transplanted lashes, hemostasis should be obtained with simple pressure, Surgicel, or topical thrombin rather than cautery to the recipient site.

Postoperative care consists of antibiotic drops. A shield should be placed over the eye so patients do not rub the grafts out at night. Pressure patches tend to distort the newly placed cilia. Sutures can be removed from the skin margins at 7 to 10 days. To remove hard crusting, the

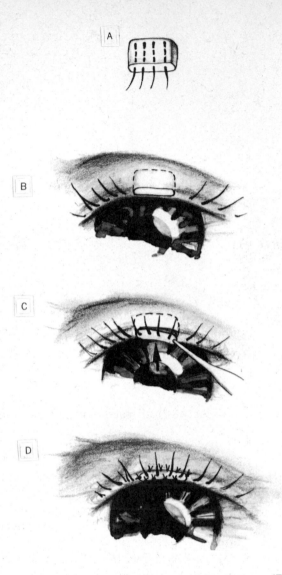

Figure 108.4 *(A) Lash segment for transplantation. (B) Recipient site prepared. (C) Lash segment placed into defect. (D) Lash graft secured with 9-0 nylon sutures.*

surgeon should cut the terminal portions of transplanted follicles. Pulling the crust with forceps might damage the graft. The cut lashes will regrow within 2 to 3 weeks.

A variation in this technique can be used when individual lashes are to be inserted. The surgeon places methylene blue dots in between the skin and tarsal plate approximately 1 mm apart at the desired recipient site. The donor strip of lashes (Fig. 108.5) is placed under the operating micro-

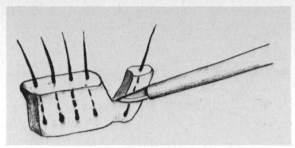

Figure 108.5 *Alternate technique of separating individual lashes.*

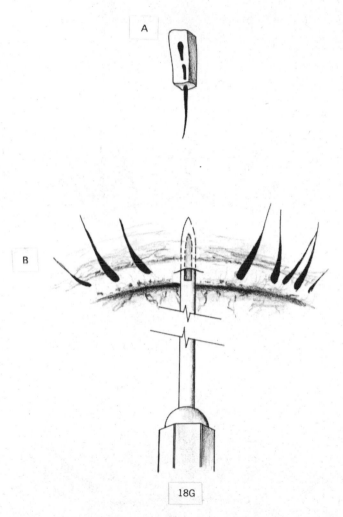

A

B

18G

Figure 108.6 *(A) Individual lash for transplant. (B) An 18-gauge needle placed into lid in the same configuration as normal lashes.*

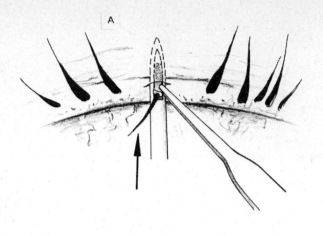

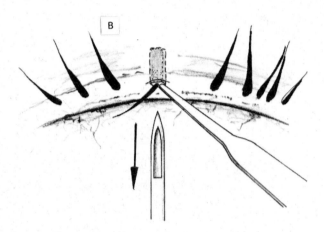

Figure 108.7 (A) Single graft inserted through needle bevel. (B) Graft fixated as needle removed.

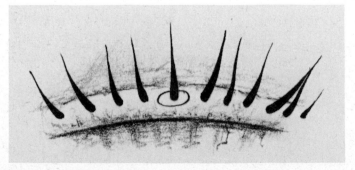

Figure 108.8 Final appearance of transplanted cilia.

scope. With meticulous dissection using a number 75 Beaver blade, individual hair follicles are prepared (Fig. 108.5).

An 18-gauge needle is pushed into the lid margin in an arching fashion up to the end of the bevel to serve as a guide for the individual donor cilia (Figs. 108.6A and B). The needle is then retracted to expose enough of the bevel to allow insertion of a single cilia using a jeweler's forcep (Fig. 108.7A). With the graft held flush against the recipient skin, the needle is removed (Fig. 108.7B). After proper alignment, the cilia can be left in the recipient site without suturing (Fig. 108.8), and postoperative care can be carried out as with strips of lashes described above. Realignment of the follicles with forceps may be necessary for several weeks. Later, individual follicles can be used to embellish a segment graft.

With this technique the surgeon can reconstruct the lash line using autogenous cilia that have appearance and function far exceeding any other transplanted hairs. The reconstructed lids have a much more normal appearance than with other methods. A 12 to 14 mm defect can be filled directly and perhaps another 7 mm reconstructed with a wedge full-thickness eyelid resection of an involved segment.

Patients should be cautioned to wear a shield at night so lash grafts will not be mechanically debreeded during sleep for several weeks.

This technique uses a rearrangement of the patient's existing lashes from inconspicuous areas into the prime cosmetic areas. Other enchancing cosmetic techniques such as permanent or temporary eyeliner can be used to supplement this procedure.

REFERENCES

1. Smith B, Cherubini T: *Oculoplastic Surgery*, ed 1. St. Louis, Mosby, 1970, pp 10, 11.
2. Reeh MJ, Beyer CK, Shannon GM: *Practical Ophthalmic Plastic and Reconstructive Surgery.* Philadelphia, Lea & Febiger, 1976, p 65.
3. Callahan MA, Callahan A: *Ophthalmic Plastic and Orbital Surgery.* Birmingham, Aesculapius, 1979, pp 77, 78.
4. Krusius FP: Transplant of living hair from the formation of lashes. *Deutsche Medizinshe Vochenschrit* 40:958, 1914.

109

Full-Thickness Eyebrow Graft

Frank P. English
Timothy D. C. Forster

INTRODUCTION

Loss of eyebrow tissue from trauma or resection of large tumors creates a problem for reconstruction, especially with a circular or oval defect. The full-thickness eyebrow graft from the contralateral eyelid technique, as described below, can be used for eyebrow reconstruction with appropriate match of skin thickness, hair texture, and eyebrow orientation.

TECHNIQUE

The surgeon should evaluate the likely donor site of the opposite eyelid for appropriate size and for proper orientation of the vibrissae such that all hair of the brow will grow in the same direction (Fig. 109.1). The donor site should be outlined with a marking pencil and incised with a large Bard–Parker blade and excised, undermining with Westcott scissors. Compression with thumb and fingers helps to produce a bloodless field during the initial incision. The graft should be taken with sufficient depth, avoiding damage to the hair roots.

After excision, the graft should be rotated so the cilia are oriented in the correct direction (Fig. 109.2). The graft should be sewn in place with interrupted 6-0 silk sutures (Fig. 109.3). If the defect extends out of the brow, the nearby hairless skin should be undermined and brought without tension in juxtaposition to the graft, and the donor site in the opposite eyelid should be closed. Excessive pressure should not be applied with a dressing. The viability of the graft can be accessed at the time of suture removal. Hair growth can be seen after some weeks into the postoperative course.

This technique provides for reconstruction of defects in the eyebrow through the proper orientation of matched tissue from the opposite eyebrow.

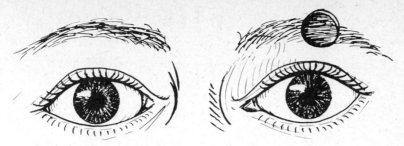

Figure 109.1   Left eyebrow defect.

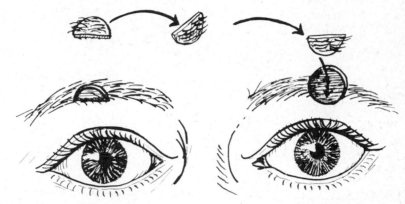

Figure 109.2   Full-thickness graft rotated for proper orientation.

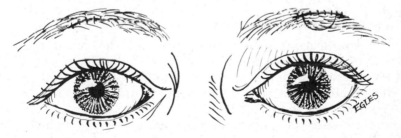

Figure 109.3   Graft secured and donor site closed. (Reprinted with permission. Ophthalmic Surgery 10:39–41, 1979.)

BIBLIOGRAPHY

English FP, Forster TDC: The eyebrow graft. *Ophthalmic Surg* 7:39, 1979.

110

Punch Hair Graft
for Eyebrow Reconstruction

Jeffrey C. Popp

INTRODUCTION

The punch hair graft technique can be used in the office as a primary procedure for reconstruction or to fill in where island flaps or strip grafts have previously failed.

TECHNIQUE

The brow region to be grafted should be outlined with a marking pen for appearance and symmetry with the opposite brow (Fig. 110.1). Recipient "punch sites" are marked with the pen with 3.5 mm between each mark for adequate spacing to avoid ischemia and possible graft failure.

By shaving the donor scalp region but leaving 1 to 2 mm of stubble, the direction of hair growth remains readily apparent. Donor and recipient sites are infiltrated with local anesthetic with epinephrine, and the recipient site is prepared using a 3.5-mm punch to remove tissue over the previous markings (Fig. 110.2).

Grafts are taken from the donor scalp site, taking care to maintain the direction of hair growth (Fig. 110.3). Excess subcutaneous fat can be trimmed, but hair follicles should not be disturbed. The donor punch grafts are gently placed into the recipient bed, maintaining the direction of the natural hair growth in a lateral direction (Fig. 110.4). Without suturing, the grafts are secured with the pressure dressing over adaptive gauze for 48 hours. Bare areas between grafts can be filled with additional grafting in as early as 3 weeks.

The punch grafts will give a "cobblestone" texture to the skin surface, which can be dermabraded once the complete brow has been reconstructed.

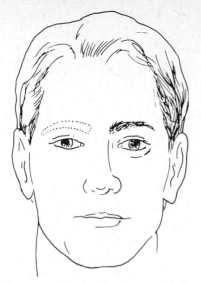

Figure 110.1 Eyebrow defect outlined.

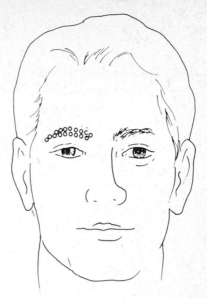

Figure 110.2 Recipient sites spaced to provide vascular supply around donor plugs.

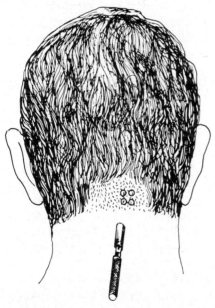

Figure 110.3 Leaving 1 to 2 mm of stubble when shaving the donor site allows for direction of hair growth to be easily determined.

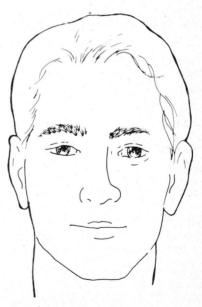

Figure 110.4 Proper orientation of donor plug stubble gives natural growth of brow hair in lateral direction.

111

Lamellar Tarsoplasty
for Correction
of Horizontal Tarsal Kink

Rodney W. McCarthy

INTRODUCTION

The tarsal kink syndrome is a severe form of congenital entropion most commonly seen in the upper lid. A marked horizontal kink encompassing the entire tarsal plate causes inversion of the lid margin and trichiasis. The child may be irritable and develop blepharospasm. The lid crease and lid fold are absent. Severe corneal ulceration may occur before establishing the correct diagnosis.

By dissecting a lamella of the abnormal tarsus, which is then sutured in reverse fashion to the tarsus, the forces of the abnormal tarsal segment can be used to correct the condition.

TECHNIQUE

The technique is designed to create a properly contoured tarsal plate (Fig. 111.1, left) from the lid with the tarsal kink (Fig. 111.1, right). The lid crease incision is made symmetric to the opposite lid, and dissection is carried through the orbicularis muscle on the levator aponeurosis inferiorly to obtain visualization of the entire tarsal plate to the level of the cilia follicles (Fig. 111.2).

With use of microsurgical techniques, a one-half thickness lamellar dissection is carried out extending from 1 mm below the superior tarsal margin inferiorly to just above the cilia follicles. The excised lamellar tissue is then reversed and repositioned in the tarsal bed to be fixed with absorbable sutures. Skin closure with crease formation is completed in the routine fashion.

The lamellar tarsoplasty is performed to reverse 50% of the vector forces that are causing the acutely angled tarsal kink (Fig. 111.3). By

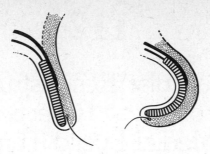

Figure 111.1 (Left) normal. (Right) Lid buckled with tarsal kink.

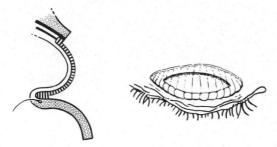

Figure 111.2 (Left) Dissection anterior to tarsus. (Right) Anterior view.

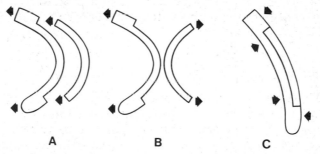

Figure 111.3 (A) Lamellar dissection. (B) Lamellar graft reversed. (C) Extreme forces neutralize tarsal kink. (Reprinted with permission. Ophthalmic Surgery 15:859–860, 1984.)

reversing the dissected lamellar tissue, equal and opposing forces are created, thereby reducing the congenital deformity. This procedure is applicable to unilateral or bilateral cases. The surgeon may apply this to any degree of kinking. Violation of the conjunctival surface is unnecessary. This procedure does not result in overcorrection.

BIBLIOGRAPHY

McCarthy RW: Lamellar tarsoplasty: A new technique for correction of horizontal tarsal kink. *Ophthalmic Surg* 15:859, 1984.

112

Canalicular Reconstruction Following Resection of Medial Eyelid Tumors

Jay Justin Older

INTRODUCTION

To excise an eyelid carcinoma completely at the medial aspect of the upper or lower eyelid, several millimeters of the lateral aspect of the canaliculus may have to be sacrificed. With a procedure to reconstruct the remainder of the canaliculus with good tear drainage, the surgeon can resect the tumor without fear of "cutting too close" to the canaliculus.

TECHNIQUE

Once the tumor has been excised and the margins read as free of tumor by microscopic examination, the canalicular reconstruction can be started. One jaw of a scissor is placed within the canaliculus, and the canaliculus is opened for about 2 mm on the posterior superior aspect (Fig. 112.1). With a small absorbable suture, such as 7-0 chromic, the cut ends of the canaliculus are sewn so that they will remain open. The anterior edge is sewn near the skin margin, and the posterior edge is sewn to the conjunctival surface of the eyelid or to an area near the caruncle.

The reconstruction of the eyelid can now be completed. If there is a large defect in the lid and a modified Hughes' procedure is required, this should be done with the medial aspect of the tarsoconjunctival flap being sewn to the tissue inferior and posterior to the remains of the canaliculus. This tissue is firm and is the extension of the medial canthal tendon. The skin surface of the reconstructed lid can now be fashioned either with a free graft or with skin advanced from the area inferior to the resected tumor.

The opened canaliculus must remain uncovered. If reconstruction can be accomplished by advancing the lateral aspect of the lid toward the medial aspect, then the tarsus in the remaining lateral part of the lid

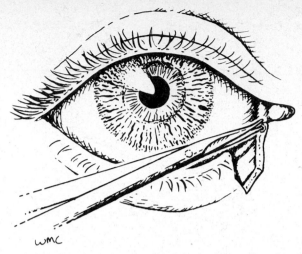

Figure 112.1 After tumor removal remaining canaliculus is incised.

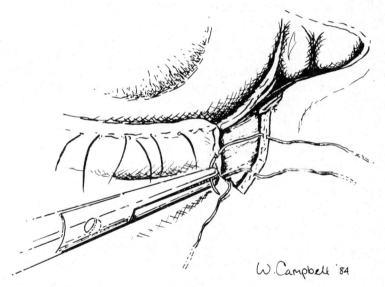

Figure 112.2 Canaliculus stitched open to drain tears.

should be tied to the extension of the inferior horn of the medial canthal tendon using absorbable sutures (Fig. 112.2). The skin margins should also be approximated leaving the open canaliculus uncovered.

Once the eyelid reconstruction has been completed, a silicone tube (size 0.012 inches inside diameter times 0.025 inches outside diameter, Storz catalog number N5941-1) is passed into the canaliculus. In some cases, the silicone tube will only pass 8 to 9 mm into the canaliculus, and, in some cases, it will pass into the lacrimal sac and perhaps even turn down toward the nasolacrimal canal.

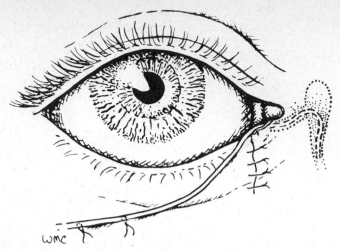

Figure 112.3 *A silicone tube in canaliculus stitched to eyelid.*

The object is to pass the tube as far as possible through the nasolacrimal system using a hand-over-hand maneuver with forceps to push the tube into the canaliculus. If this maneuver is unsuccessful, then the tube can be attached to the back of a Quickert probe, passed through the remains of the canaliculus, through the nasolacrimal canal, and out the nose. Metal probes with silicone tubing attached, such as the Crawford intubation set are commercially available.

After the probe is brought out the nose, the tube is cut free of the probe and pulled back so that the tube end is within the nasolacrimal canal. The part of the tube which extends beyond the canaliculus onto the face is then stitched to the adjacent eyelid using interrupted 6-0 silk sutures on a sharp needle (Fig. 112.3). The suture is passed through the skin and around the tube, and the tube is tied firmly to the skin.

If a small enough needle is used, the needle may be passed through the tube, and in this way it can attach the tube to the skin. The end of the tube may be tied in a knot to prevent the unlikely possibility of the tube migrating into the canaliculus as sutures pull loose. The tube is left in place for 1 to 2 weeks and then removed.

BIBLIOGRAPHY

Kraft SP, Crawford JS: Silicone tube intubation in disorders of the lacrimal system in children. *Am J Ophthalmol* 94:290, 1982.

Older JJ: Treatment of the lacrimal excretory system after resection of medial canthal and eyelid tumors. *Ophthalmic Surg* 10:29, 1979.

Quckert MH, Dryden RM: Probes for intubation in lacrimal drainage. *Trans Am Acad Ophthalmol Otolaryngol,* 74:431, 1970.

113

Medial Conjunctival Reconstruction

Peter A. Rogers

INTRODUCTION

Large defects of the medial conjunctiva that occur following excision of lesions such as malignant melanoma of the semilunar (Fig. 113.1A) fold cause difficulty in reforming adequately the medical cul-de-sacs of the upper and lower eyelids. Free conjunctival grafts can provide coverage, but fixation of the graft to form the medial fornix presents a difficult problem.

By recessing the medial bulbar conjunctiva from the limbus as in strabismus surgery, the cul-de-sacs can be reformed with bulbar conjunctiva and the donor defect covered with a free grafts or adjacent bulbar conjunctiva.

TECHNIQUE

Figure 113.1B shows the defect to be constructed. A peritomy is performed at the medial conjunctiva with two relaxing incisions carried medially from near the superior and inferior limbus. The conjunctiva between the limbus and lateral edge of the defect is undermined thus allowing the conjunctival edge to be approximated to the most medial cut edge of conjunctiva. The undermined flap of conjunctiva from the limbus moves medially leaving a defect over the limbus and medial rectus muscle (Fig. 113.1C).

The original defect is closed with sutures of 6-0 plain catgut, and the conjunctiva immediately lateral to the suture line is "tucked in" to provide the cul-de-sacs of the medial ends of the upper and lower lids.

Two methods work well to close the donor defect on the globe. A free conjunctival graft from the superior supratarsal area can be sutured to the conjunctival and episclera (Fig. 113.1D). Or, the edges of the conjunctiva can be brought together over the medial rectus muscle with the limbal area left to granulate (Fig. 113.1E).

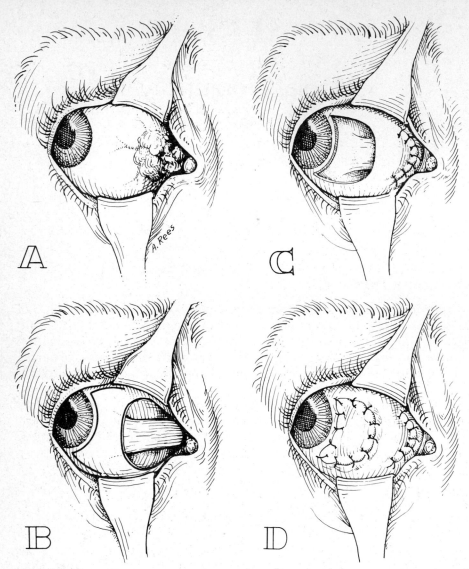

Figure 113.1   (A) Medial conjunctival lesion to be excised. (B) Peritomy to advance conjunctiva over medial defect. (C) Defect closed creating bare area on globe. (D) Donor site covered with free conjunctival graft.

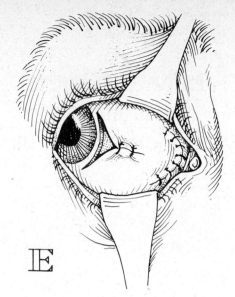

(E) Alternatively: direct closure.

114

Lateral Canthal Reconstruction with Periosteal Flaps

Murray A. Meltzer

INTRODUCTION

Methods to reconstruct the lateral canthus generally involve soft tissue manipulation, which provides unstable long-term results, or techniques that use involved drilling and wiring techniques at the lateral canthus. Using crossed strips of periosteum from the lateral orbital rim, the lateral canthus can be reconstructed with a natural appearance and contour.

TECHNIQUE

With stretching of the lateral canthal tendons, shortening of the horizontal fissure with rounding of the lateral canthus can occur (Fig. 114.1). A repair can be achieved by performing a generous canthotomy and exposure of the periosteum of the lateral orbital rim. Methylene blue should be used to outline two flaps (5 × 10 mm) of periosteum based posteriorly into the orbit. The flaps should angle outward and upward as shown (Fig. 114.2) in the shape of a "Y" with a strip of intact periosteum remaining between the arms of the "Y." The flaps should be incised and freed. Next, the flaps should be crossed and fIxed to the remnants of lateral canthal tendon or tarsal plate with permanent sutures (Fig. 114.3). A central fixation suture placed where the two flaps are crossed (Fig. 114.4) is passed through the strip of intact periosteum at the lateral orbital rim to tighten the new lateral canthal tendon.

With the periosteal flaps based posteriorly and crossed, a normal posterior upward pull is provided to the lower lid and a downward inward pull provided to the upper lid.

Postoperatively, a normal canthal position and angle will be established using these firm strips of periosteum (Fig. 114.5). The technique avoids extensive dissections and intricate wiring or bone fixation, which may otherwise be required to provide a lasting result.

368

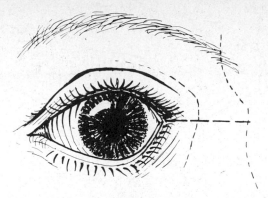

Figure 114.1 Medial displacement and rounding of the lateral canthus.

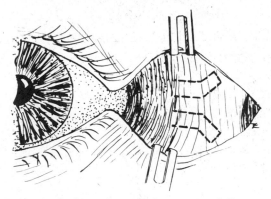

Figure 114.2 Posteriorly based angled periosteal flaps.

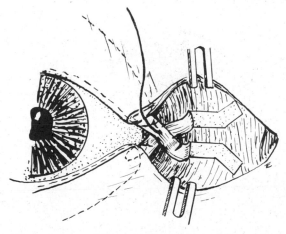

Figure 114.3 Flaps are mobilized, crossed, and fixed to lateral lid segment.

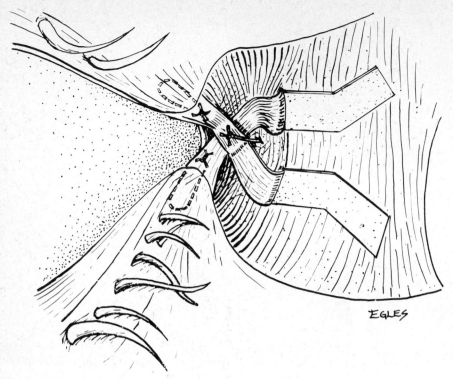

Figure 114.4 Fixation of flaps.

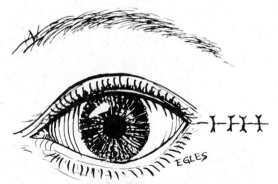

Figure 114.5 Normal position and angle of reconstructed canthus.

115

Tarsal Pedicle Flap for Lower Eyelid Reconstruction

Charles R. Leone, Jr.
John V. Van Germet

INTRODUCTION

The traditional Mustarde method of lower eyelid reconstruction (1,2) uses a temporal-zygomatic skin flap and nasal septal cartilage with nasal mucosa to provide the anterior and posterior layers of the new eyelid (3).

The use of a tarsal pedicle flap for lower eyelid reconstruction (4) avoids the necessity of taking nasal septal cartilage, and the flap acts as a hinge to hold up the temporal part of the flap that might otherwise sag downward as frequently has been a problem at the lateral canthus.

TECHNIQUE

To reconstruct the defect, a temporal flap is fashioned from the lateral canthus following the extension of the curve of the lower eyelid over the zygomatic arch toward the ear. The lid defect should be created as shown (Fig. 115.1, left). The flap is undermined to rotate easily into the defect with the incision taken as far toward the ear as necessary.

To create the tarsal pedicle flap, the upper eyelid is everted. An incision splits the lateral 2.5 to 3 mm of the upper eyelid is carried to the superior tarsal border. The horizontal aspect of the flap begins 2 mm from the lid margin, cutting full-thickness tarsus as far medially as necessary to fill the lower lid defect. This incision is carried then vertically 4 mm, then back horizontally to the lateral canthus creating a flap similar to a sideways letter "T" with a conjunctival attachment to the superior cul-de-sac.

The tarsal flap is separated from the overlying orbicularis muscle and the vertical part of the flap pulled into the lower eyelid defect and sutured through the skin flat with a double-armed 4-0 silk suture over a silicone

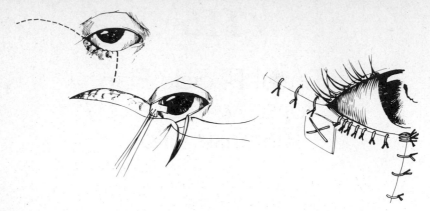

Figure 115.1 T-shaped tarsal pedicle flap from upper eyelid for lower eyelid reconstruction.

peg or sutured to the conjunctival remanant in the inferior cul-de-sac with interrupted 6-0 chromic catgut (Fig. 115.1, center). The horizontal arm is connected to the tarsus of the medial lid segment as well as the conjunctiva of the inferior cul-de-sac with interrupted 6-0 chromic catgut with the knots on the anterior surface. Skin edges are sutured to the marginal aspect of the tarsal graft with interrupted 6-0 silk sutures. The tarsal defect in the upper eyelid is left unsutured.

A buried 4-0 silk suture is used to suspend the temporal skin flap to the periosteum above the level of the lateral canthus, and the remainder of the skin closure is carried out with 5-0 silk (Fig. 115.1, right). Skin sutures are removed in 7 days, and the double-armed silk vertical hinge suture is removed from the tarsus in 12 days.

Despite surgical shortening of the horizontal fissure, little difference in appearance can be appreciated between the two fissures. This procedure provides an upward curvature of the lateral aspect of the lower eyelid with a sharp lateral canthal angle, two problems that are very difficult to avoid with the Mustarde technique.

REFERENCES

1. Mustarde JC: Repair and reconstruction in the orbital region. Baltimore, Williams & Wilkins, 1966, pp 116–162.
2. Mustarde JC: Problems in eyelid reconstruction. *Ann Ophthalmol* 4:883, 1974.
3. Leone CR Jr: Nasal septal cartilage for eyelid reconstruction. *Ophthalmic Surg* 4:68, 1974.
4. Leone CR Jr: Tarsal pedicle flap for lower eyelid reconstruction. *Arch Ophthalmol* 95:1423, 1977.

116

Modification of the Hughes Flap to Prevent Upper Eyelid Complications of Entropion, Retraction, and Loss of Lashes

Wendell L. Hughes

INTRODUCTION

The Hughes flap can be used as a dependable method to reconstruct even total lower eyelid defects without complications of late lower lid contraction, as seen in horizontal sliding flaps. The complications of this flap usually arise from the internal layer from the upper lid: permanent loss of upper eyelid lashes, retraction of the upper eyelid, and entropion of the upper lid.

The surgeon can avoid these complications by using the modifications in the Hughes flap, as described below.

TECHNIQUE

The original Hughes flap technique provides a tarsal conjunctival layer by splitting the lid midway between the anterior and posterior borders with the incision carried superiorly to include the Müller's muscle as a vascular base for the flap (Fig. 116.1A, left). The root bulbs of the lashes are frequently injured as they can extend into the substance or even surface of the tarsal plate. Splitting the lid margin can lead to an inward contraction of the upper lid margin causing entropion and irritation after separation of the Hughes flap (Fig. 116.1A, right). These modifications avoid the problems mentioned above.

First, with the lid everted, an oblique incision should be made through the tarsus beginning at the conjunctival margin and coming to the anterior surface of the tarsus approximately 3 mm above the lid margin (Fig.

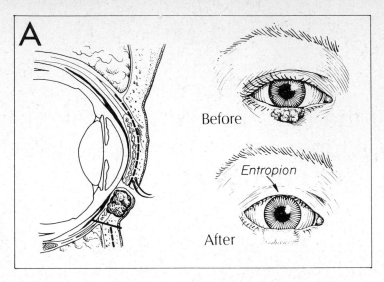

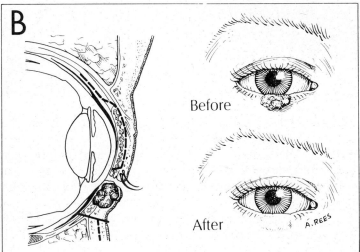

Figure 116.1 *Hughes flap (A) modified to avoid complications (B).*

116.1B, left). This incision leaves a thin border of tarsus to be joined at the lower fornix conjunctiva providing a smoother union to complete the inner layer of the reconstructed lower lid. The incision inside the upper lid as opposed to splitting the gray line provides stability to the upper lid and prevents entropion. Also, the lash follicles are not involved, thus preventing loss of upper lid lashes (Fig. 116.1B, right). Cementing the lashes upward against the skin of the upper lid helps to ensure a normal direction of the lash root.

As another important modification, the surgeon should fashion the tarsoconjunctival flap such that the dissection, on reaching the superior tarsal plate, should include only conjunctiva and not the Müller's muscle.

374

The incision is extended upward in a plane between the conjunctiva and Müller's muscle, which can be facilitated by putting a lid plate into the upper conjunctival fornix. The incision should be far enough to allow the tarsoconjunctival flap to extend without tension into the lower lid defect. The conjunctiva can be easily retracted into the defect, but conjunctiva and muller's cannot.

When the Müller's muscle is left attached to the tarsoconjunctival flap, lid retraction can result at the time of separation (Fig. 116.1A, right). When only conjunctiva attaches to the superior portion of the flap, the lid maintains a normal position without retraction (Fig. 116.1B, right). Fashioning the flap section too narrow horizontally is better than one too wide to provide a tight lower lid rather than one with sagging laxity.

The technique described above allows the surgeon to rebuild a functional, cosmetically pleasing lower lid avoiding problems in the upper eyelids, such as retraction, entropion, or loss of lashes.

BIBLIOGRAPHY

Hughes WL: A new method for rebuilding a lower lid: Report of a case. *Arch Ophthalmol* 17:1008, 1937.

Hughes WL: Total lower lid reconstruction: Technical details. *Trans Am Ophthalmol Soc* 74:321, 1976.

117

Semicircular Skin Flap for Reconstruction

Allen M. Putterman

INTRODUCTION

Reconstruction of large defects in the eyelids generally requires skin grafts. With the semicircular skin flap technique, defects of upper and lower eyelids approaching a 50% loss of eyelid skin can be closed satisfactorily without subsequent ectropion.

The technique uses the geometric principle that the distance in a semicircle exceeds that of a straight line. The semicircular skin flap provides an abundance of skin as the small flap straightens and slides to fill the defect.

TECHNIQUE

Figure 117.1 (top) shows the outline of the defect that will be created after removal of the tumor. To provide skin coverage, an infralash incision is drawn from the nasal aspect of the ellipse closest to the eyelid margin and across the eyelid within 2 mm of the lid margin to the lateral canthus. At this point a semicircular line is then drawn from the temporal aspect of the first line, curving in a convex-upward position for lower eyelid skin replacement. (A convex-downward configuration can be used for upper eyelid defects).

The semicircle should extend to the temporal end of the eyebrow and come down laterally to a point on a horizontal level with the lateral canthus.

After local infiltration of 2% lidocaine with epinephrine (1:100,000) for anesthesia and hemostasis, the skin incision is performed. A sharp-pointed scissors is used to undermine the skin from the underlying orbicularis oculi muscle in a temporal and nasal direction to the tumor excision, including the lateral canthal semicircle. To facilitate dissection and prevent skin buttonholing, the surgeon should observe the scissor blades through the translucent skin.

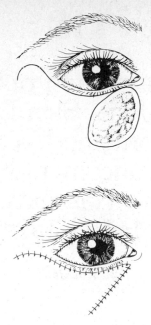

Figure 117.1 Large defect from tumor (above) reconstructed with semicircular skin flap (below). (Putterman AM: Semicircular skin flap in reconstruction of nonmarginal eyelid skin defects. Am J Ophthalmol 84:708–710, 1977. Published by The American Journal of Ophthalmology. Copyright by The Ophthalmic Publishing Company.)

First, the elliptical defect from the tumor is closed with 6-0 black silk suture. Then the flap is closed with 6-0 black silk from nasal to temporal eyelid margin, continuing with the semicircular area (Fig. 117.1, bottom).

If the wound seems to close with a great deal of tension, interrupted rather than continuous sutures can be used.

Tension can be further relieved with 4-0 black silk mattress sutures tied over cotton pledgets in areas of excessive stress. A light pressure dressing should be applied for 24 hours, and skin sutures should be removed in 5 to 7 days.

BIBLIOGRAPHY

Putterman AM: Semicircular skin flap in reconstruction of nonmarginal eyelid skin defects. *Am J Ophthalmol* 84:708, 1977.

118

Reconstruction of Large Nasal-Jugal Skin Defects with Combined Temporal Advancement Flap and a Nasolacrimal Free Graft

M. Kim Jack

INTRODUCTION

With defects extending past the nasal-jugal fold, the lateral canthal flap cannot bring in skin of the proper thickness. The dermal-epidermal thickness of the area extending down the nose varies from the eyelid skin with a thickness of 1 mm to nasal skin as thick as 3 mm. The nasal-jugal furrow demarks the boundary between the thin skin and subcutaneous tissues of the lid and the thick skin and subcutaneous tissue of the nose and cheek (Fig. 118.1).

Defects in this area, consequently, require flaps and grafts of skin that match the adjacent tissue according to the skin thickness. The technique below avoids the disadvantage of distant forehead flaps or the mismatch of skin from adjacent sliding flaps.

TECHNIQUE

A large defect crossing the nasal-jugal furrow can be reconstructed by first mobilizing a lateral semicircular skin flap (Fig. 118.2) to cover the upper portion with thin skin. To close the remaining portion, an adjacent "Lazy S" nasal-labial graft can be rotated into the remaining defect (Fig. 118.3). With the rotational flap in place, the donor defect from below can be closed and the transposition secured with dental roll and sutures (Fig. 118.4).

378

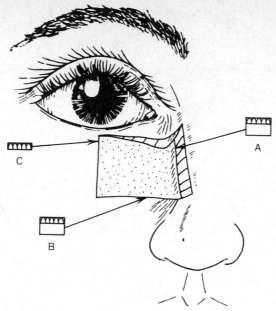

Figure 118.1 Nasal-jugal defects involve skin with different thicknesses.

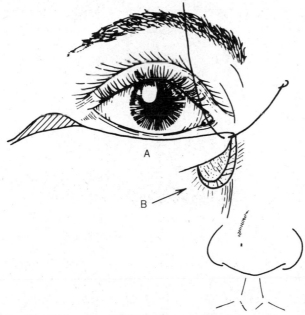

Figure 118.2 Semicircular skin flap mobilized to cover defect in thin skin.

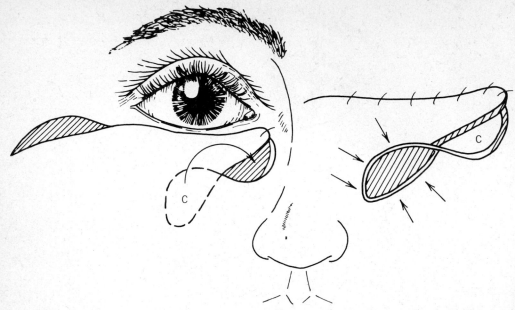

Figure 118.3 Lazy-S nasal-labial graft rotated to match thicker skin.

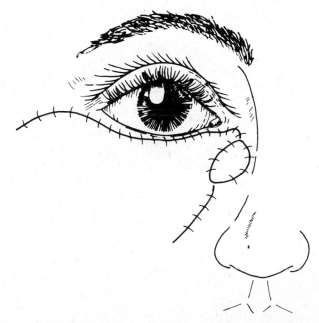

Figure 118.4 Closure of defect and Lazy-S defect. (Reprinted with permission. Ophthalmic Surgery 11:392–394, 1980.)

This flap should be used with lesions crossing the nasal-labial furrow. Mobilizing the thin skin of the eyelid and rotating the thicker skin of the cheek solves the problem of skin mismatch and avoids extensive procedures previously used for reconstructive reasons.

BIBLIOGRAPHY

Jack MK: Reconstruction of a large nasal-jugal skin defect utilizing a combined temporal advancement flap and a nasolacrimal free graft. *Ophthalmic Surg* 11:392, 1980.

Putterman AM: Semicircular skin flap and reconstruction of eyelid nonmarginal skin defects. *Am J Ophthalmol* 84:708, 1977.

Smith B: Eyelid Surgery. *Surg Clin N Am* 39:10, 1959.

Tenzel RR: Reconstruction of the central one half of an eyelid. *Arch Ophthalmol* 93:125, 1975.

119

Reconstruction with Subcutaneous-Base Triangular Skin Flaps

David H. Saunders

INTRODUCTION

Direct closure of circular defects after the removal of skin cancer, such as basal cell carcinoma, results in a puckered appearance. Elliptical excisions can be used, but at the price of wasting normal tissue. Inadequate skin closure will result in problems such as punctal ectropion, brow distortion, or wide depressed scars in the lateral canthal area.

Free grafts can be used to cover defect, but a second surgical site is required and the color match may not be perfect. The defect can be allowed to granulate, but at the price of prolonged recovery and the risk of unpredictable contraction.

The technique described below provides for immediate reconstruction of round or oval defects without any supporting skin flap. The defect is closed with triangular-shaped skin with a subcutaneous base supported by a random blood supply for the skin.

TECHNIQUE

The lesions are removed to obtain free margins under frozen-section control. The typical circular defect (Fig. 119.1) can be closed with one or two subcutaneous-based skin pedicles with subcutaneous blood supply. The triangles are marked on the perimeter of the circles in the direction of normal skin lines and incised with a number 15 blade without disturbing the subcutaneous vascular pedicle.

The flaps are partially undermined, advanced into the circular defect, and sutured to the opposite perimeter (single triangle), or the opposite triangle. The remaining defect is closed, as shown in Figure 119.1.

This technique provides for immediate closure of the typical circular defect using a V-to-Y approach supported by a subcutaneous pedicle,

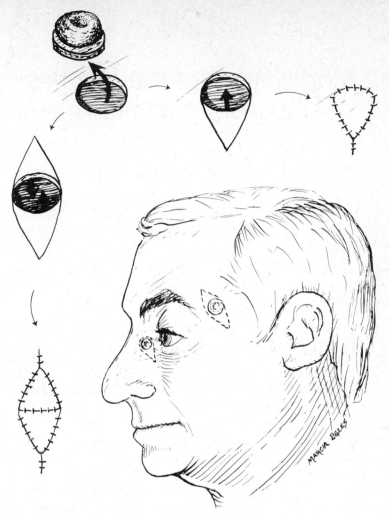

Figure 119.1 *Defects reconstructed with triangular skin flaps nourished by subcutaneous blood supply.*

which results in a good cosmetic appearance when directed within the appropriate skin lines.

BIBLIOGRAPHY

Barron JN, Emmett AJJ: Subcutaneous pedicle flaps. *Br J Plast Surg* 18:51, 1965.

Emmett AJJ: The closure of defects by using adjacent triangular flaps with subcutaneous pedicles. *Plast Reconstr Surg* 59:45, 1977.

Saunders DH, Shannon GM: Subcutaneous-based triangular skin flaps. *Ophthalmic Surg* 11:437, 1980.

Trevaskis AE, Remple J, Okunski W, et al: Sliding subcutaneous pedicle flaps to close circular defects. *Plast Reconstr Surg* 46:455, 1970.

120

Modification of the Hughes Tarsoconjunctival Flap

Norman Shorr
Joel E. Kopelman

INTRODUCTION

The Hughes procedure, as described by Wendell Hughes, uses a tarsoconjunctival advancement flap from the upper eyelid to reconstruct the lower eyelid. Many authors, including Hughes (1,2) recommend that Müller's muscle attachments to the superior border of the tarsus be preserved and that Müller's muscle be simultaneously advanced with the tarsoconjunctival flap to maintain an adequate blood supply for the flap.

Failure to sever Müller's muscle at time of construction of the advancement flap may lead to complications (Fig. 120.1) such as (1) upper eyelid retraction after tarsoconjunctival graft separation (2) upper eyelid notching or (3) upper eyelid entropion. We describe a technique to avoid these complications yet maintain viability of the flap.

TECHNIQUE

The tarsal component of the tarsoconjunctival flap is outlined with the inferior margin approximately 2 mm from the eyelid margin. A scalpel blade is used to incise the tarsal component (Fig. 120.2) and the tarsus is then dissected from the overlying levator aponeurosis in the pretarsal space (Fig. 120.3).

The width and height should correspond to the defect before the excision of a lesion. The wound edges will retract apart after the lesion is excised suggesting a wider piece of tarsus than necessary. Too wide a flap causes laxity and sagging of the reconstructed lower eyelid.

A lateral cantholysis with semicircular advancement flap can be used to reduce the size of the defect to be reconstructed.

The tarsoconjunctival flap is then dissected superiorly between the Müller's muscle and conjunctiva beginning at the superior tarsal margin.

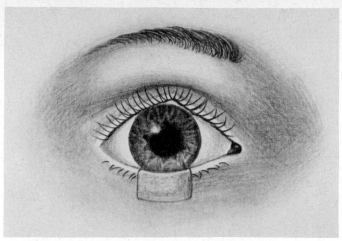

Figure 120.1 Upper eyelid notching, retraction, and entropion after Hughes flap reconstruction of lower eyelid.

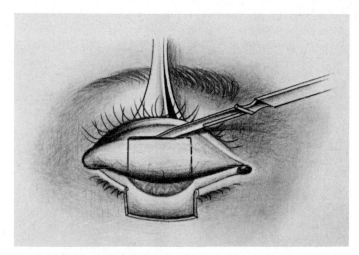

Figure 120.2 Hughes flap incised.

All strands of Müller's muscle should be dissected from the conjunctival portion of the tarsoconjunctival flap. The tarsoconjunctival flap should lie in the defect without tension.

Tarsus can then be sutured to the conjunctival edge of the lower eyelid defect (Fig. 120.4). A free full thickness skin graft is then placed over the tarsoconjunctival flap (Figure 120.5).

In profile (Fig. 120.6), the tarsoconjunctival flap has been advanced, and the Müller's muscle has been severed and retracted from the original attachment at the superior tarsal margin.

The upper eyelid is now placed on an inferior stretch, secured to the cheek with horizontal mattress sutures (Fig. 120.7) to facilitate adequate

385

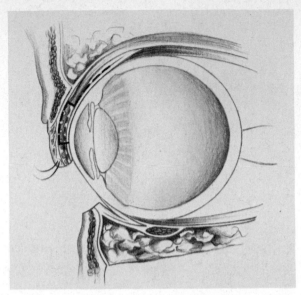

Figure 120.3 Sagittal section showing flap should include conjunctiva, but not Müller's muscle.

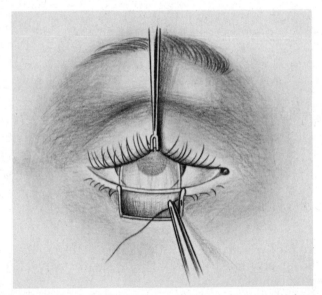

Figure 120.4 Tarsus attached into defect.

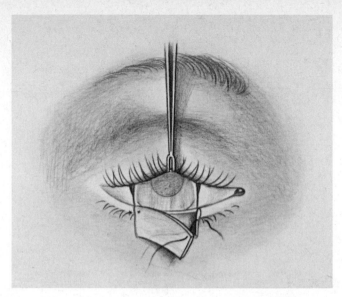

Figure 120.5 *Free skin graft over tarsoconjunctival flap.*

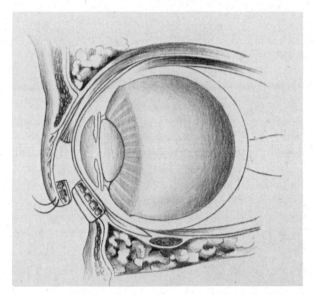

Figure 120.6 *Flap initially supported by vascularity of conjunctiva.*

retraction of Müller's muscle, to inhibit movement of the upper eyelid, and to minimize traction on the tarsoconjunctival flap.

The eyelid can be opened in the examining chair without anesthesia when the flap is divided with scissors.

By dissecting Müller's muscle free from the tarsus at the original procedure, a good functional and cosmetic eyelid results without necessity of reoperation to correction notching, upper lid entropion, or eyelid retraction.

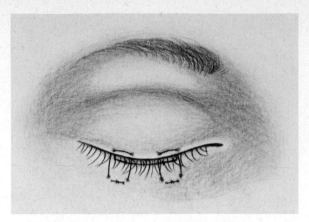

Figure 120.7   Closure with upper eyelid placed on stretch.

REFERENCES

1. Cies WA, Bartlett RE: Modification of the Mustarde and Hughes methods of reconstructing the lower lid. *Ann Ophthalmol* 7:1497, 1975.
2. Hughes WL: Eyelid reconstruction, in Silver B (ed): *Ophthalmic Plastic Surgery Manual*, ed 2. San Francisco, American Academy of Ophthalmology and Otolaryngology, 1964, p 71–74.

121

Reconstruction of the Medial Canthal Eyelid with Free Tarsoconjunctival Graft and Nasal-Based Pedicle Skin-Muscle Flap

Charles R. Leone, Jr.
Stanley I. Hand, Jr.

INTRODUCTION

Medial canthal defects are more difficult to repair than lateral defects because of the lack of available tissue at the medial canthus. A temporal rotation flap leaves a lateral area without tarsal support against the globe unless additional reconstruction or mucous membrane covering is performed in the lateral eyelid area. The Hughes procedure works satisfactorily, but it requires the eye to be closed until the eyelid flap is separated.

A tarsal-conjunctival free flap and skin-muscle pedicle flap, as described in the technique below, allow for immediate reconstruction of the medial canthal area without extensive manipulation of the lateral canthus or grafts from distant sites, such as the nose or ear cartilage. A free tarsal-conjunctival graft is placed for the internal lamellar nourished by a pedicle of skin muscle flap. A free skin graft is used to close the defect created by the pedicle flap.

TECHNIQUE

The upper lid should be everted over a Desmarres retractor, and a free tarsal conjunctival graft 4 mm wide corresponding at a length and size of the defect should be removed from the upper lid (Fig. 121.1). The lower edge of the graft should be at least 3 mm from the eyelid margin to provide adequate tarsal support and prevent upper lid entropion. The upper defect is left unsutured.

389

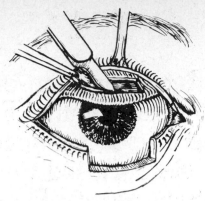

Figure 121.1 Free tarsoconjunctival graft from upper eyelid to fill defect.

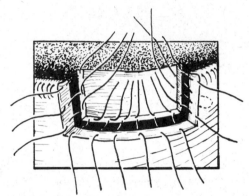

Figure 121.2 Graft sutured into defect.

The tarsal graft, with the conjunctival surface toward the eye, is secured with a 4-0 Dacron suture to the lower arm of the medial canthal tendon or with 6-0 chromic catgut to any remnant of the tarsus, such that the superior edge of the tarsal graft is level with the eyelid margin. Sutures are used to attach the inferior portion of the graft to the conjunctiva in the inferior cul-de-sac with knots tied on the anterior surface to avoid rubbing against the cornea (Fig. 121.2). A graft too tight against the globe can be trimmed to avoid postoperative sag.

The skin beyond the medial aspect of the defect forms the base of the pedicle flap to be rotated into the defect (Fig. 121.3). An outline can be drawn slightly larger than the defect. To be filled, the flap with orbicularis is excised and rotated upward to cover the tarsal-conjunctival graft. The skin is sutured to the tarsal-conjunctival graft with 6-0 silk to create the new eyelid margin (Fig. 121.4) and the lateral aspect of the flap sutured to the lateral eyelid segment. A full-thickness postauricular skin graft can be placed in the defect created by the transfer of the pedicle flap to the eyelid margin (Fig. 121.5).

390

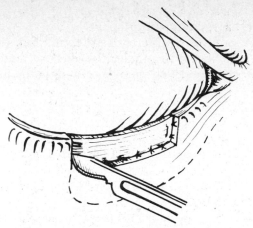

Figure 121.3 Skin flap mobilized to provide vascular supply for free tarsoconjunctival graft.

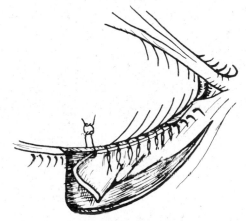

Figure 121.4 Skin flap secured into defect.

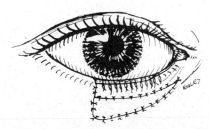

Figure 121.5 Free skin graft used to cover defect created by skin flap. (Leone CR Jr, Hand SI Jr: Reconstruction of the medial canthal eyelid with free tarsal-conjunctival graft and nasal based pedicle skin muscle flap. Am J Ophthalmol 87:797–801, 1979. Published by The American Journal of Ophthalmology. Copyright by The Ophthalmic Publishing Company.)

Small stab incisions can be made in the graft to allow for drainage. The graft should have only slight redundancy.

This technique for lower eyelid reconstruction confines the reconstruction to the local area, and it eliminates the need for temporal flaps or an eyelid sharing procedure, which require occluding the fissure for several weeks.

BIBLIOGRAPHY

Leone CR Jr, Hand SI Jr: Reconstruction of the medial eyelid. *Am J Ophthalmol* 87:797, 1979.

Mustarde JC: Repair and reconstruction in the orbital region. Baltimore, Williams & Wilkins, 1966, pp 116–147.

Smith B.: Eyelid reconstruction, in Sol DB (ed): *Management of Complications in Ophthalmic Plastic Surgery*. Birmingham, Aesculapius, 1976, pp 226–228.

Tenzel RR: Reconstruction of the central one-half of an eyelid. *Arch Ophthalmol,* 93:125, 1975.

122

Eyelid Reconstruction with Augmented Pedicle Flap

Martin Bodian

INTRODUCTION

Most procedures to reconstruct major lower eyelid defects require that the lids be sewn together for an extensive period or that flaps be supplemented with grafts such as chrondo-mucosa. Techniques that work well for smaller defects may not be applicable to large lower lid defects.

With the technique below, a single-stage augmented pedicle flap can be used to reconstruct a total defect of the lower lid without the necessity of additional mucosal grafting.

TECHNIQUE

To reconstruct the lower eyelid defect, a protective lens is inserted and lateral canthotomy directed posteriorly for 4 mm. At this point, a semicircular 15 mm in diameter, based on a line projected from the lateral canthus to the top of the ear, is incised. In a similar manner, a second incision from the lower edge of the incision is made slanting slightly downward from the defect toward the lower earlobe with a second semicircle 15 mm in diameter beneath and somewhat lateral to the one on the upper lid (Fig. 122.1, top).

The entire flap should be undermined and enlarged as needed to allow advancement to cover the defect. As the flap advances, the semicircles will flatten to augment the flap. The flap should be anchored to the periosteum with tension sutures placed at the lateral orbital rim to permit the flap to cover the defect with a minimum of tension. Mattress sutures are passed medially to fix the flap to the medial edge of the defect and pass through bolsters. With the protective contact lens removed, modified Frost sutures are placed to prevent retraction, and the wounds are closed (Fig. 122.1, lower).

Postoperative wound care should include antibiotic ointment, Telfa

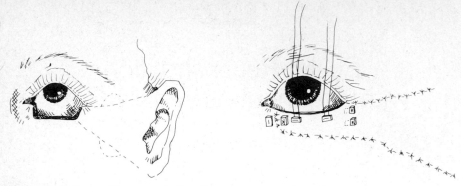

Figure 122.1 *(Top) Pedicle flap augmented with 15-mm semicircles starting 4 mm from lateral canthus. (Below) Augmented pedicle flap advanced into defect. Incision lines become straightened. (Bodian M: Extensive lid reconstruction using an augmented pedicle flap. Ann Ophthalmol 15:35–37, 1983.)*

pads, and semipressure eye dressings for 48 hours. Subsequently, the eye may be left open until the skin sutures are removed at approximately 4 days and the tension sutures at approximately 10 days.

With any suggestion of vertical retraction, the lid should be massaged in a rotary fashion for 5 minutes three times daily, starting as early as 3 weeks postoperatively when the wound edges are firmly healed. Mucous membrane grafts are not necessary to line the reconstructed lid, as epithelium will resurface the posterior portion of the flap in 2 to 3 weeks.

The semicircles are formed to augment the pedicle flap. By 3 to 6 months postoperatively the skin incisions are relatively straight and inconspicuous.

This procedure allows the surgeon to obtain a single-stage reconstruction of the patient's lower eyelid without closing the eyelids for protracted periods or using complicated tarsal, nasal, or bucal mucous membrane grafts.

BIBLIOGRAPHY

Bodian M: Extensive lid reconstruction using an augmented pedicle flap. *Ann Ophthalmol* 15:35, 1983.

Bodian M: Protective contact lens for eyelid surgery. *Am J Ophthalmol* 68:148, 1969.

Leone C Jr, Van Gemert JV: Lower eyelid reconstruction with upper eyelid transpositional grafts. *Ophthalmic Surg* 11:315, 1980.

Tenzel RR, Stewart WB: Eyelid reconstruction by the semicircle flap technique. *Trans Am Acad Opthalmol* 85:1164, 1978.

123

Avoiding Notch in Upper Eyelid Repair

Ralph E. Wesley

INTRODUCTION

Repair and reconstruction of the upper eyelid are particularly critical since the lid margin passes over the globe repeatedly during each blink and closure. This technique avoids lid notching and trichiasis, which are both unsightly and discomforting to the patient.

TECHNIQUE

In closing eyelid lacerations that involve partial loss of the tarsus or in the resection of tumor, the cut edges of the tarsus should extend perpendicularly from the lid margin for the entire vertical border of the tarsus (Fig. 123.1, left). When the tarsal edges are brought together in this manner, the lid margin will be smooth and the lashes correctly oriented.

When a slanting incision (Fig. 123.1, middle) or partial thickness tarsal incision (Fig. 123.1, right) is performed during tumor resection or lid repair, the closure will buckle or twist the tarsus to form a lid notch, a distorted eyelid, and misdirected lashes.

By proper sectioning of the tarsal plates, distortion of the eyelid can be avoided (Fig. 123.1, left). In eyelid reconstruction or tumor resection, the tarsal plate must be sectioned vertically in a perpendicular manner for the entire vertical length of the tarsal plate to provide for a smooth closure. Figure 123.1, middle, shows improper angle tarsal excision causing notching. Figure 123.1, right, shows partial tarsal excision results in buckling and notching.

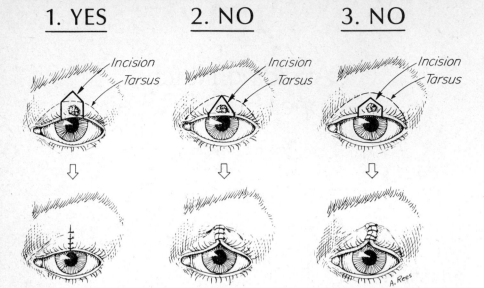

1. YES   2. NO   3. NO

Figure 123.1 Perpendicular incisions completely through vertical tarsus (1) avoid buckling and notching caused by angled (2) or partial thickness (3) incisions.

124

Prevention of Entropion
in the Cutler–Beard Procedure

Richard P. Carroll

INTRODUCTION

The Cutler–Beard procedure can be used to reconstruct complete upper eyelid defects using a full-thickness flap from the opposing lower eyelid while preserving the margin of the donor eyelid. Since the flap contains little or no tarsus, shrinkage of the posterior lamellar after separation can sometimes result in cicatricial entropion with ocular irritation from fine cilia or keratinized tissue on the margin rubbing against the eye.

This technique for separation of the Cutler–Beard flap and for the use of ear cartilage within the flap helps to prevent entropion in patients after upper eyelid reconstruction.

TECHNIQUE

The Cutler–Beard procedure uses a full-thickness flap from the lower lid for upper eyelid reconstruction (1). To preserve the lower lid margin, the horizontal incision is made full thickness at the base of the lower tarsus to spare the inferior marginal artery. The vertical incisions are then extended down toward the cheek, and the flap is mobilized to come under the bridge of lower lid margin to be sutured into the defect.

Sclera (2) has been used as a tarsal substitute, but ear cartilage offers the advantage of avoiding late contraction, which can occur with eye bank sclera. The flap is formed (Fig. 124.1A) to fill the defect and split between the anterior and posterior lamellars. Posterior lamellar is sewn into the defect and a graft of ear cartilage sewn in as a tarsal substitute as previously described with scleral grafts (2) (Fig. 124.1B). Once the ear cartilage has been attached to the tarsal remnants and levator aponeurosis, the skin muscle flap can be advanced and sewn into the defect (Fig. 124.1C).

Full-thickness autogenous ear cartilage appears to be superior to preserved sclera in avoiding postoperative shrinkage and subsequent entro-

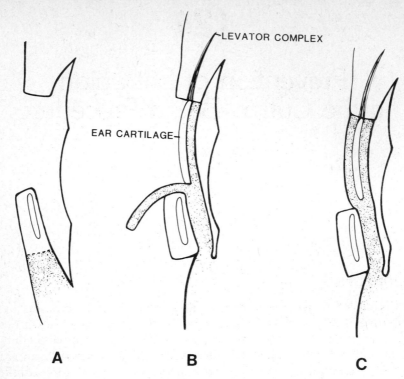

LEVATOR COMPLEX

EAR CARTILAGE⌐

A   B   C

Figure 124.1   *Ear cartilage graft in Cutler–Beard flap.*

pion. Ear cartilage has made excellent graft material in other eyelid reconstruction (3). The postoperative edema noted with scleral grafts has not
occurred in patients with autogenous ear cartilage.

Care in separating the flap can also help to prevent entropion. When
separating the flap, a beveled (Fig. 124.2A) rather than straight incision
should be made for the separation. A lip of conjunctiva (Fig. 124.2B) can
then be wrapped around the reconstructed lid margin such that mucous
membrane rather than keratinized epithelium would be in contact with
the globe.

These modifications and technique offer the surgeon an opportunity to
provide comfort for patients after reconstruction of the upper eyelid with
Cutler–Beard flap.

REFERENCES

1. Cutler NL, Beard C: A method for partial and total upper lid reconstruction.
   Am J Ophthalmol 39:1, 1955.
2. Wesley RE, McCord CD Jr: Transplantation of eye bank sclera and the Cutler–
   Beard method of upper eyelid reconstruction. *Ophthalmol* 87:1022, 1980.
3. Baylis HI, Rosen N, Neuhaus RW: Obtaining auricular cartilage for reconstructive surgery. *Am J Ophthalmol* 93:709, 1982.

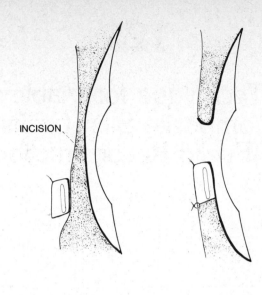

INCISION

A   **B**

Figure 124.2   Angled incision to avoid entropion.

125

Technique for Viable Composite Skin Grafts in Eyelid Reconstruction

Allen M. Putterman

INTRODUCTION

In traumatic, congenital, or surgical defects of the upper eyelid that are too large to reconstruct by direct closure with canthotomy or cantholysis or lacking adjacent tissue necessary for the Cutler–Beard technique, a composite graft must be used.

Because the free, full-thickness composite graft has no blood supply and must rely on vascularization from the surrounding eyelid, a high failure rate occurs. The viability of free grafts comes from small buds of vascularized tissue that penetrate from an overlying or underlying flap just as a free skin graft over the orbicularis muscle receives its blood supply from buds of blood vessels growing in from the orbicularis muscle.

This technique increases the viability of composite eyelid grafts via vascularization from overlying and underlying flaps. This is accomplished by altering the composite graft to a skin component and a tarsal-conjunctival-margin component. The skin graft is placed against the orbicularis muscle, and the tarsal-conjunctival-margin component is placed against a skin flap.

TECHNIQUE

The surrounding 1-mm edge of the upper eyelid coloboma is excised with a number 11 Bard–Parker blade to provide a raw edge for the composite graft to rest against (Fig. 125.1A, left). The size of the composite graft, which is circumscribed with a marking pen on the opposite upper eyelid, is equivalent to the defect in the colobomatous upper eyelid when the nasal and temporal eyelid remnants are brought as close as possible to each other with slight tension (Fig. 125.1A, right).

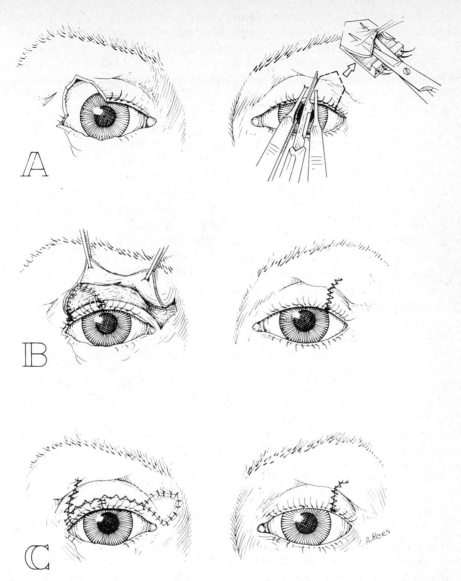

Figure 125.1 (A) Free composite graft is taken to fill right eyelid defect. Skin removed from graft to be used on right lid. (B) After composite graft is secured, skin-muscle flap is mobilized to provide vascular support. (C) Skin from composite graft is used to cover defect created nasally by mobilization of skin-muscle flap.

A number 15 Bard–Parker blade is used to make a skin incision 2 mm above the eyelashes over the larger segment of remaining eyelid, beginning at the edge of the coloboma and extending to the opposite extreme of the eyelid segment. An oblique skin incision is then made from the end of the supralash incision, angulated slightly away from the coloboma site. The skin is then undermined from the orbicularis muscle over the eyelid segment with a sharp-pointed iris scissors (Fig. 125.1B, left). Observing the points of the scissors beneath the translucent skin facilitates dissection of the skin flap from the orbicularis muscle without skin penetration.

The composite full-thickness graft is then taken from the opposite upper eyelid by grasping the eyelid margin on each side of the marked line with two forceps and penetrating the eyelid about 5 mm from the margin (Fig. 125.1A, right). A slicing motion then severs the eyelid margin. This method provides a smooth, square, sharp cut through the margin and aids in approximation of the eyelid later in the procedure. A similar cut is then made at the site of the other edge of the composite graft. A Westcott scissors if used to create vertical and then oblique cuts from the superior aspect to remove a full-thickness pentagon of the upper eyelid that matches the coloboma.

The composite graft is then divided into two sections (Fig. 125.1A, right). A number 15 Bard–Parker blade is used to incise the skin 2 mm above the cilia across the graft. The skin is undermined from the orbicularis muscle and placed on a 4 × 4 piece of gauze soaked in saline solution. The orbicularis muscle is then undermined from the levator aponeurosis, adherent to anterior tarsus and is excised and discarded.

The tarsal-conjunctival-margin graft is then sutured into the coloboma site (Fig. 125.1B, left). Three 6-0 black silk sutures unite the temporal eyelid margin of the graft to the temporal eyelid margin of the coloboma. One suture passes through the squared corner where tarsus meets conjunctiva, a second suture passes through the gray line, and a third through the first row of eyelashes closest to the gray line. These sutures are then tied in triplicate, and the two eyelash suture ends are tied over the four internal suture ends. When all six ends are severed, they point away from the cornea.

The nasal eyelid margin of the graft is then sutured to the nasal coloboma in the same way. The superficial tarsus and levator aponeurosis of the graft are then sutured to the superficial tarsus and levator aponeurosis of the eyelids surrounding the graft with interrupted 6-0 Dexon sutures. The skin above the eyelid margin of the graft is sutured to surrounding skin with interrupted 6-0 black silk sutures.

The skin flap is then brought over the composite graft and sutured with interrupted 6-0 black silk sutures to the graft and surrounding skin (Fig. 125.1C, left). In this way, the flap provides a blood supply in contact with the graft.

By sliding the skin flap over the composite graft, a skin defect is created at the opposite end of the eyelid. This is covered with the skin graft that was separated previously from the composite graft (Fig. 125.1C, left). The skin graft, which now lies against a vascularized bed of orbicularis muscle, is sutured to surrounding skin with interrupted 6-0 black silk sutures.

If direct closure of the composite graft donor site (Fig. 125.1B, right, and 125.1C, right) is hampered by excessive tension of the opposing flaps, a lateral canthotomy and cantholysis can be performed. The closure is then made with three 6-0 black silk sutures in the eyelid margin, similarly placed to those used to unite the composite graft to surrounding eyelid margin. Several superficial tarsal and levator aponeurosis 6-0 Dexon sutures unite the eyelid above the margin, and the skin and orbicularis muscle are closed with a continuous 6-0 black silk suture.

A light pressure dressing is applied over the reconstructed eyelid. The donor eyelid is left without a dressing. The skin sutures are removed 5 to 6 days postoperatively, and the eyelid margin sutures are removed 11 to 14 days postoperatively.

BIBLIOGRAPHY

Callahan A: Free composite lid graft. *Arch Ophthalmol* 45:539, 1954.

Cutler NL, Beard C: Reconstruction of upper lid. *Am J Ophthalmol* 39:1, 1955.

Fox SA: Autogenous free full-thickness eyelid grafts. *Am J Ophthalmol* 67:941, 1969.

Putterman AM: Viable composite grafting in eyelid reconstruction. *Am J Ophthalmol* 85:237, 1978.

Youens WT, Westfall C, Barfeld F, et al: Full-thickness lower lid transplant. *Arch Ophthalmol* 77:226, 1967.

126

Sliding Tarsal Flap in Lateral Eyelid Reconstruction

Ralph E. Wesley

INTRODUCTION

Lateral upper eyelid defects create special problems in reconstruction. The bridge flap can be used from the lower lid but requires closure of the eyelid. Horizontally, sliding skin flaps frequently contract causing lateral exposure. Direct closure may provide coverage, but frequently results in ptosis.

With the sliding tarsal flap, a normal eyelid can be reconstructed with tarsus and conjunctiva on the posterior aspect, creating good function and appearance to the reconstructed eyelid.

TECHNIQUE

To reconstruct a lateral defect (Fig. 126.1A) the eyelid should be everted and a tarsoconjunctival flap slightly smaller than the defect created (Fig. 126.1B). A horizontal incision should be made full-thickness through the tarsus 3 to 4 mm behind the lid margin to prevent entropion, and the vertical incision should be carried superiorly past the upper border of the tarsal plate.

As with the Hughes flap, the Müller's muscle should be dissected from the upper border of the tarsus so that only conjunctiva attaches to the superior tarsus. The flap should be anchored laterally with a permanent suture at the normal level of the lateral canthus with the position directed posteriorly to the orbital rim (Fig. 126.1C).

The medial aspect of the tarsal flap should be closed to the laeral cut edge of the normal lid (Fig. 126.1D), and then a skin graft placed on the outer surface of the tarsal conjunctival flap (Fig. 126.1E). A temporary nylon suture holds the lower lids down during the first postoperative week to help stabilize the flap.

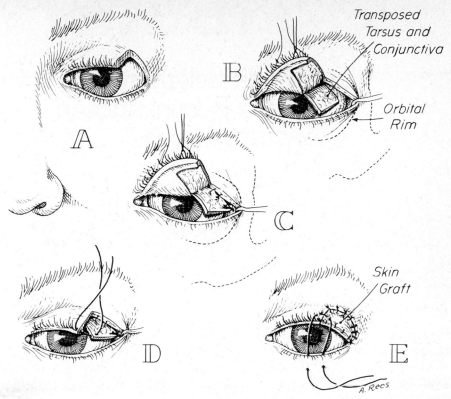

Figure 126.1 *Upper lid defects too large for direct closure reconstructed using tarsoconjunctival flap posteriorly and skin graft anteriorly. Sliding tarsal flap attached only to conjunctiva, not to Müller's muscle.*

By forming a sliding tarsal flap attached only by conjunctiva, the lid will heal without contractive forces caused by leaving Müller's muscle attached, and yet avoids ptosis from direct closure.

The skin graft should be left 1 mm from the lid margin so that mucous membrane rather than keratinized epithelium forms the margin in contact with the cornea.

127

Eye Bank Sclera and Cutler-Beard Reconstruction of Upper Eyelid

Ralph E. Wesley

INTRODUCTION

Upper eyelid defects, including the total upper eyelid, can be reconstructed with the Cutler–Beard bridge flap technique. Since the flap includes no tarsus from the lower eyelid, the lid margin may be unstable, resulting in entropion. The flap can contract vertically, causing exposure. The flap can thin with a less than desirable appearance.

Transplanting sclera into the flap provides for better stability and cosmesis in upper eyelid reconstruction.

TECHNIQUE

To reconstruct the upper eyelid defect, a flap should be drawn on the lower eyelid 4 to 5 mm below the lid margin with vertical incisions extending down onto the cheek (Fig. 127.1A). A full-thickness incision should be carried through the lower eyelid and the flap freed well down onto the cheek.

Normally, at this point, the flap is passed under the bridge of tissue and fixated into the defect. Instead, the conjunctiva should be separated from the skin muscle portions of the flap. The conjunctiva should be passed under the defect and sewn in place with a running 6-0 plain catgut suture (Figure 127.1-B).

A piece of eyebank sclera should be fashioned to fit the defect and sewn medially and laterally to the edges of the tarsal plates or canthal tendons and superiorly to the levator aponeurosis with 6-0 Vicryl (Fig. 127.1C). Finally, the remaining skin muscle is brought under the bridge and sewn into the defect with interrupted 7-0 silk sutures (Fig. 127.1D).

At 6 weeks later the flap can be separated and the remnants of the flap replaced in the lower lid (Fig. 127.1E).

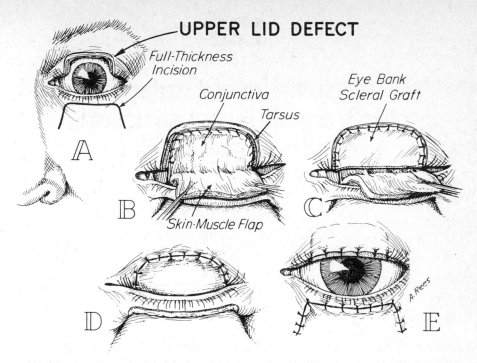

UPPER LID DEFECT

Full-Thickness Incision

Conjunctiva

Tarsus

Eye Bank Scleral Graft

Skin-Muscle Flap

A. Rees

Figure 127.1 *Scleral graft placed into Cutler–Beard flap to add substance and lid margin stability to reconstructed upper eyelid.*

The implantation of sclera provides greater stability and durability to the reconstructed upper eyelid.

BIBLIOGRAPHY

Cutler NL, Beard C: A method for partial and total upper lid reconstruction. *Am J Ophthalmol* 39:1, 1955.

Smith B, Obear M: Bridge flap technique for large upper lid defects. *Plast Reconst Surg* 38:45, 1966.

Wesley RE, McCord CD Jr: Transplantation of eye bank sclera in the Cutler–Beard method of upper eyelid reconstruction. *Ophthalmology* 87:1022, 1980.

128

Split-Level Grafts for Vertical Reconstruction of the Upper Eyelid

Bernice Z. Brown

INTRODUCTION

Burns, trauma, irradiation, complications of cosmetic surgery, and severe inflammation, such as herpes zoster, can cause a full-thickness vertical shortening of the upper eyelid with cosmetic and functional deformity. Most methods of eyelid reconstruction are designed for horizontal insufficiency and cannot be adapted to vertical upper eyelid inadequacy with an intact eyelid margin. Other methods elongate only the anterior or posterior lamella, but not both.

With the split-level full-thickness eyelid grafts of skin and mucous membrane, each graft has a vascular bed for viability of the graft and vertical elongation of the upper eyelid.

TECHNIQUE

Figure 128.1 illustrates the principles of this technique. The upper eyelid should be split horizontally (Fig. 128.1A) and separated (Fig. 128.1B) such that grafts can be placed at different levels of the eyelid and supported by separate vascular beds (Fig. 128.1C). Since this technique is usually employed in eyelid shortened vertically by cicatricial conditions, the grafts undergo contraction and require a few millimeters of extra lengthening with this procedure.

The affected eyelid (Fig. 128.2A) should be everted over a Desmarres retractor. A horizontal incision should be made completely through the tarsal surface approximately 5 mm above the eyelid margin (Fig. 128.2B). With the retractor removed and a 4-0 mattress suture through the lid margin, a horizontal skin incision is made across the upper eyelid above the superior tarsal border (Fig. 128.2C) with a number 15 blade. In cases in which the eyelid cannot be everted, the external incision should be made

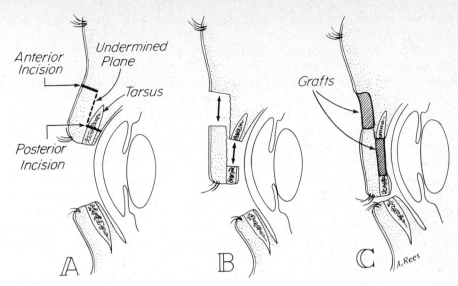

Figure 128.1 Lid split so each graft is on a vascular bed.

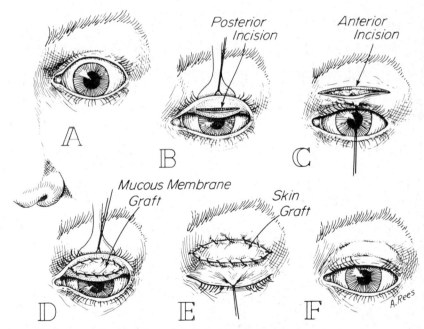

Figure 128.2 Split-level vertical lid lengthening.

first: After retraction of the skin edge, the second transtarsal incision can be made.

Sharp Westcott scissors should be used to undermine the skin and orbicularis superiorly and inferiorly to release traction bands holding the eyelid in retracted position. The lower internal eyelid incision is then joined with the upper external skin incision. (Figs. 128.1A and B).

With the upper eyelid everted, a full-thickness graft, such as buccal mucous membrane, nasal chondral mucosal, ear cartilage, or homologous tarsal graft should be sutured into the posterior incisions between the cut edges of the tarsal conjunctiva with a continuous 6-0 plain catgut suture (Fig. 128.2D). Externally, with the lid retracted downward, a retroauricular full-thickness skin graft can be placed into the anterior incision with interrupted or running sutures (Fig. 128.2E).

Marginal sutures or temporary tarsorrhaphy for 1 week help keep the lid on stretch to prevent retraction. The skin graft should be extended with Xeroform gauze or eye pad.

This technique produces the vertical elongation of the eyelid (Fig. 128.2F), which cannot be accomplished as easily and effectively by any other single-stage procedure.

BIBLIOGRAPHY

Brown BZ, Beard C: Split-level full-thickness eyelid graft. *Am J Ophthalmol* 87:388, 1979.

McCord CD Jr, Wesley R: Reconstruction of the upper eyelid and medial canthus, in McCord CD Jr (ed): *Oculoplastic Surgery*. New York, Raven, 1981, p 185.

FACIAL NERVE DISORDERS

PART X

129

Coronal Flap in Treatment
of Blepharospasm

Ralph E. Wesley

INTRODUCTION

Extirpation of the orbicularis muscle is the safest, most effective surgical treatment for benign essential blepharospasm. Brow and eyelid incisions have been used to remove orbicularis muscle to eliminate or reduce the incapacitating, uncontrolled squeezing of the eyelids. However, brow incisions can leave noticeable scars and contraction of the subcutaneous scars, in some cases, can make brow incisions especially unsightly.

The coronal technique eliminates brow contracture and hides the incision at the hairline while allowing the surgeon generous access to the procerus, corrugator, and superior orbital portions of the orbicularis muscle in treating blepharospasm.

TECHNIQUE

In patients with blepharospasm, the bicoronal incision can be drawn at the hairline (Fig. 129.1) or placed back inside the hairline. Under general or local anesthesia the incision is infiltrated with 1:100,000 epinephrine with 2% lidocaine for vasoconstriction, as well as to the areas of muscle extirpation.

The incision is carried full-thickness to the skull, centrally into the temporalis fascia to the lateral segments, with beveling of the incision to prevent loss of hair follicles. Neurosurgical Raney clips can be applied to the wounds for hemostasis, though use of a Shaw heated scalpel eliminates the need for clips. The flaps should then be undermined to the supraorbital rims out to the root of the helix of the ear to avoid the superfical temporal artery and allow adequate exposure of the supraorbital rim.

The flap will usually separate rapidly from the forehead with a minimum of bleeding using blunt dissection. With the flap rotated down-

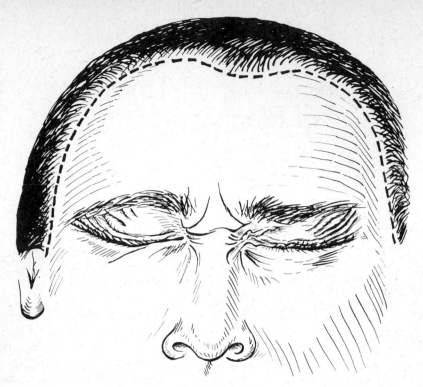

Figure 129.1 *Cornal incision for blepharospasm.*

ward, the supraorbital neurovascular bundles can be identified, and more medially, the corrugator and proceurus muscles can be excised to eliminate central spasm (Fig. 129.2). The flap provides access to the superior orbicularis muscle, which should be excised. In addition, a small amount of periosteum centrally may be removed to provide a firm adhesion of the brow to the orbital rim replacement of the flap.

Once hemostasis has been obtained, the flap can be replaced and sutured with staples.

To accomplish the rest of the operation, an incision is made in the lid fold out to the lateral canthus, as well as a subciliary incision to provide access to remove the preseptal, pretarsal, and orbital orbicularis muscle (Fig. 129.3). Through the skin incision, a repair of disinserted levator aponeurosis can be accomplished using 6-0 Vicryl sutures. Many patients have stretched retractors of the upper lid due to constant squeezing (Fig. 129.4).

To correct any laxity of the lower lid, the lateral lid can be resected full-thickness, as described in Chapter 20 (Fig. 129.5) and reattached to the orbital rim with a 4-0 vicryl suture to prevent any postoperative sagging or ectropion.

Figure 129.6 shows the patient after closure of both the coronal flap and the skin incisions.

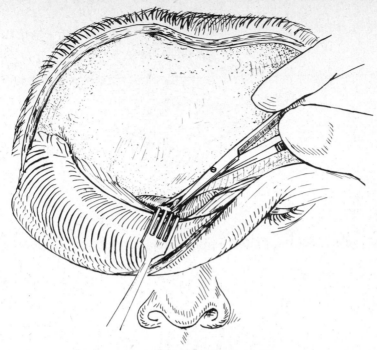

Figure 129.2 *Coronal flap rotated inferiorly to remove procerus and corrugator muscles.*

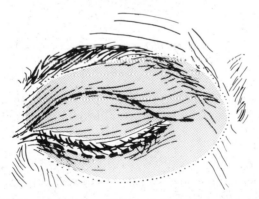

Figure 129.3 *Upper and lower lid incisions to remove orbicularis muscle shown in shaded area.*

This provides an effective exposure to reduce or eliminate blepharospasm through extirpation of the orbicularis muscle. Complications include frontal anesthesia from damage or removal of branches of the frontal nerve, hemorrhage, orbital edema, and retraction of the tissues. The most common complication, however, with most blepharospasm surgery is failure to remove enough orbicularis muscle thus leaving some residual spasm.

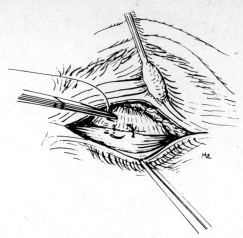

Figure 129.4 *Repair of levator aponeurosis defect from blepharospasm.*

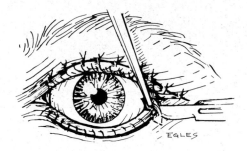

Figure 129.5 *Laxity of lower lid repaired.*

The hairline incision is nearly always inconspicuous, and closure with surgical staples speeds the operation and produces a nice cosmetic result.

BIBLIOGRAPHY

Gillum WN, Anderson RL: Blepharospasm surgery: An anatomical approach. *Arch Ophthalmol* 99:1056, 1981.

McCord CD Jr, Shore J, Putman JR: Treatment of essential blepharospasm: A modification of exposure for the muscle stripping technique. *Arch Ophthalmol* 102:269, 1984.

416

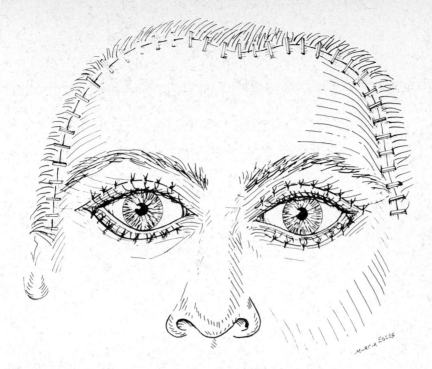

Figure 129.6   Closure of eyelid and coronal incisions.

130

Eyelid Closure from Temporalis Muscle/Fascia Sling in Facial Palsy

Ralph E. Wesley

INTRODUCTION

Patients with facial palsy and keratitis sicca may not receive adequate closure from a lateral tarsorrhaphy. The cerclage procedure and palpebral spring methods can provide relief but have the complication of extrusion and infection of the foreign material, which increases with longer and longer follow up.

Tight closure can be accomplished in patients with facial palsy using temporalis fascia attached to a strip of temporalis muscle as a sling in the upper and lower eyelids. The patient can activate closure by chewing. This method allows for permanent correction to facial palsy since foreign materials need not be implanted.

TECHNIQUE

With local or general anesthesia, an incision should be carried down into the temporal region to the temporalis fascia (Fig. 130.1A). With the fascia exposed, the strip of sling should be drawn with methylene blue. The fascia should be incised but leaving the base still attached superiorly (Fig. 130.1B). Next, an incision is made just above the superior attachment carried through to the temporalis muscle (Fig. 130.1C), which can then be elevated from the temporalis fossa.

A horizontal incision should be made at the lateral canthus, and the complex of temporalis muscle and fascia can be tunneled through to the lateral canthus (Fig. 130.1D).

With the medial canthal tendon exposed by a vertical incision at the medial canthus, a wright fascia needle can be used to pass the strips of fascia through the upper and lower lids (Fig. 130.2A). The fascia should be passed beneath the external head of the medial canthal tendon (Fig.

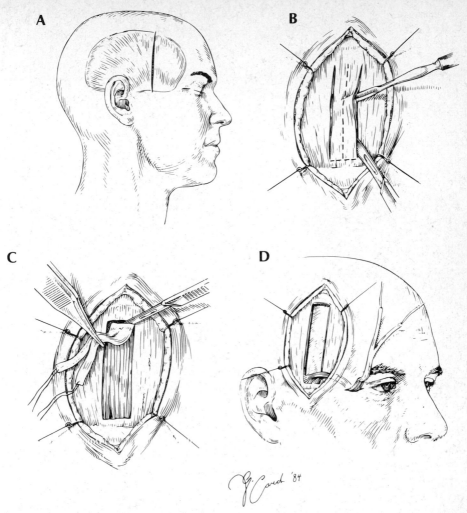

Figure 130.1 *Temporalis muscle with fascia attached for greater length.*

130.2B) and then fixed with permanent sutures after adjusting the tension to provide for tight closure of the eyelid (Fig. 130.2C).

Postoperatively, the patient can activate eyelid closure with a chewing motion on the involved side. The closure can be adjusted postoperatively, but rarely is too tight a closure obtained.

Over the years, the fascia does not extrude, but can loosen. Fixation with permanent sutures at both the medial and lateral canthus reduces the risk of subsequent extrusion. An incision in the upper and lower lids facilitates passage in two strokes and provides access for a permanent suture to be placed for fixation of the fascia to the upper and lower tarsal plates in the midsection of the lid.

This technique allows for a dynamic rather than a static sling procedure of the eyelids. Patients seem to develop a super tentorial control

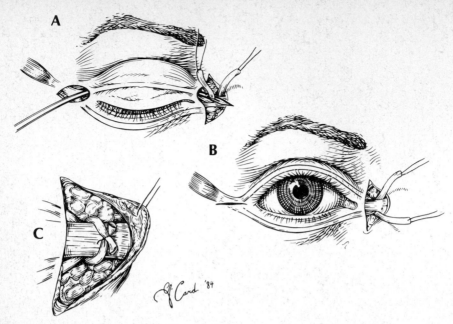

Figure 130.2 Fixation of fascia for dynamic eyelid sling.

mechanism such that eyelid closure can be accomplished without consciously thinking about the action.

131

Silicone Cerclage in Facial Palsy

Ralph E. Wesley

INTRODUCTION

Patients with exposure keratitis and ocular irritation from facial palsy that cannot be relieved with lateral tarsorrhaphy have generally been treated with a silicone cerclage procedure. The cerclage provides tighter closure than the lateral tarsorrhaphy. But, with time, extrusion of the spring has been a problem.

With the technique for medial and lateral canthal fixation below, patients can obtain relief from the facial palsy with a greatly reduced chance of silicone cerclage extrusion.

TECHNIQUE

With either local or general anesthesia, a weak epinephrine solution should be injected into the medial and lateral canthus and upper and lower lids for hemostasis. A vertical incision should be made at the medial canthus and carried to the external head of the medial canthal tendon. At the lateral canthus, a vertical incision should be carried to the lateral orbital rim at the level of the lateral canthal tendon.

While protecting the eye, two drill holes are placed through the lateral orbital rim horizontally just above and below the lateral canthal tendon (Fig. 131.1A). Using a disposable eyelet needle, the silicone is passed in a figure 8 looping configuration through the deep heads of the medial canthal tendon, which can then be fixed with permanent suture (Fig. 131.1B).

A Wright fascia needle is used to pass the silicone from the medial incision to the lateral canthal incision. The pass through the lower incision should be within 1 mm of the lid margin. A lower pass will result in a tarsal ectropion. The upper silicone should be passed higher, being several millimeters from the lid margin (Fig. 131.1C). For easier passage from

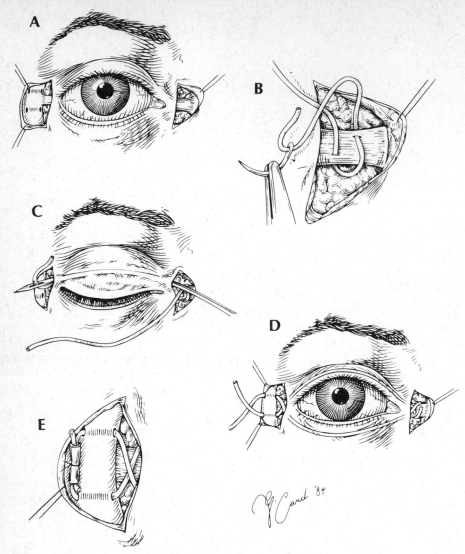

Figure 131.1 *Silicone cerclage for eyelid closure in facial palsy. Fixation with permanent suture at medial canthus and cross-fixation through bone at lateral canthus reduce incidence of extrusion.*

the medial to lateral incisions, one or two incisions can be made along the pathway so that the passage can be made in one or two shorter steps rather than one large passage.

At the lateral canthus, the lower strip should be placed in the upper drill hole and the upper strip in the lower to provide a cross-action pulling the upper lower lid inward and upward for the normal contour, and vice versa for the upper lid (Fig. 131.1D). For final fixation, the silicone should be passed through a Watzke sleeve.

The sling should be adjusted to provide 1 to 2 mm of lagophthalmos. Then a permanent stitch should be tied around the Watze sleeve for permanent fixation of the silicone cerclage (Fig. 131.1E).

Postoperatively, the patient will normally have 1 to 2 mm of lagophthalmos, but will have dramatically improved closure over the preoperative position. Should adjustment of the silicone be required, the lateral canthal incision can be opened and the sling tightened or loosened after removing the suture around the Watske sleeve.

Complications can include eyelid malposition, infection, granuloma, and extrusion.

Generally, the tighter the sling the greater the chance of extrusion.

This technique greatly reduces chances of extrusion due to the deep permanent fixation at the medial canthus and the inward and crossing fixation to the bone at the lateral canthus.

132

Palpebral Spring for Lagophthalmos due to Facial Nerve Palsy

Robert E. Levine

INTRODUCTION

Some patients with lagophthalmos and exposure keratitis from facial nerve palsy cannot obtain adequate closure with a procedure such as the lateral tarsorrhaphy or the Silastic cerclage. For these patients, the palpebral spring provides much tighter closure of the eyelids. In addition, the palpebral spring provides a more cosmetic and functional approach to the eye problem than does tarsorrhaphy.

TECHNIQUE

The spring should be fashioned before surgery, making a loop in 0.010 inch stainless steel orthodonic wire. With one round-nosed plier to bend and a second pair of pliers to fixate the wire, a loop at the fulcrum should be formed approximately 5 mm in diameter. The loop should be as flat as possible. The posterior portion of the loop will be the arm of the spring resting on the periosteum of the orbital rim. The anterior extension will be the lower arm, to be positioned in the upper eyelid overlying the tarsal plate. A curve should be placed in the arms of the spring, which conform to the contour of the lid. One curve should be in the frontal plane, allowing the upper arm of the spring to conform to the curvature of the orbital rim and for the lower arm to conform to the contour of the upper eyelid. A second curve should be made anterior/posteriorly for the upper arm of the spring to fit the orbital rim and for the lower spring to fit the curvature of the globe below.

   With ocular protection from a scleral shell, local anesthetic with epinephrine should be injected into the midtarsus of the upper lid and at the lateral orbital rim. Only the minimum amount of infiltration anesthesia should be used, so as to prevent lid akinesia that might interfere with evaluation of lid function.

The separation of the arms of the spring in the closed position should be approximately one and a half times the separation when the lids are opened. With severe lagophthalmos, the ratio can be increased to two. Intraoperatively, reducing the tension of the spring is easier than increasing tension. Consequently, the arms should initially be too far apart rather than too close together.

To insert the spring, a 1-cm incision should be made slightly superior to the midtarsus, about 5 mm medial to the center of the upper lid, lying parallel to the lid margin. Dissection is carried to the anterior surface of the tarsus. A 2-cm incision should be made over the lateral orbital rim, with dissection carried to the periosteum.

A blunted 22-gauge spinal needle should be passed in a slightly inferior direction from the medial incision at the midtarsus in a plane between the anterior surface of the tarsus and the orbicularis oculi. The needle is directed to pass 2 mm superior to the lashes in the lateral extent of the upper lid, emerging at the lateral orbital rim incision.

The under surface of the upper lid should be checked to ensure that the tarsus has not been inadvertently perforated. The stylet should be removed and the end of the previously prepared spring passed into the needle. The needle is withdrawn, bringing the spring into position (Fig. 132.1A).

A permanent suture, such as 4-0 mersilene, should be placed through the fulcrum of the spring and secured to the periosteum of the orbital rim. An extra bite of periosteum should be taken before tying the stitch. The spring should be made so that the fulcrum is placed as far laterally as practical on the orbital rim.

With the scleral shell removed, the spring contour should be checked with the eye opened and closed. Ideally, the spring should be positioned so the lower arm moves slightly posteriorly on opening the lid to accommodate normal lid movement in that direction. Two additional 4-0 mersilene sutures are used to secure the fulcrum, taking an additional bite of periosteum with each stitch.

Loops should be formed in the upper and lower ends of the wire with the orthodonic pliers. The superior loop should lie at the upper end of the lateral incision, and the inferior loop should lie about 5 mm medial to the center of the upper lid. To allow for smooth contour, the loop in the lower arm should be directed superiorly and the excess wire cut (Fig. 132.1B). Each loop should be closed so that no sharp free end could possibly perforate the tissues.

With precise placement, pressure on adjacent tissues is minimal to prevent any point that might lead to extrusion or migration. To secure the lower lid, a piece of 0.2-mm thick Dacron patch, which had been folded in a Gelfoam press and placed in a steam autoclave, is cut and placed around the wire. The crease is directed toward the lid margin. The piece should

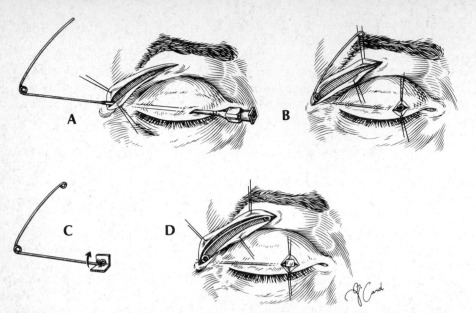

Figure 132.1 *Palpebral spring for lagophthalmos from facial palsy. (Reprinted with permission from House WF, Luetje CM: Acoustic Tumors, vol II. Baltimore: University Park Press, 1979, p 135.)*

be approximately 5 mm wide and 10 mm long (Fig. 132.1C). The Dacron is secured to the loop of the spring by a nylon 8-0 suture tied internally. The Dacron patch can be held in position in the upper lid by closing overlying tissues meticulously with vertical mattress sutures and interrupted skin sutures of 6-0 Tri-Con.

Final tension in the spring can be accomplished by varying the position of the upper arm or bending the wire with two instruments. The upper arm should be secured to the periosteum with three 4-0 mersilene sutures, again taking an extra bite of periosteum with each stitch.

A final inspection of the spring should be made with the patient seated and supine and tension adjusted as needed. Slight overcorrection is preferred.

The lateral wound can be closed with 5-0 plain catgut sutures deeply and with interrupted or running 6-0 Tri-Con sutures for the skin. Ophthalmic antimicrobial ointment and a moderate pressure dressing should be placed and removed the next day. Swelling should resolve over the following week, at which time the skin sutures can be removed.

Spring adjustments can be made by injecting a local anesthetic and making an incision above the lower arm of the spring adjacent to the fulcrum to expose 0.5 cm of wire. Tension on the wire can be adjusted with two pliers and the wound closed with one or two sutures.

Adjustments may be required to fine tune the spring or to reduce tension as facial nerve function returns. In patients with satisfactory return of facial function, the spring can be removed. Patients with permanent facial paralysis generally tolerate the spring well for many years when meticulous attention to detail is paid initially.

Problems with the spring can include extrusion, migration, breakage, infection, and requirement for postoperative adjustment. Patients selected for this procedure must, therefore, be followed carefully while the spring is in. The secure closure, simulated blink, and relief of exposure keratitis that can be provided with this technique make the results gratifying.

BIBLIOGRAPHY

Guy CL, Ranshoff J: The palpebral spring for paralysis of the upper eyelid in facial nerve paralysis. *J Neuro Surg* 29:431, 1968.

Levine RE, House WF, Hitselberger WE: Ocular complications of seventh nerve paralysis and management with palpebral spring. *Am J Ophthalmol* 73:219, 1979.

Levine RE: Management of the eye after acoustic tumor surgery, in House WF, Luetje CM (eds): *Acoustic Tumors: Management.* Baltimore, University Park Press, 1979, vol 2, pp 105–149.

Morel–Fatio D, Lalardrie JP: Le ressort palpebral: Contribution a l'étude de la chirurgie plastique de la paralysie faciale. *Neuro-Chir* 11:303, 1965.

133

Lid Suture for Exposure of Keratitis

Ralph E. Wesley

INTRODUCTION

The unconscious patient, or one with a facial palsy, in the intensive care unit has a high risk for the development of corneal ulceration. With exposure and drying of the cornea, *Pseudomonas* can proceed to form a corneal ulcer no longer restrained by the epithelial barrier.

Taping the eyes shut can frequently provide protection, but the eyelid suture technique allows for a tighter closure and easier access for nursing personnel to administer medication.

TECHNIQUE

Ideally, the upper lid should be anesthetized with local anesthetic and a 4-0 monofilament suture placed through the upper lid and tied (Fig. 133.1A). The suture should be pulled down onto the lower lid for tight closure of the eyelids. A one-half inch Steri-strip should be applied over the monofilament suture, the suture draped superiorly, and a second strip of tape applied for additional strength (Fig. 133.1B).

As the suture is taped, the patient should close both eyes. Once the tape is applied, the eyelid should not open at all when the opposite eye opens.

With this technique, the patient's eye can be protected while providing access for medications or observation.

In patients with facial palsy, the suture can be left open during the day and taped close for protection at night.

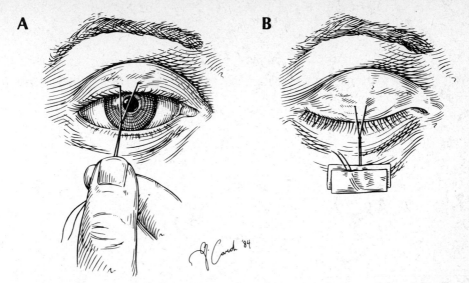

Figure 133.1 Eyelid suture secured with Steri-strips provides tight closure, but allows for ocular examination in patients with facial palsy or unconscious patients with exposure.

ORBITAL DISORDERS

PART XI

134

Repair of Prolapsed Lacrimal Glands

Byron Smith
Richard L. Petrelli

INTRODUCTION

The lateral horn of the levator aponeurosis divides the lacrimal gland into orbital and palpebral lobes. Relaxation of suspensory ligaments can cause an unsightly bulging unilateral or bilateral mass in the lacrimal fossa, especially in patients with blepharochalasis.

Performing a blepharoplasty will not rid the patient of this unsightly mass. With the technique below, the surgeon can repair the herniated lacrimal gland and perform a biopsy in selective cases.

TECHNIQUE

The skin should be incised through the superior tarsal fold (Fig. 134.1A) and undermined deep to the orbicularis muscle. The dissection should be carried upward to the temporal two-thirds of the superior orbital rim where the attachment of the orbital septum to the periorbita is exposed and incised 2 mm below the orbital rim. The orbital rim periosteum should not be disturbed.

With pressure on the globe, the lacrimal gland will protrude through the incision (Fig. 134.1B). The gland can be recognized by its pinkish gray color and the firm consistency in contrast to orbital fat, which appears yellow and soft. Excessive fat can be removed, but absolute hemostasis is mandatory. A biopsy of the anterior margin of the lacrimal gland can be performed, and the defect can be closed with a secure, absorbable suture.

The gland should be suspended into its normal position by passing a double-armed suture through the anterior margin (Fig. 134.1C) with a whip stitch so the suture will not pull out of the glandular tissues when the suture is tied.

Two needles of the 4-0 chromic should now be used inside the upper

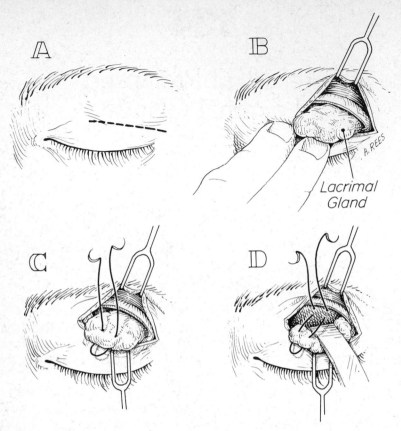

Figure 134.1   *Repair of prolapsed lacrimal gland.*

orbital rim (Fig. 134.2A). The needles are passed from within the orbit forward through the periosteum of the anterior portion of the lacrimal fossa.

A nasal speculum can be used to expose the fossa and recipient area into which the suture is placed. As the suture is pulled up and tied securely, the lacrimal gland will be mobilized and fixed back into the lacrimal fossa (Fig. 134.1D and Fig. 134.2B).

The orbital septum can be closed with interrupted 4-0 catgut sutures. Excess skin and redundant orbicularis muscle can be excised. The skin can be closed with a continuous suture of 5-0 nylon, and a light pressure dressing can be applied.

This procedure allows the surgeon to biopsy the lacrimal gland and secure the gland back into its original position. Hemostasis is mandatory; otherwise, the gland will continue to bleed. The suture through the lacrimal gland should be tied before passing the double-arms back out through the periosteum, otherwise slippage can occur. The orbital septum should be closed securely to prevent reherniation of the gland.

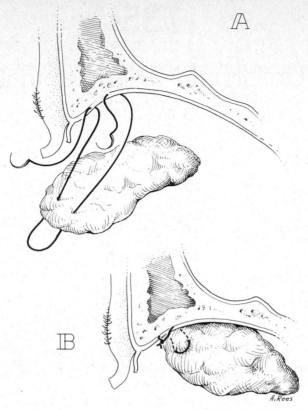

Figure 134.2 Fixation of lacrimal gland inside orbital rim.

BIBLIOGRAPHY

Smith B, Petrelli R: Surgical repair of prolapsed lacrimal glands. *Arch Ophthalmol* 96:1132, 1978.

135

Unilateral Medial Canthal
Wiring Technique

Charles K. Beyer

INTRODUCTION

Fractures of the medial orbital wall can create a lateral displacement of the medial canthus by the outward pull of the orbicularis muscle. The canthus loses its angular shape and becomes more rounded, and the horizontal fissure narrows producing telecanthus. Epicanthal folds arise from an overlapping of the nasal skin into the medial canthal area from the posterior displacement of the nasal, bony skelton. Transnasal wiring may be required to correct bilateral deformities such as blepharophimosis or bilateral nasal fractures.

With this procedure, the surgeon can correct unilateral medial canthal fracture or tendon deformities with a single incision and a procedure technically less difficult than transnasal wiring.

TECHNIQUE

Protective lenses are inserted into each eye. A gull-wing incision is made over the involved medial canthus with dissection carried to the underlying angular artery and vein, which are cauterized or tied as needed (Fig. 135.1A). The periosteum is stripped from the nasal bone and posterior lacrimal crest to the lacrimal bone for wide exposure. The entrapped bony fragments in the ethmoid region behind the posterior lacrimal crest should be mobilized carefully and removed.

Next, a dacryocystorhinostomy should be performed. Nasolacrimal bone irregularities anterior to the lacrimal crest should be smoothed and reduced with a high-speed dental burr.

Then, 3 to 4 mm from the anterior lacrimal crest two holes are drilled through the nasal bone 1 cm apart for 30-gauge stainless steel wire to be placed into the bony perforations and brought out behind the anterior lacrimal crest (Fig. 135.1B). The wire is then passed through the medial

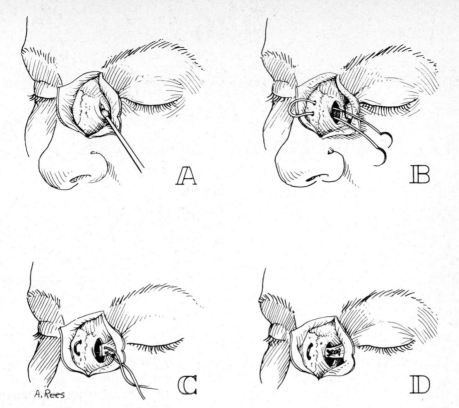

Figure 135.1 *Unilateral transnasal wiring.*

canthal tendon with curved needles (Fig. 135.1C) and twisted tightly to bring about the appropriate medial canthal tendon (Fig. 135.1D). The skin can then be closed using standard techniques.

This technique allows the surgeon to easily perform the equivalent of a unilateral transnasal wiring without an incision on the uninvolved side.

BIBLIOGRAPHY

Beyer CK, Fabian RL, Smith B: Naso-orbital fractures, complications, and treatment. *Ophthalmology* 89:456, 1982.

Beyer CK, Smith B: Naso-orbital fractures: Their complications and treatment, in Tessier P, Callahan A, Mustarde JC, Salyer KE (eds): *Symposium on Plastic Surgery in the Orbital Region.* St Louis, Mosby, 1976, pp 107–112.

Beyer CK, Smith B: Naso-orbital fractures, complications and treatment. *Ophthalmologica* 163:418, 1971.

Converse JM, Smith B: Naso-orbital fractures and traumatic deformities of the medial canthus. *Plast Reconstr Surg* 38:147, 1966.

Smith B, Beyer CK: Naso-orbital fractures and traumatic deformities of the medial canthus. *Plast Reconstr Surg* 38:147, 1966.

136

The Inferior Fornix Orbital Approach with Lateral Cantholysis

James L. Moses
Clinton D. McCord, Jr.

INTRODUCTION

The oculoplastic surgeon needs access to the inferior orbit to treat several disorders: blow-out fractures with significant enophthalmos and/or restriction of extraocular muscle movements; orbital rim fractures; anophthalmic sockets with contracture and fat absorption requiring inferior orbital volume augmentation to enhance the fullness of the orbit to correct enophthalmos, hypoophthamos, and superior sulcus deformities, and exophthalmos, requiring inferior medial and/or lateral orbital decompression.

Traditional exposure of the inferior orbit has been made via a subciliary incision or an incision directly over the orbital rim. The subciliary incision carried beneath the orbicularis oculi muscle can lead to ectropion or lid retraction. The incision directly over the orbital rim can leave an unsightly scar.

Previous procedures attempting to enter the inferior orbit through a conjunctival approach provided limited exposure due to tension exerted by the medial and lateral canthal tendons.

The exposure of the inferior orbit, as described below, through the inferior fornix conjunctiva with lateral canthotomy and cantholysis provides broad visualization of the lateral, inferior, and medial orbit without producing ectropion or a visible scar.

TECHNIQUE

A skin incision at the lateral canthal angle bisects the lateral canthal tendon (Fig. 136.1). Traction sutures are placed through the lower lid and

438

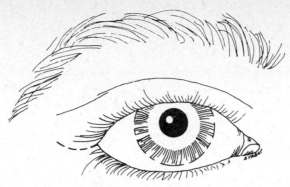

Figure 136.1 *Lateral canthal incision.*

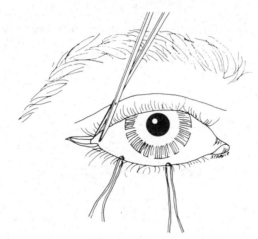

Figure 136.2 *Cutting inferior remnants of the lower lateral canthal tendon.*

a pointed Westcott scissors is used to incise remnants of the inferior limb of the lateral canthal tendon (Fig. 136.2) allowing the lower lid to swing freely outward. The inferior fornix can be fully visualized (Fig. 136.3).

With a Westcott scissors or a number 15 Bard–Parker blade, an incision is carried through the conjunctiva and inferior lid retractors (Fig. 136.4). The incision should be carried down to the orbital rim, exercising care to make sure the skin is not folded inward causing a "buttonhole" through the skin surface. With the incision carried to the inferior orbital rim, the anterior aspects of the incision are retracted with rake retractors.

A periosteal incision just internal to the most superior aspect at the inferior orbital rim (Fig. 136.5) allows the periosteum to be elevated from the orbital floor with a Freer or Tenzel periosteal elevator. The contents of the orbit can be suspended with a malable orbital retractor (Fig. 136.6).

With this exposure, an inferior orbital fracture can be reduced and supporting elements placed. With orbital decompression for thyroid exophthalmos, the orbital floor on each side of infraorbital nerve can be

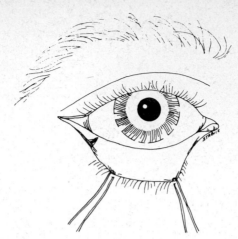

Figure 136.3 *After inferior canthototomy, lid swings down to expose lower fornix.*

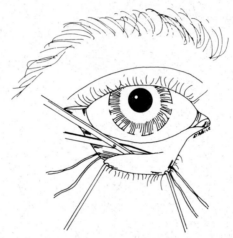

Figure 136.4 *Incision through conjunctiva and lower lid retractors to inferior orbital rim.*

removed and the periosteum elevated medially upward along the ethmoid sinus for further decompression. The periosteum can then be stripped from the orbital rim laterally in the initial incision to provide for removal of the lateral orbital wall for a third wall decompression, if needed.

In cases involving inferior rim fractures, periosteum can be removed from the rim to allow for placement of stainless steel wires. In cases of anophthalmos, augmentation material such as (methylmethacrylate) can be placed posteriorly in the inferior orbit to push the implant upward and outward thus correcting a sunken superior sulcus.

At the completion of the procedure, the periosteum may be closed and the conjunctiva reapproximated with a running 6-0 Vicryl suture. The inferior limb of the lateral canthal tendon is reformed using a permanent

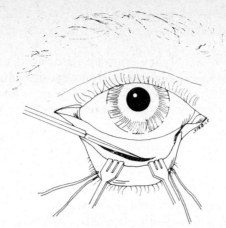

Figure 136.5 Retraction periosteal incision at orbital rim.

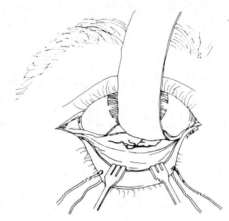

Figure 136.6 Orbital contents elevated for visualization of floor fracture.

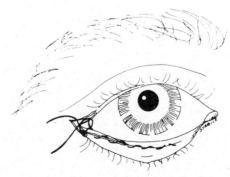

Figure 136.7 Closure of conjunctiva and lateral canthal tendon. (Reprinted with permission. Ophthalmic Surgery 10:59–63, 1979.)

suture, such as 4-0 Polydek or mersilene (Fig. 136.7). If correction of lower lid laxity is desired, a portion of the lower lateral lid can be resected before this closing.

The skin is closed with a few simple or running sutures. The small lateral canthal incision is hidden readily in natural skin lines.

This technique provides the ophthalmic plastic and orbital surgeon wide access to the inferior orbit without producing ectropion or cicatricial deformities.

BIBLIOGRAPHY

McCord CD Jr, Moses JL: Orbital fractures, in McCord CD Jr (ed): *Oculoplastic Surgery*. New York, Raven Press, 1981, pp 243–255.

McCord CD Jr: Surgical approaches to orbital disease, in McCord CD Jr (ed): *Oculoplastic Surgery*. New York, Raven Press, 1981, pp 285–311.

McCord CD Jr: Orbital fractures, in Silver B (ed): *Ophthalmic Plastic Surgery*, ed 3. San Francisco, American Academy of Ophthalmology, 1977, pp 282–286.

McCord CD Jr, Moses JL: Exposure of the inferior orbit with fornix incision and lateral canthototomy. *Ophthalmic Surg* 10:53, 1979.

137

Medial Canthal Tendon Fixation in Transnasal Wiring

Ralph E. Wesley

INTRODUCTION

Transnasal wiring can reestablish the normal canthal angle and position of the medial canthal tendon in cases of severe nasal orbital fractures and telecanthus from blepharophimosis. Transnasal wiring initially reestablishes a normal canthal position and angle, but the results frequently deteriorate as the wire slowly cuts through the medial canthal tendon.

TECHNIQUE

Long-term results are dramatically improved with a permanent suture, such as 4-0 Polydek, passed through the upper and lower medial canthal tendons and then tied to the wire (Fig. 137.1A) instead of passing the wire directly through the medial canthal tendon.

Each separate suture is tied around the 26-gauge transnasal wire before final tightening (Fig. 137.1B). Once the wire is tightened in the usual fashion, the normal canthal angle will be reestablished.

With this additional step, the permanent suture will not "cheese wire" through the medial canthal tendon, yet the strength and nonreactivity of the steel is used.

BIBLIOGRAPHY

Callahan A: Surgical correction of the blepharophimosis syndrome. *Trans Am Acad Ophthalmol Otolaryngol* 77:687, 1973.

McCord CD Jr: The correction of telecanthus and epicanthal folds. *Ophthalmic Surg* 11:446, 1980.

Smith B, Beyer CK: Medial canthoplasty. *Arch Ophthalmol* 82:3448, 1969.

443

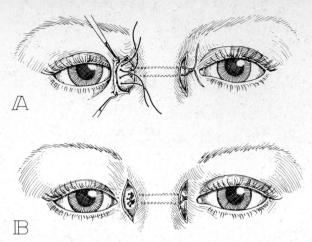

Figure 137.1 Long-term results of transnasal wiring improved by passing permanent sutures through the upper and lower canthal tendons to be secured to the wire, rather than by passing the wire directly through the medial canthal tendon.

138

Transcranial Superior Orbital Approach to the Orbit

Joseph C. Maroon
John S. Kennerdell

INTRODUCTION

The lateral microorbitotomy can provide exposure for tumors located in the superior, temporal, or inferior orbital compartments, as well as those in the lateral orbital apex. A medial approach can be applied to medially located orbital tumors that do not extend to the apex. Lesions involving intracranial extension and those located in the orbital apex or deep medial orbital compartment have traditionally required a craniotomy, removing the frontotemporal bone with preservation of the superior orbital rim.

The frontotemporal approach can involve considerable difficulty when dealing with large tumors deep in the apex or when attempting to repair a transected anulus of Zinn. The brain must be retracted to provide adequate visualization.

Using the transcranial superior orbital approach described below, the surgeon can obtain access to intracranial or deep orbital tumors, with the best visualization of orbital contents and with minimal retraction of the brain.

TECHNIQUE

Using a bicoronal skin incision a few millimeters behind the hairline just anterior to the tragus of the ear on the affected side, extending approximately to the superior temporal line on the opposite side (Fig. 138.1, upper left), the entire frontal flap and temporalis muscle is elevated with subperiosteal dissection (Fig. 138.1A). The supraorbital nerve should be elevated with subperiosteal dissection, or if encircled in the supraorbital rim by bone it should be freed with a small osteotome.

With blunt dissection, the subpericranial dissection is carried into the

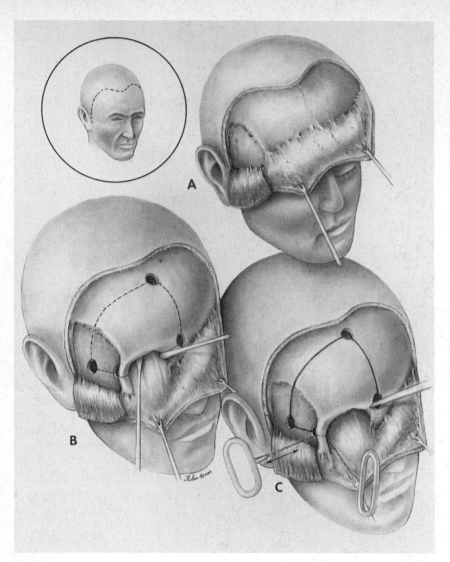

Figure 138.1 *Improved access to posterior orbit and tumors with intracranial extension. (A) Coronal flap. (B) Bone flap outlined. (C) Gigli saw used to cut flap. (D) Elevating bone flap. (E) Flap includes orbital roof. (F) Remaining bone on posterior orbital roof to be removed with rongeurs. (G) Wide exposure of orbital apex from above. (Maroon JC. Kennerdell JS: Surgical approaches to the orbit, indications and techniques.* J Neurosurg *60:1226–1235, 1984.)*

orbit displacing the periosteum from the orbital roof. The lateral periorbita should be separated from the frontal portion of the zygomatic bone. The temporalis muscle should be dissected from the anteriormost portion of the temporalis fossa down to the zygomaticotemporal suture line (Fig. 138.1B).

446

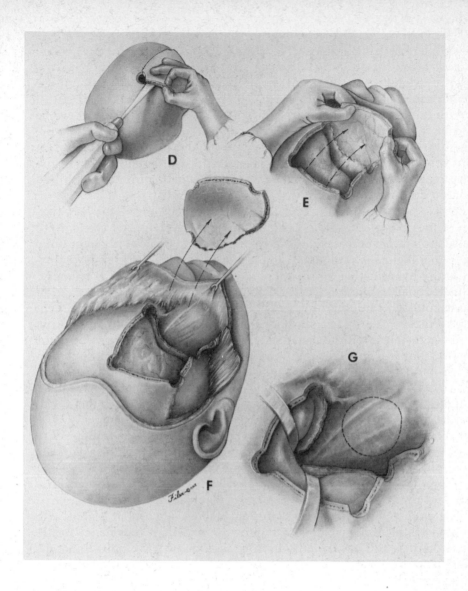

Usually a five-hole bone flap is prepared. The first hole is placed in the temporal fossa anteriorly to expose the lateral wall of the orbit as well as the intracranial compartment. The second hole lies above the glabella, which usually perforates the frontal sinus. Two to three additional holes are placed at the surgeon's discretion.

The zygomatic arch is transected by passing a Gigli saw from the anterior temporal burr hole into the lateral orbit above the dissected periorbital fascia (Fig. 138.1C). Standard saw cuts should connect the remaining burr holes. An osteotome could be used to transect the anterior, medial, orbital ridge from the glabellar burr hole into the orbit, taking care not to extend too far posteriorly, which might interrupt the trochlear strut.

The bone flap can be elevated by standard technique (Fig. 138.1D). The only bone remaining untransected is the thin superior orbital roof, which usually breaks posteriorly allowing the entire superior orbital ridge, superior orbital roof, and frontal bone to be removed in one piece (Figs. 138.1D and E).

With minimal retraction on the dura, small bone-biting rongeurs can be used to remove the remaining portion of the orbital roof, including the bone over the optic canal (Fig. 138.1F and G). Out-pouching of orbital fat from rents in the periorbita from elevation of the bone flap create no complication. Standard precautions are taken if the frontal sinus and ethmoid sinus are opened during elevation of the flap.

For lesions extending intracranially, this approach allows for visualization of the optic nerve and chiasm for possible involvement. Optic nerve transection or decompressive palative surgery can be performed for optic nerve meningiomas. Tumors in the orbital Apex can be approached extradurally by retracting the levator and superior rectus muscles laterally.

Interorbital exploration can be facilitated by microdissection techniques and self-retraining intraorbital retraction provided by the Greenburg retractor.* Three to four blades may be used to retract the brain in addition to the interorbital contents. The anatomic relationship of the ethmoid sinuses medially and the pneumatized anterior clinoid processed laterally should be kept in mind to prevent persistent CSF leaks.

Closure of the wound requires a water-tight dural repair. The frontal, ethmoid, and sphenoid sinuses should be closed by impacting them with muscle, and then oversewing with pericranium and dura. The bone, with roof intact, should be replaced and the bone flap secured with fine-gauge wire. An orbital roof prosthesis is unnecessary. Methyl methacrylate cranioplastic plugs are placed in all of the burr holes except those under the temporalis muscle. The skin is closed in the usual fashion with a subgaleal drain left for 24 hours. A tarsorrhaphy is not required.

This approach provides access for removal of deep orbital lesions with possible intracranial extension with an excellent cosmetic result. Enophthalmos can occur, but within a week or two, becomes unnoticeable. Pulsating proptosis has not occurred using this technique. CSF leaks and extraocular disturbances have been avoided.

BIBLIOGRAPHY

Maroon JC, Kennerdell JS: Surgical approaches to the orbit: Indications and techniques: *J Neuro Surg* 60:1226, 1984.

Kennerdell JS, Maroon JC: Microsurgical approach to intraorbital tumors. Technique and instrumentation. *Arch Ophthalmol* 94:1333, 1976.

*Greenburg retractor manufactured by the Codman Company, Randolph, Massachusetts.

139

Four-Wall Orbital Decompression for Severe Dysthyroid Exophthalmos

John S. Kennerdell
Joseph C. Maroon

INTRODUCTION

Most often orbital decompression for dysthyroid exophthalmos is performed for apical decompression of an optic neuropathy or to reduce exophthalmos for corneal or cosmetic reasons. Most decompressions are accomplished by allowing the orbital tissues to expand into the ethmoid and maxillary sinuses (two-wall decompression) and removing the lateral orbital wall (a three-wall decompression).

In patients with such severe dysthyroid exophthalmos that the eyes are displaced 30 mm forward and/or develop a 10 mm difference between sides, the standard methods may not provide relief. With the four-wall decompression technique described below, an experienced neuro-ophthalmic orbital team can provide maximum decompression of the optic nerve and reduction of exophthalmos.

TECHNIQUE

Under general anesthesia, the subcutaneous tissue and temporalis muscle over the lateral wall of the orbit should be infiltrated with 10 cc 2% lidocaine with 1:100,000 epinephrine for hemostasis.

A straight 30-mm incision is made from the lateral canthus toward the top of the ear (Fig. 139.1A) and carried down to the temporalis fascia and the periosteum of the zygoma. The subcutaneous tissue should be undermined over the periosteum of the lateral zygoma to the superior and inferior orbital rims. The periosteum of the zygoma should be incised along the lateral orbital rim with a cutting electrocautery. A linear incision should extend back into the temporalis muscle to create a T-shaped opening in the periosteum. With a periosteal elevator, the temporalis

449

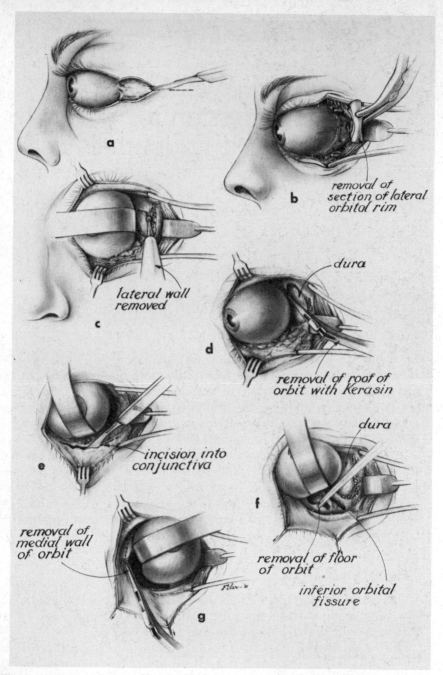

Figure 139.1 Four-wall orbital decompression in severe dysthyroid exophthalmos.

muscle belly and the periosteum should be elevated from posterior aspect to the zygoma.

With the periorbita elevated, a Striker saw is used to make boney cuts through the zygoma angled posteriorly through the superior and inferior orbital rims (Fig. 139.1B). The lateral orbital rim can be broken away with a large rongeur. The posterior lateral orbital wall is removed with a rongeur and the sphenoid wing partially removed with the Hall air drill (Fig. 139.1C) down to the level of the dura of the temporal lobe (Fig. 139.1D). The superior orbital periosteum is dissected free from the roof with a periosteal elevator and the lateral posterior roof removed with rongeurs. Viewing the CT scan in the operating room helps the surgeon to avoid the frontal sinuses.

An inferior canthotomy is performed and the incision carried through the inferior conjunctival cul-de-sac to the inferior orbital rim as far medially as the lacrimal punctum (Fig. 139.1E). With the inferior periorbita elevated and the inferior orbital neurovascular bundle identified, a Hall air drill is used to make a small opening in the orbital floor. Rongeurs are used to remove the orbital floor lateral and medial to the neurovascular bundle (Fig. 139.1F). With the globe elevated, the medial orbital wall should be removed posteriorly as far as visibility allows (Fig. 139.1G). The posterior inferior lamina papyracea can be manually broken inward toward the midline with the surgeon's index finger.

Several periorbital incisions to allow fatty prolapse increase the decompression. The inferior conjunctiva should be closed with running 6-0 Dexon suture. The canthi can be approximated with 4-0 Dexon, which is also used to close the lateral periorbita to the periosteum of the zygoma and to close the temporalis fascia and approximate the wound edges.

The piece of bone removed from the lateral wall can be replaced to allow for accurate Hertel readings postoperatively. The posterior portion of the bone should be trimmed and only the anterior rim replaced before closing the periosteum. This provides a boney rim for Hertel measurements but does not replace bone, which might interfere with the orbital decompression.

The final skin closure is accomplished with a running 6-0 mild chromic suture. Steri-strips are placed over the wound for reinforcement, and Maxitrol ointment is applied to the eye and wound. A soft dressing has been used to provide evenly distributed pressure over the orbit. The patients are treated postoperatively with IV and oral steriods.

The four-wall decompression with removal of the orbital roof is not recommended in patients over 65 years of age due to the thin, incompetent nature of the dura, which may lead to cerebral spinal fluid leaks. This method of decompression, while required rarely, can provide reduction of proptosis in the range of 10 to 17 mm.

BIBLIOGRAPHY

Kennerdell JS, Maroon JC: An orbital decompression for severe dysthyroid exophthalmos. *Ophthalmology* 89:467, 1982.

140

Calvarial Bone Grafting with Vascularized Bone Flap

Joseph G. McCarthy

INTRODUCTION

Calvarial bone grafts can be used for boney reconstruction in the perior-bital area (Chapter 141). Patients with soft tissue recipient sites of poor quality, for example, scar tissue and Treacher–Collins syndrome, have reduced bone survival. By using a muscle-fascial-periosteal pedicle with the calvarial bone flap, the greatest degree of bone survival can be obtained.

TECHNIQUE

A supra-auricular plane through a coronal incision can be used to provide access to the temporalis fascia and temporal line. An Asch metal template is placed over an appropriate area in the peridural-frontal calvaria above the temporal line but behind the hairline. The skeletal portion of the flap should be above the temporal line and at an anterior position toward the lateral wall of the orbit to provide sufficient flap length during transfer (Fig. 140.1). The skull has greater thickness at this point.

After the site and dimensions of the donor bone have been selected, the overlying soft tissue of galea and pericranium should be incised at a distance several millimeters beyond the boney portion of the flap. The temporalis fascia and muscle should then be outlined and incised. The boney portion of the flap can incorporate the outer table or, in special situations, a full-thickness calvarial flap when additional volume is required.

The relatively narrow pedicle incorporates the main trunk of the superficial temporal vessels.

The Dexon sutures are inserted from the pericraniofascial layer through holes in the bone to prevent disassociation of the soft tissue pedicle from the bony portion of the flap. The gap in temporalis muscle can be filled by

452

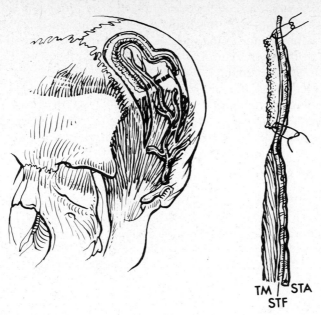

Figure 140.1 (Left) Bone flap attached to superficial temporal artery should be harvested where the bone is most thin, as marked by dashed line. (Right) TM (temporalis muscle), STF (superficial temporal fascia), and STA (superficial temporal artery).

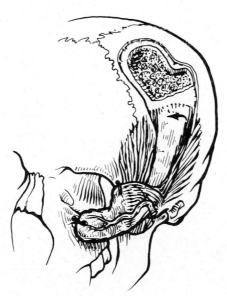

Figure 140.2 Defect filled with calvarial bone-vascular flap. Arrow shows donor defect closed by direct approximation. (McCarthy JG, Zide BM: The spectrum of calvarial bone grafting: Introduction of the vascularized calvarial bone flaps. Plast Reconstr Surg 74:10–18, 1984.)

approximating the fascial edges along the defect after the posterior nonflap portion of the muscle has been mobilized and rotated anteriorly. Contour restoration at the donor site can be performed using either split calvarial bone from the peridural area or a small amount of methacrylate applied with fine-mesh wiring.

Generally, the donor bone and composite flap can be transferred easily to the periorbital and zygomatic regions (Fig. 140.2). With this technique, the frontal branch of the facial nerve is at risk, but the volume of bone transferred appears to be the highest of any calvarial grafting techniques.

BIBLIOGRAPHY

McCarthy JG, Zide BM: The spectrum of calvarial bone grafting: Introducting of the vascularized calvarial bone flap. *Plast Reconstr Surg* 74:10, 1984.

Zins JE, Whitaker LA: Membranous versus endochondral bone autographs: Implications for craniofacial reconstruction. *Surg Forum* 30:521, 1979.

141

Single-Table Calvarial Bone Graft

Joseph G. McCarthy

INTRODUCTION

Problems arise from traditional sources of bone grafts. Tibial bone grafts have a high risk of pathologic fracture. Rib grafts can cause an irregular washboard effect. Grafts from the ilium involve a second operative site with significant morbidity and postoperative discomfort.

With the use of calvarial bone grafts for periorbital reconstruction, a single donor site allows for the harvesting of grafts of adequate size and contour, minimum postoperative morbidity and discomfort, and a camouflaged scalp donor scar (1).

TECHNIQUE

With a coronal incision, the template is placed over the calvaria to find a donor site with the appropriate size and contour to match the defect (Fig. 141.1A and B). A large round burr is used to outline the template to the depth of the inner cortex indicated by bleeding from the diploic space. Additional outer cortex should be removed along the periphery to provide access for osteotomes (Fig. 141.1C).

Curved and straight osteotomes are progressively advanced through the diploic space to remove the outer table (Fig. 141.1D). The graft can then be wired into the boney defect (Figure 141.1E).

Since the bone has been harvested from a portion of the calvaria covered by hair-bearing scalp, the defect should not be conspicious. With the passage of time, the palpable defect becomes less obvious. This technique involves the removal of the outer table while leaving the inner table of the skull intact. Membranous calvarial bone grafts (2) have better volume survival when compared to grafts of endochondral origin. This technique allows the surgeon to use a single operative site to provide a bone graft of the desired size and contour. The main disadvantage is the relatively small amount of bone transferred when using only the outer table.

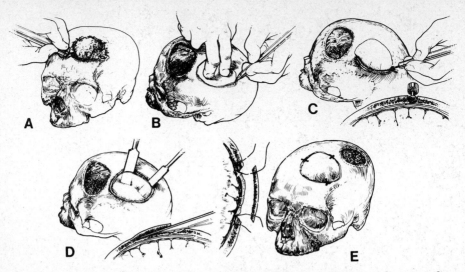

Figure 141.1 *(A) Freshening periphery of defect. (B) Template used to outline donor site with desired contour. (C) Round burr cuts to depth of inner table. Pear-shaped burr used to provide access for osteotome. (D) Outer table elevated. (E) Graft secured. Note donor site hidden beneath hear bearing scalp. (McCarthy JG, Zide BM: The spectrum of calvarial bone grafting: Introduction of the vascularized calvarial bone flaps. Plast Reconstr Surg 74:10–18, 1984.)*

REFERENCES

1. McCarthy JG, Zide BM: The spectrum of calvarial bone grafting: Introduction of the vascularized calvarial bone flap. *Plast Reconstr Surg* 74:10, 1984.
2. Zins JE, Whitaker LA: Membranous versus endochondral bone autographs: Implications for craniofacial reconstruction. *Surg Forum* 30:521, 1979.

142

Medial Canthal
Tendon Repositioning

John B. Mulliken

INTRODUCTION

With hydrocephalus (1) the orbit can enlarge relative to the globe causing anterior displacement of the adnexa and a relative enophthalmos. With the lids and lacrimal drainage anteriorly displaced, the patient may experience chronic epiphora and ocular irritation.

The technique of medial canthal tendon repositioning reapproximates the ocular adnexa to the globe and closes the soft tissue defect in cases of orbital disparity in a manner not possible by simple transnasal wiring.

TECHNIQUE

The surgeon should make a vertical 1.5-cm incision over the insertion of the medial canthal tendon (Fig. 142.1). The medial canthal tendon and a cuff of periosteum should be released with sharp dissection (Fig. 142.2). Proceeding posteriorly with subperiosteal dissection, the deep heads of the preseptal muscles and lacrimal sac are freed from the lacrimal fossa. A hole should be drilled in each medial orbital wall at the site of the desired canthal attachment.

A 3-0 polypropylene suture is placed through one medial canthal tendon, and a curved awl is used to pass the suture transnasally to the opposite tendon (Fig. 142.3). The two tendons are tied together as they are guided into the medial wall openings and retropositioned approximately 15 mm or an amount such that the puncta will rest against the globes. This shortens the horizontal dimension of the palpebral fissure and widens the angle of each medial canthus.

The skin defect created by the retropositioning of the medial canthal tendon can be closed with a rhomboid rotation flap from the nasal region (Figs. 142.4 and 142.5).

This procedure can eliminate ocular irritation and epiphora by the repositioning of the lacrimal drainage and ocular adnexa to the globe.

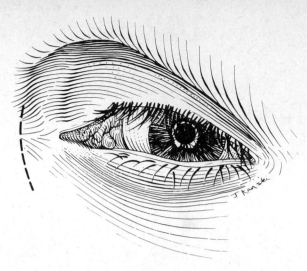

Figure 142.1 *Incision over anteriorly displaced medial canthal tendon.*

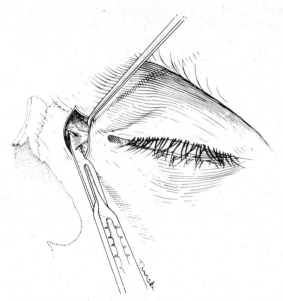

Figure 142.2 *Medial canthal tendon and periosteum reflected.*

This avoids more involved reconstructive procedures such as osteotomies to reduce the size of the orbital cavities or procedures to increase the periorbital soft tissue volume by the addition of alloplastic material.

REFERENCES

1. Mulliken JB, Boger WP III. Correction of anteriorly displaced medial canthus by tendon retro positioning. *Am J Ophthalmol* 92:846, 1981.

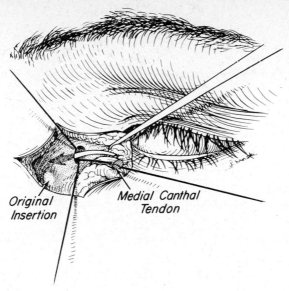

Original Insertion

Medial Canthal Tendon

Figure 142.3   Medial canthal tendon suture passed transnasally.

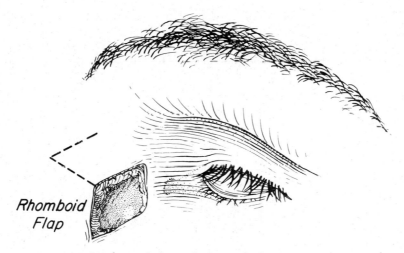

Rhomboid Flap

Figure 142.4   Soft tissue defect after canthal repositioning.

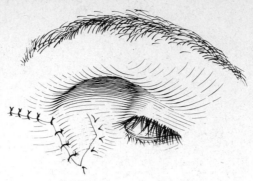

Figure 142.5 *Closure with rhomboid flap. (Mulliken JB, Boger WP, II: Correction of anteriorly displaced medial canthus by tendon retro positioning. Am J Ophthalmol 92:846–850, 1981. Published by The American Journal of Ophthalmology. Copyright by The Ophthalmic Publishing Company.)*

143

Microfibrillar Collagen for Hemostasis in Orbital Surgery

Robert E. Kalina

INTRODUCTION

Persistent bleeding during ophthalmic plastic or orbital procedures makes surgery more difficult and may lead to complications. Conventional methods of hemostasis are difficult to apply to tissues which are highly vascular, friable, or inaccessible areas deep in the orbit. The technique below uses microfibrillar collagen hemostat (MCH), an absorbable agent prepared from purified bovine corium collagen, to obtain hemostasis in these problem situations.

TECHNIQUE

The MCH accelerates the coagulation of blood by producing adhesion and aggregation of platelets to produce a physiologic, true fibrin clot. MCH can be used in normal patients as well as those on heparin or who have taken aspirin. The material is ineffective in patients with thrombocytopenia or intrinsic coagulation disorders such as hemophilia.

MCH is usually applied with dry forceps to prevent sticking to anything moist, including gloved fingers. Delivery into the orbit or other inaccessible areas is usually unsatisfactory with usual techniques.

A disposable plastic 10-cc syringe is modified by cutting off the tip (Fig. 143.1). The plunger is removed and MCH packed loosely into the syringe until approximately one-half to two-thirds full. The plunger is reinserted and the contents pressed into a wafer (Fig. 143.2).

Immediately before application of the MCH wafer, the operative site should be blotted dry. This modified syringe with compressed MCH provides a convenient system for placement of MCH directly at the site of deep orbital hemorrhage (Fig. 143.3). Pressure over the MCH wafer for a short time provides best results. Once hemostasis has been achieved,

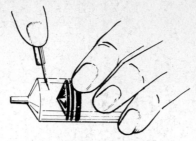

Figure 143.1 Cutting end from 10-cc syringe.

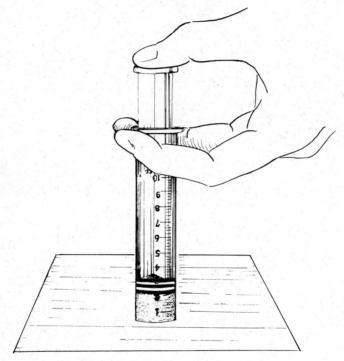

Figure 143.2 MCH compressed into a thin wafer.

excess MCH should be teased away to leave only a thin layer over the affected area.

This material can be used in enucleation, orbital and ophthalmic plastic surgery, without apparent adverse effects. MCH offers the surgeon a valuable tool for hemostasis working in inaccessible cavities or in patients with bleeding disorders from anticoagulation (heparin/aspirin).

BIBLIOGRAPHY

Allavie JJ, Kalina RE: Microfibrillar collagen hemostat in ophthalmic surgery. *Ophthalmology* 88:443, 1981.

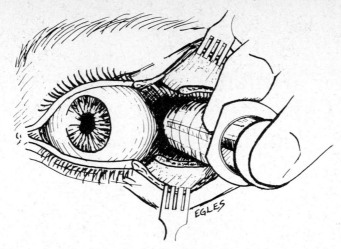

Figure 143.3   MCH applied to orbital bleeder for hemostasis.

Cobden RH, Thrasher EL, Harris WH: Topical hemostatic agents to reduce bleeding from cancelous bone: A comparison of microcrystalline collagen, thrombin, and thrombin-soaked gelatin foam. *J Bone Joint Surg* (AM) 58:70, 1976.

Mason RG, Read MS: Some effects of a microcrystalline collagen preparation on blood. *Haemostasis* 3:31, 1974.

Vistnes LM, Goodwin DA, Tenery JH, et al: Control of capillary bleeding by topical application of microcrystalline collagen. *Surgery* 76:291, 1974.

Zucker MB: The functioning of blood platelets. *Sci Am* 242:86, 1980.

144

Anterior Approach
to Optic Nerve Decompression
in the Optic Canal

N. Branson Call

INTRODUCTION

Blunt anterior head trauma with fractures and/or hemorrhage into the optic canal or expanding sphenoid wing meningiomas that compress the optic nerve are difficult to treat. Megadose steroids have been used with some success when the optic nerve decompression is due only to edema. Surgical decompression through a frontal craniotomy is especially dangerous in a patient who has suffered head trauma and has cerebral hemorrhage.

This technique describes decompression of the optic nerve through an anterior transethmoidal approach from the medial orbit.

TECHNIQUE

Under general endotracheal anesthesia, a 2-cm incision is made, 1 cm medial to the medial canthus, in a vertical direction. Using traction sutures for exposure and hemostasis, the medial canthal tendon is avulsed and tagged. The lacrimal sac is removed from the lacrimal sac fossa, and the medial orbital wall is infractured, with total removal of the anterior and posterior ethmoid air cells and mucosa (Fig. 144.1). Care is taken to preserve the anterior and posterior ethmoidal arteries and lacrimal sac fossa. Using the operating microscope, gentle retraction of the medial periorbita exposes the medial rim of the optic canal, with the optic nerve, surrounded by periorbita, entering it.

The sphenoid sinus is then entered through the posterior ethmoid sinus, and the medial lip of the optic canal is gently infractured into the sphenoid sinus with a Cottle periosteal elevator (Fig. 144.2). With illumination and magnification from the operating microscope, the optic nerve

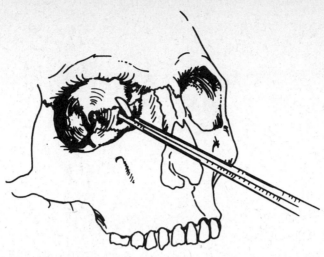

Figure 144.1 *The medial orbital wall is removed, followed by total anterior and posterior ethmoidectomy. The ethmoidal arteries and the lacrimal sac fossa are preserved.*

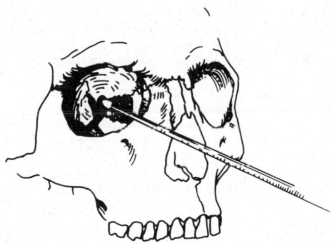

Figure 144.2 *After the sphenoid sinus has been entered, the medial wall of the optic canal is gently infractured until thickened bone is encountered (6–10 mm).*

itself is not touched. Care is taken to preserve and avoid the ophthalmic artery, which runs along the inferior aspect of the optic canal. Thickened bone at the posterior aspect of the optic canal marks the end of the dissection.

An anterior nasal ethmoidostomy is then created to place a thin rubber catheter stent. The medial orbital wall is then reconstructed with a thin silicone sheet, similar to the repair of a blowout fracture (Fig. 144.3). The

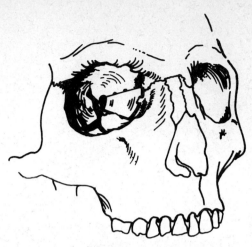

Figure 144.3 *The medial orbital wall is reconstructed with a sheet of silicone. It can be wedged into position with a tongue of silicone under the posterior lacrimal crest.*

medial canthal tendon is resutured into position with the preplaced suture, and the wound is closed in the usual fashion. Postoperative antibiotics are given for 3 days. Systemic steriods may be used. The nasoethmoidal stent is removed in 1 to 2 weeks.

Anterior optic nerve decompression of the optic canal can be used as an adjunct to megadose steroids in patients with optic canal fractures or hemorrhage. Although the injury to optic nerve is sometimes irreversible, the morbidity of decompression is low enough that the potential advantages of surgical decompression are great. Good results have been obtained, particularly if the vision is not already NLP. This same approach can be used to decompress the optic nerve in cases of progressive compression of the optic nerve by sphenoid wing meningioma, usually after the neurosurgeon has debulked the tumor from a craniotomy approach.

BIBLIOGRAPHY

Anderson RL, Gross CE, Panje WR: Optic nerve blindness following forehead trauma. *Ophthalmol* 89:445, 1982.

Fukado Y: Results in 400 cases of surgical decompression of the optic nerve. *Mod Probl Ophthalmol* 14:474.

Ramsey JH: Optic injury and fracture of the canal. *Br J Ophthalmol* 63:607, 1979.

Index

Numbers in *italics* refer to illustrations.

Epicanthus inversus, in blepharophimosis, 307

Epicranium, preparation in temporalis muscle transfer, 160, *162*

Epiphora:
  and correction of punctal malposition, 194, *195, 196*
  treatment of, 150–151, *152*

Ethmoidectomy, in optic nerve decompression, 464, *465*

Ethmoidostomy, anterior nasal, in optic nerve decompression, 465–466, *466*

Eversion:
  of upper eyelid, 282, *282*
  controlled recession, 333, *334*

Excision:
  of distichiasis follicles, 101–102, *102*
  eyelid lesions and, 21, *22*
  of lashes, for lower eyelid trichiasis, 99, *100*
  nasally, of abnormal-appearing skin, 61–62, *62–63*
  of skin elipse, for entropion correction, 95, *96*
  subconjunctival chalazion technique, 3, *4, 5*
  of triangular skin-muscle, lower lid blepharoplasty and, 50–52, *51*

Exposure keratitis:
  eyelid suture technique and, 428, *429*
  inferior, conjunctival advancement flap for, 283, *284–285*
  and lateral tarsorrhaphy technique, 10, 11
  and suture tarsorrhaphy system, 324–326
  tape application in, 12, *13*

Extended lower lid blepharoplasty, for blepharochalasis, 64–65, *65*

External tarsoaponeurectomy, and upper eyelid ptosis repair, 290–294

Extraocular muscle force, transmission to fornices, 264, *266, 267*

Eye bank, sclera from, 406–407

Eyebrow:
  full thickness graft for, 356, *357*
  ptosis of, brow fixation and, 85, *86–89, 89*
  punch hair graft for, 358, *359*
  suspension of, for blepharoptosis, 304–306

Eye examination, bandages allowing, 34–35, *35*

Eyelashes:
  excision of, for lower eyelid trichiasis, 99, *100*
  loss of, Hughes flap modification and, 373–375
  reconstruction of, *see* Cilia transplantation

Eyelid:
  bandages for, 34–35, *35*
  cicatricial diseases of, 130
  contour defects of, 315–318
  contralateral, eyebrow graft from, 356, *357*
  facial palsy and, 418–420
  flaccid, epiphora treatment from, 150–151, *152*
  horizontal shortening procedure for, 157–159
  lateral:
    in cilia transplantation, 349, *350*
    reconstruction of, 404–405
  medial canthal, reconstruction of, 389–392
  normal anatomy of, *148*
  oriental:
    and occidental compared, 48
    surgical correction of, 47, *48, 49*
  resection of, for undercorrected blepharoptosis, 315–318
  surgery of, *see* Blepharoplasty
  suspension of, for blepharoptosis, 304–306
  tumor of, canalicular reconstruction and, 362–364
  see also Lower eyelid; Upper eyelid

Eyelid crease:
  adjustable silicone rod frontalis sling and, 301–303
  eyelid resection and, 316, *317*
  formation of, 47, *48, 49*
  levator muscle isolation and, 297, *298*
  tarsoaponeurectomy and, 291, *291*
  and upper eyelid retraction, 338, *339*

Eyelid fold, creation of, 307, *308–310*

Eyelid lesions, biopsy techniques for, 21, *22*

Eyelid punctum, *see* Punctum

Eyelid retraction:
  controlled recession and, 333–337
  and Hughes flap reconstruction, 384, *385*
    modification of, 373–375
  and lateral tarsorrhaphy technique, 10, 11
  levator aponeurosis lengthening and, 343–345
  pedicle tarsal rotation flaps and, 338–342
  see also Lower lid retractors

Eyelid sling, 418–420

Eyelid suture technique, in unconsciousness, 428, *429*

Eyelid turgor, testing for, 139, *140*

Eye pads, bandaging technique with, 34, *35*

Sutures (*Continued*)
   in Fasanella-Servat procedure, 271–273
      for corneal irritation prevention, 274,
         275–276
   and first knot maintenance, 29–30, *30*
   Frost, *see* Frost suture
   in horizontal shortening procedure, *158,*
      159
   imbricating, for senile entropion repair,
      110, 110, *111*
   intermarginal, grafting and, 132, *133*
   in Jones glass tube placement, 216–217,
      218
   lateral canthal tendon tuck, *140,* 141
   in lower eyelid reconstruction, 371–372,
      372
   in medial canthal plication, 142–143,
      143
   in medial canthal tendon repositioning,
      457, 459, 460
   in modified lateral tarsorrhaphy, 40–41,
      40
   myoconjunctival, prosthetic motility
      and, 264, *266*
   in palpebral spring insertion, 425–426
   in prolapsed lacrimal gland repair,
      433–434, *434, 435*
   pull-out, *see* Pull-out suture
   in punctal malposition correction, *195,*
      196
   and repair of entropion, 93–94
   in right-angle technique to elongate
      fascia, 288, *289*
   in semicircular skin flap eyelid
      reconstruction, 376–377
   for sliding tarsal flap, 404–405
   in socket reconstruction, 256, *257*
   tarsal rotation, ectropion repair with,
      153–156
   for tarsoconjunctival graft, *390,* 390
   for temporalis muscle transfer, 259
   in trapdoor incision closure, 102, *103*
   unconsciousness and, *428, 429*
   in upper-lid entropion correction,
      104–105, *105*
   Weiss, 125, *128*
   zygomaticotemporal line of, *446,* 446
Suture tagging, in dacryocystorhinostomy,
   177, *178*
Suture tarsorrhaphy:
   for keratopathy, 324–326
   Steri-strips for, 14, *15*
Symblepharon ring, 327
Syndrome:
   Stevens-Johnson, 130
   tarsal kink, 360–361, *361*
   Treacher-Collins, 452

Tape:
   for ectropion correction, 137, *138*
   and lagophthalmos reduction, 12, *13*
Tarsal ectropion, 147, *148–149*
Tarsal kink syndrome, reconstruction in,
   360–361, *361*
Tarsal pedicle flap, for lower eyelid
   reconstruction, 371–372
Tarsal polishing, for cicatricial diseases of
   eyelids, 130–132, *131*
Tarsal rotation sutures, ectropion repair
   with, 153–156
Tarsoaponeurectomy, external, and upper
   eyelid ptosis repair, 290–294
Tarsoconjunctival flap:
   reconstruction using, 384–388
   trapdoor type, for distichiasis, 101–102,
      102, 103
Tarsoconjunctival graft, medial canthal
   eyelid reconstruction with, 389–392
Tarsoplasty, lamellar, and horizontal tarsal
   kink correction, 360–361, *361*
Tarsorrhaphy, *see* Lateral tarsorrhaphy;
   Suture tarsorrhaphy
Tarsus:
   blepharophimosis and, 307, *309*
   and chalazion surgery, 3, *4, 5*
   chalazion surgery and, *7, 8*
   graft from, for upper entropion
      correction:
      contralateral, 116, *117*
      ipsilateral, 114–115, *115*
   and horizontal tarsal kink correction,
      360–361, *361*
   and lateral tarsorrhaphy, 10, *11*
   lower eyelid reconstruction and, 371–372
   notching and, 395, *396*
   pedicle flaps from, 338, *340*
   and senile entropion repair, 108, *110,* 110
   sliding tarsal flap and, 404–405, *405*
   upper, biopsy of, 18, *19–20*
   and upper-lid entropion correction, 104,
      105
   vertical buckling of, 327–330
Tear drainage, *see*
   Conjunctivodacryocystorhinostomy
Telecanthus:
   in blepharophimosis, 307, *308*
   transnasal wiring and, 443, *444*
Temporal advancement flap, for
   reconstruction of naso-jugal skin
   defects, 378, *379–380,* 381
Temporalis fascia sling, and temporalis
   muscle, 418–419, *419, 420*
Temporalis muscle:
   and autogenous dermis-fat orbital
      implantation, 258–261

in calvarial bone grafting, 453
and recurrent involution ectropion
    correction, 160–161
  exposure of, 161
  preparation of, 162
  transposition of, 163
and temporalis fascia sling, 418–419,
    419, 420
Tendon, see Lateral canthal tendon; Medial
    canthal tendon
Tenon's capsule:
  and autogenous dermis-fat graft, 258–261
  in double-sphere implantation
    technique, 245, 246, 247
Tenon's cavity:
  dermis-fat graft and, 248, 250
  ocular prosthesis motility and, 264, 265
Tenotomy hook, use in
    dacryocystorhinostomy, 203, 205
Thermal cautery, see Cautery
Thigh, as graft donor site, 248, 250
Thinning, imbricating sutures with, 110,
    112
Threading, of fascia latae strips, 277, 278
Tightening, of lateral canthal tendon, 53, 54
Tissue:
  excision of, in clothesline procedure,
    314
  orbital soft, reconstruction of, 248–252
  subcutaneous, removal of, 27, 28
Transconjunctival biopsy, with disposable
    skin punch, 18, 19–20
Transcranial superior orbital approach,
    445–448
Transnasal wiring:
  medial canthal tendon fixation in, 443,
    444
  unilateral, 437
Transplantation:
  of cilia, see Cilia transplantation
  of sclera, 406–407
  see also Implantation
Trapdoor incision, 101–102, 102, 103
Trauma, and punctal malposition, 194
Treacher-Collins syndrome, 452
Trephine skin punch, eyelid lesions and,
    21, 22
Triangular skin flaps, subcutaneous-base,
    reconstruction with, 382–383, 383
Triangular skin-muscle excision, lower lid
    blepharoplasty and, 50–52, 51
Trichiasis, lower lid, lash excision for, 99,
    100
Tubing:
  Silastic, 198–200
  silicone, see Silicone intubation
  see also Jones glass tube placement

Tuck, in lateral canthal tendon, 139, 140,
    141
Tumor:
  excision of, 25, 26
    medial conjunctival reconstruction
      after, 365
    medial eyelid, canalicular reconstruction
      and, 362–364
    orbital, access to, 445–446, 446
    and semicircular skin flap eyelid
      reconstruction, 376–377
Turgor, of eyelid, testing for, 139, 140

Ulceration, corneal, and eyelid suture
    technique, 428
Unconsciousness, lid suturing and, 428,
    429
Unilateral transnasal wiring, 437
Upper eyelid:
  blepharoplasty for, coronal brow lift and,
    73
  controlled recession of, 333–337. See
    also Eyelid retraction
  Cutler-Beard procedure and, 397–398,
    399
    with eye bank sclera, 406–407
  entropion of, see Entropion, of upper
    eyelid
  eversion of, 4-0 silk traction sutures for,
    281, 282
  Hughes flap modification and, 373–375
  notching of, following Hughes flap
    reconstruction, 384, 385
  ptosis of, external tarsoaponeurectomy
    for, 290–294
  split-level grafts for, 408, 409, 410
  see also Eyelid
Upper eyelid fascia latae frontalis
    suspension, lasso technique with,
    279, 280
Upper tarsus:
  biopsy of, 18, 19–20
  tarsoaponeurectomy and, 291, 293

Vacutainer, vacuum drain and, 16, 17
Vacuum drain, 16, 17
van Graeffe muscle hook, ostium stenosis
    and, 174, 175
Vascular bed, temporalis muscle transfer
    for, 258, 259
Vascularized bone flap, calvarial bone
    grafting with, 452, 453, 454
Vein grafting, and nasolacrimal
    reconstruction, 225–228
Vertical reconstruction, of upper eyelid,
    408, 409, 410